SEXUALITY
AND ITS DISCONTENTS

SEXUALITY
AND ITS DISCONTENTS

MEANINGS, MYTHS & MODERN SEXUALITIES

JEFFREY WEEKS

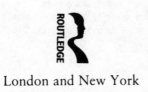

London and New York

First published in 1985
by Routledge & Kegan Paul Ltd
Reprinted 1985 and 1986

Reprinted 1989 and 1991 by Routledge
11 New Fetter Lane, London EC4P 4EE

Simultaneously published in the USA and Canada
by Routledge – a division of
Routledge, Chapman and Hall, Inc.
29 West 35th Street, New York, NY 10001

Set in Sabon, 11 on 12pt
and printed in Great Britain
by Butler & Tanner Ltd, Frome, Somerset

Library of Congress Cataloging in Publication Data

Weeks, Jeffrey, 1945–
Sexuality and its discontents.
Bibliography: p.
Includes index.
1. Sex. 2. Sex (Psychology) 3. Sexual ethics
I. Title.
HQ21.W38 1985   306.7   84–27725

British Library Cataloguing in Publication Data

Weeks, Jeffrey
Sexuality and its discontents:
meanings, myths & modern sexualities
1. Man. Sexuality. Sociological perspectives
I. Title
306.7

ISBN 0–415–04503–7

For Chetan, Micky and Angus,
and in memory of Geoff

CONTENTS

Preface   *ix*

Acknowledgments   *xi*

PREFACE

Few topics evoke so much anxiety and pleasure, pain and hope, discussion and silence as the erotic possibilities of our bodies. Throughout the Christian era, as Susan Sontag has observed, sex has been treated as a 'special case'. Since at least the eighteenth century it has also been the focus simultaneously of 'scientific' exploration and political activity. This book asks whether, as a result of all this concern, we are any more sure today than we were in the reputed Dark Ages of the last century about the 'real' meaning of sexuality. Over a hundred years of theoretical debate and sex research, social morality crusades and radical oppositions, definitions and self-definition, have produced a crisis of sexual values in which many fixed points have been radically questioned and where contending forces battle for the future of sexuality. The aim of the book is to show the historical, theoretical and political forces that have created the framework of this crisis of sexual meanings.

The book begins with an examination of our current 'discontents', of which the rise of a new 'Moral Right' is a potent sign, to show how the crisis is rooted in a sexual and sexological tradition which has ascribed an inflated importance to sexuality. This 'sexual tradition' is the subject of the second section, which explores the valiant endeavours of those scientists of desire and philosophers of sex, the sexologists of the past century, to locate the truth of sexuality in 'Nature'. 'Nature', I suggest, in fact had little to do with it. This is followed by a critical examination of the tradition of psychoanalysis, which has a latent power to disrupt the naturalism and essentialism of the sexological tradition and to challenge our conceptions about the relationship between identity and desire. The book closes with an examination of the theories and practice of the new social movements of recent years, especially the feminist, lesbian and gay movements who have organised around questions of identity, desire and choice to challenge the certainties of the past, and take us beyond the boundaries of sexuality. What does this mean for the future of the science of sex—and of sexual politics?

This book is itself the product of the recent revolution in theoretical and political perspectives which it describes and analyses, the major result of which has been to further our understanding of the *historical* invention of 'sexuality' over recent centuries. From this starting point, the book seeks to analyse the complex historical interactions between sexual theory and sexual politics over the past century, in order to question the neutrality of sexual science and to challenge its hegemonic claims. In particular, what are the meanings of such concepts as 'identity', consent and choice if we reject the idea of a 'true sex'? These themes contribute to another task, an understanding of the sexual present, a peculiar combination of old oppressions and new opportunities, and of contending moral and political positions. By linking our present discontents to a clear understanding of the past and a realistic hope for the future, I hope to contribute to a more rational and optimistic vision of the subject of sex than is currently on offer from either right or left.

ACKNOWLEDGMENTS

This book covers a good deal of ground and many people have helped me negotiate its sometimes treacherous contours. None of them, of course, are responsible for any pitfalls I may have landed in. For support of various kinds, material, moral, intellectual, emotional and practical I warmly thank: Henry Abelove, Alan Bray, Sue Bruley, Wendy Burns, Jane Caplan, George Chauncey, Emmanuel Cooper, Barry Davis, Mattias Düyves, Simon Emmerson, Mary Evans, Elizabeth Fidlon, John Gagnon, Bob Gallagher, Sue Golding, Gert Hekma, Michael Ignatieff, Joe Interrante, Jonathan Katz, Caradoc King, Jane Lewis, John Marshall, Mary McIntosh, David Morgan, Barbara Philp, Ken Plummer, Colin Pritchard, Ellen Ross, Gayle Rubin, Raphael Samuel, Barbara Taylor, Rosemary Ulas, Judith Walkowitz, Simon Watney, Elizabeth Wilson.

Rosalind Coward, Janet Sayers and 'anonymous others' read parts or all of the book in draft and gave me helpful (and improving) comments. I am very grateful for their supportive interest (and I exculpate them from any blame).

Janet Parkin showed her usual impeccable judgment in interpreting my handwriting, and in transforming it into legible typescript. She has my warmest thanks.

I owe an enormous debt to my students at the University of Kent at Canterbury. They sat through my lectures and seminars, endured my speculations, were polite in their interjections and objections, and provided enormous stimulation. Without them ...

As I was completing this book Geoff Horton was fighting an overwhelming illness from which he died. His courage gave me new insights into human endurance, and I honour his memory.

Micky Burbidge, Angus Suttie and Chetan Bhatt gave me domestic warmth and support, and I am more than grateful. I dedicate the book to them, and to the memory of Geoff.

Finally: when I published my last book my young nieces,

Karen and Sîan, asked me to mention them in the next. I do so now, with pleasure and affection—and with the hope that one day they will find this book enlightening and useful (a hope I extend to all my readers).

PART ONE

Sexuality and its discontents

... in modern civilised life sex enters probably
even more into *consciousness* than hunger.

EDWARD CARPENTER, *Love's Coming of Age*

CHAPTER 1

Introductory: the subject of sex

> Since Christianity upped the ante and concentrated on sexual behaviour as the root of virtue, everything pertaining to sex has been a 'special case' in our culture, evoking peculiarly inconsistent attitudes.
>
> SUSAN SONTAG, *Styles of Radical Will*

> ... we reaffirmed that the most important organ in humans is located between the ears.
>
> CAROLE S. VANCE, *Diary of a Conference on Sexuality* 1982

Sexuality as a 'special case'

Sexuality is as much about words, images, ritual and fantasy as it is about the body: the way we think about sex fashions the way we live it. We give a supreme importance to sex in our individual and social lives today because of a history that has assigned a central significance to the sexual. It has not always been so; and need not always be so.

We live, as the British feminist Sue Cartledge once suggested, between worlds, between a world of habits, expectations and beliefs that are no longer viable, and a future that has yet to be constructed.[1] This gives to sexuality a curiously unsettled and troubling status: source of pain as much as pleasure, anxiety as much as affirmation, identity crisis as much as stability of self. Sex exists today in a moral vacuum. In the resulting confusion and uncertainty there is a temptation to retreat into the old verities of 'Nature' or to search for new truths and certainties, a new absolutism. I want in this book to reject both paths—to offer instead a clarification of the real, complex but resolvable problems that confront us. We do not

3

need a *new* morality: rather we should seek ways of living which recognise different beliefs, desires—and moralities.

We tend to see sexuality as a protean force, drawing on the resources of the body, providing the energy for myriad manifestations of desire, and having unique effects. But the more we explore this 'special case' of sex, the more variegated, ambivalent and wracked by contradiction it seems. There is, I would argue, no simple relationship between 'sex' and 'society' (nor a simple 'sex' or 'society'), no easy fit between biological attributes, unconscious fantasy and desire, and social appearance and identity. The mediating elements are words and attitudes, ideas and social relations. The erotic possibilities of the human animal, its generalised capacity for warmth, intimacy and pleasure, can never be expressed 'spontaneously' without intricate transformations; they are organised through a dense web of beliefs, concepts and social activities in a complex and changing history. We cannot hope to understand sexuality simply by looking at its 'natural' components. These can only be realised and given meaning through unconscious processes and via cultural forms. 'Sexuality' is a historical as well as a personal experience.

For this reason, this book is about ways of thinking about sex, about the ideas, meanings and myths that sketch the outline of our sexual lives. It is concerned with the categories of thought, the inventions of the mind, that have organised the way we think and live our sexuality. It is preoccupied with the ways in which we *have* thought of sex in order to see alternative ways of thinking about and realising our erotic needs and desires.

Sexuality today is, perhaps to an unprecedented degree, a contested zone. It is more than a source of intense pleasure or acute anxiety; it has become a moral and political battlefield. Behind the contending forces—liberals and radicals, libertarians and the resurgent forces of social purity, the activists and the apathetic—lie contrary beliefs, and languages, about the nature of sex: sex as pleasure, sex as sacrament, sex as source of fulfilment, sex as fear and loathing. These issues are fought out on a terrain which is constantly extending, through the commoditisation of sexual pleasures, the spiralling expansion of potential desires, even the proliferation of new sex-related dreads and diseases, and is simultaneously characterised by the emergence of new social movements and sexed subjectivities. The subject of sex has moved to centre stage in contemporary political and moral discourse. Through it we are expected to express our subjectivity, our sense of intimate self, our 'identity'. Through its grids of definition we are subjected to the operations of power, fixed in a world which tries to form us, but which we could re-form.

There is a struggle for the future of sexuality. But the ways we respond to this have been coloured by the force of the accumulated historical heritage and sexual traditions out of which we have come: the Christian organisation of belief in sex as sacramental and threatening, the libertarian belief in sex as subversive, the liberal belief in sex as source of identity and personal resource, all rooted in a mélange of religious, scientific and sexological arguments about what sex is, what it can do, and what we must or must not do. We are weighed down with a universe of expectations. Sexuality could be a potentiality for choice, change and diversity. Instead we take it as a destiny, and all of us, women and men, homosexual and heterosexual, young and old, black and white, are held in its thrall, and pay its expensive dues.

Sexuality as history and politics

This is the final book in what has become an unplanned, informal trilogy of works, concerned with the social organisation of sexuality. It is entirely self-contained in itself, but at the same time it takes up, develops and occasionally revises, themes set forth in the earlier books. This body of work was sparked off by the emergence at the end of the 1960s and early 1970s, in America, Europe and elsewhere, of the feminist, lesbian and gay movements. Its form was shaped by the vicissitudes of sexual politics as the utopian aspirations of the late 1960s gave rise to the disillusion of the late 1970s and early 1980s. But throughout there have been three organising preoccupations: with the question of sexual identity, with the relations between the sexual and the social, and with the limiting and defining effects of the existing scientific, moral and political discourses on sexuality. The first book, *Coming Out*, grew out of my own involvement in the gay movement.[2] Its explicit concern was with the emergence and effects of the campaigns for homosexual rights and freedom. Its implicit, and guiding, involvement was with the whole issue of sexed identity—with the historical variability and mutability of sexual identity in general and the gay identity in particular. My starting point was the rejection of any approach which assumed the existence, across cultures and across time, of a fixed homosexual person. On the contrary, I argued then, as I argue now, that the idea that there is such a person as *a* 'homosexual' (or indeed *a* 'heterosexual') is a relatively recent phenomenon, a product of a history of 'definition and self-definition' that needs to be described and understood before its effects can be unravelled.[3] There is no *essence* of homosexuality whose historical unfolding can be illuminated. There are only changing patterns in the organisation of desire whose specific configuration can be decoded. This, of course, propels us into a whirlwind of deconstruction—for if the gay identity is of recent provenance, what of the heterosexual identity? And what of the fixity we ascribe to our gender placings, our masculinity and femininity? 'Nature', I suggest, can explain little of these.

This belief led, easily enough, to the second set of preoccupations: with the social ordering and regulation of sexuality, with the historical and social side of the process I have defined as one of definition and self-definition. This was the subject of my second book, *Sex, Politics and Society*.[4] The period covered by the book—roughly the period of industrial capitalism—indicates the initial aim of the study: to demonstrate the relationship between the triumph of capitalist social relations and the social control of sexuality. Its final form, however, is rather different as its organising ideas changed. The history of sexuality is a complex one; its propelling force cannot be reduced to the effects of a single set of relations. Sexuality as a contemporary phenomenon is the product of a host of autonomous and interacting traditions and social practices: religious, moral, economic, familial, medical, juridical. Capitalist social relations do certainly set limits and pressures on sexual relations as on everything else; but a history of capitalism is not a history of sexuality. The exact nature of the relationship—the complex mediations, the partial and ever-changing articulations, the proliferation of social interventions and the intricate forms of resistance—needs to be understood through concrete historical investigations, not assumed because of a strict adherence to a macro-historical masterplan.

Amongst the most crucial forms of mediation are the categories, concepts and languages which organise sexual life, which tell us what is 'good' or 'bad', 'evil' or 'healthy', 'normal' or 'abnormal, 'appropriate' or 'inappropriate' behaviour. These too have a complex history—but the chief guardians of these definitions during this century have been the 'sexologists', the scientists of sex, the arbiters of desire. Amongst my earliest pieces of writing on sexual matters was an article on the great English sexologist, Havelock Ellis.[5] This present book examines, in more detail, as one of its major themes, the social role and effects of such sexologists. My task is not to blame them as the 'onlie begetters' of current ways of thinking about sex. I would distance myself from any view which sees the sexologists as no more than agents for hidden social imperatives, whether of 'social control' or of 'modernisation'; or as apologists for the sexual status quo; or even as encoders of oppressive sexual values.

Sexology has never been a unified discipline; its participants have never expressed a single intellectual perspective; and its effects have never been unilinear or gone unchallenged. Sexual ideas alone do not create the sexual world. Nevertheless the high priests of sexual theory *have* contributed to the world we inhabit: they offered ideas and often practical help to reforming, and not so reforming, activity; they promoted the belief that sex was of crucial importance to individual health, identity and happiness; they marketed many a handbook and often a technique or two to attain the joys of sex; they gave a scientific credence to often dubious political positions; and they set an agenda for sexual change which, to a remarkable degree, has been completed. Their work has been appropriated, deployed, utilised and occasionally distorted in a variety of social arenas and forms. They cannot be blamed individually or even perhaps collectively for the world we live in. We are, after all, actors in that world. But their legacy is one that needs to be exhumed, re-examined and probably rejected before we can write a new agenda.

Possibly the most potent of their legacies is what is now generally known as 'sexual essentialism'. Throughout this book I shall challenge ways of thinking which reduce a phenomenon to a presupposed essence—the 'specific being', 'what a thing is', 'nature, character ... substance ... absolute being' (*Oxford English Dictionary*)—which seeks to explain complex forms by means of an identifying inner force or truth. The sexologists have spent a great deal of their energies in seeking the 'truth of sex'—in biology usually, in the instinct, the chromosomes and hormones, the DNA, the genes, or less often, but powerfully, in psychic energy or unconscious compulsions. The belief that sex is an overpowering force which the social/moral/medical has to control is an old and deeply rooted one, and central to the western, Christian traditions (though not invariably to others). Sexologists worked to give this a scientific basis and concern. The result has been, I believe, disastrous, because it has always made the battle for, or against, this sexual force the chief focus of sexual writing. Within such a Manichean perspective it has been impossible to confront, let alone answer, key questions—about identity, pleasure, power, choice—which bedevil the domain of sex. Certain questions have not been posed because they could not be asked within the old frame of reference.

To hack away at the old structures of meaning is relatively easy, and certainly necessary. To find a new one is less so. It is this which makes recent radical theoretical and political developments so important. The critique by contemporary sociologists of the 'hydraulic model' of sexuality, the belief that sex is like a gushing stream whose force can be given full reign, or dammed, left to roam free or channelled into harmless byways, has forced us to rethink the certainties of existing *social* definitions of sexuality; while the studies inspired by the new social history have underlined the *historical* nature of the importance we assign to the sexual.[6] A large part of the stimulus for this new historical approach has come from the work of the modern women's movement. Most crucially, feminism has disinterred the male assumptions behind the hydraulic model itself. Many contemporary feminists have noted the absence of a language for female sexuality except in terms of the male model. The rupture that feminism proposes both with traditional ways of thought and with well-established political practices—the assertion of the power of female desire in all its forms against masculinist assumptions and practices—has had a profoundly disturbing impact on the politics of sex, as on other areas.

This in turn has contributed to a redefinition of the nature of power and politics in the modern world. 'Power' no longer appears as a homogeneous force which can be straightforwardly expressed or captured. Power, like the politics around it, can be seen as mobile, heterogeneous, insistent and malleable, giving rise to various forms of domination, of which the sexual is one, and producing constant forms of challenge and resistance, in a complex history.

My previous books, like this one, have been cast in the form of historical investigations. This is partly, no doubt, the product of a specific academic training and intellectual predilection. But, more significantly, I believe, a historical approach can be seen as having a relevant political purpose behind it. It is noticeable that many of the most important contributions to radical political analyses in recent years have been in the form of historical investigation—whether of working-class, black or women's oppression and subordination.

But there can be no easy way of reconciling 'history' and 'politics'. There have been three characteristic approaches in the attempt to marry the two, each of which has definite political effects.[7] The first is 'history as a lesson'. Here the emphasis is on learning from the past in order to understand the present, and provide guidelines for the future. Tempting as it sounds as a strategy, the problem with this is that it assumes a transparent and homogeneous past whose warnings can simply be read off. Unfortunately, 'history' never moves along a single tramline. Its structure is always fractured, its discontinuities as evident as its continuities. More crucially, how can we know that we know the past? The past, as the novelist put it, is a foreign country. Its languages can baffle the most agile translator.

The second approach offers us 'history as exhortation'. The most characteristic note here is the adjuration of the class, or nation, or gender, or oppressed minority to listen to its past, to find in its buried glories the moral example and histories of resistance to give us strength in present difficulties, to rescue, as E.P. Thompson powerfully put it, the downtrodden from the 'enormous condescension' of posterity, and of historians.[8] At its best this strategy can evoke lost worlds of struggle, investigate hidden byways, reassess the way we see the development to the present. It recovers from the victors the pain, work and aspirations of the vanquished. It challenges us to challenge their defeat and looks to their triumph. But at its worst it can provide only a consoling myth, a false hope, an unrealistic reading of the present based on a false image of the past and an unrealisable hope for the future.

The third way is to see 'history *as* politics'. This involves understanding the fundamental connections of history and politics, to grasp the ways in which the past has a hold on, organises and defines, the contemporary memory. The aim here is to understand 'the present' as a particular combination of historical forces, to find out how our current political dilemmas have arisen, to provide a historical perspective on political decisions, and to see the present *as* historical.

Each of the first two approaches has been deployed in the construction of histories of women and of sexual minorities; and often these methods have had their desired effects. There is now a rich library on the struggles of women, and a growing one on the living of homosexuality.[9] But it is the third approach which seems to me most appropriate intellectually and politically to the investigation of sexuality today.

If, as I want to suggest, the sexual only exists in and through the modes of its organisation and representation, if it only has relevant meaning via cultural forms, then no search for a founding moment of oppression, nor glory in past struggles around it, can contribute to an analysis of its current hold on our thought, action and politics. What is needed is a history of the historical present as a site of definition, regulation and resistance. History and politics on this reading are not uneasy bedfellows: they are essential partners.

Sexuality and the politics of choice

For this reason, the next chapters, Chapters 2 and 3, look in more detail at the historical present, the mobile ensemble of power and struggles which have shaped this book, posed the questions it presents, and the politics it is a response to. I suggest that the current controversies about sexuality stem from a crisis in the concept of the 'sexual revolution', and of the very idea of 'sexual liberation'. But more than this, they indicate a faltering in the meaning of 'sexuality' itself. I try to show here how sexuality has been shaped by an intricate web of concepts and belief that organise attitudes and political response—but which are now, in varying ways, in crisis. This has provided fertile soil for the rise of fervent new moralisms.

This is followed in Part 2 by an analysis of the 'sexual tradition' which has provided the reservoir of ideas and the legitimation for current attitudes. The section is devoted to a study of sexology and the ways of thinking about sex which have dominated the past hundred years or so—and still structure our responses today. Chapter 4 examines the importance of sexology in insisting upon the privileged role of sex in expressing 'the natural'. Chapter 5 explores in more detail the theoretical and political consequences of posing the central question of sexuality as an 'eternal duel' between the 'unruly energy' of sex and the constraints of 'society', and takes up the challenge to this uneasy contest by exploring the relevance of recent critiques of sexual essentialism, and the certainties of the 'sexual tradition'. My aim here is not to dismiss sexology and all its works. Many sexologists were brave supporters of what they regarded as the truth. Their work contains insights which we need to retain—and expand. The problem lies in the reliance placed on *their* truths, at the expense of the alternative truths dramatised by the appearance on the historical stage of new sexual identities and movements. We need to learn from these pioneers, not be enslaved by them.

One such pioneer, Freud, is a haunting presence and a powerful point of reference throughout these chapters. The third section is devoted to an investigation of the challenge posed by psychoanalysis and the theory of the 'unconscious' to the sexological tradition. The psychoanalytic tradition, however distorted it has been by moralistic assertions, does offer, I believe, major insights into the possibility of a non-essentialist theory of sexuality and gender. Chapter 6 is concerned, therefore, with the complex relationship of Freud to sexology, and the radical theory of desire that emerges from this crucial, creative encounter. Chapter 7 looks at the political consequences of this theory of desire, placing Freud and orthodox psychoanalysis against the so-called 'Freudian left' and more recent challenges to psychoanalytic rigidities. My aim here is to show that identity is not a simple product of desire, that the flux of potentialities is greater than sexological categories would imply, and that the field of sexuality is wider than our rigid orthodoxies have proposed. The final section of the book, Part 4, returns us to the present, to the dilemmas at the heart of those contemporary debates which try to break with the orthodoxies: dilemmas about identity, pleasure, choice. Chapter 8 tackles, with particular reference to feminist and gay contributions to the question, the issue of identity and the problems presented by the emergence of new sexual definitions, subjectivities, styles, and subcultures. Chapter 9 looks at the moral and political problems posed by the plethora of choices which now face us as sexual beings. In particular, there is an investigation of the touchstone issues of pornography, intergenerational sex, sex as power and as play. Finally, the book closes with a political and polemical conclusion, with the aim not of foreclosing debate but of suggesting issues that should be central to it. These chapters are contributions to the development of what I call a 'radical pluralist' position, whose advocacy is the ultimate purpose of this book. It is a perspective built on the range of sexual possibilities, not on their denial.

I realise that such a circular organisation of the material—starting in the present, going back to the past, and then steaming back to today and perhaps tomorrow may at first sight seem unconventional and disconcerting. But to disrupt fixed assumptions is precisely one of my intentions. My purpose is not to offer a comprehensive history of sexual ideas as such, but to show how we in this contradictory present are locked into a living history which we must understand before we can escape from it.

I belong to a generation which hoped for a great deal from the 'sexual revolution' and what was called 'sexual liberation'. For many, sexual freedom seemed to offer not only an expansion of areas of private choice but also a (perhaps *the*) key to wider social transformation. As I write, however, my bookshelves are beginning to groan with the wordy products of those who have hastily, often in pain and anguish, sometimes with lucrative publishing contracts, retreated from that particular battlefield. Sexual freedom, it seems, far from being an opportunity, was a delusion, a god that failed.

If we over-invest hope in a golden idol we are bound to get disillusioned. But there is something astir more dangerous than the simple clearing away of a veil of illusions. The retreat from any rational idea of sexual freedom and sexual change feeds into the deepening conservatism of our time—has in fact been essential to it—and the apostasy now is just as overindulgent and destructive as the glorification of sexual excess was then. I cannot help thinking about the many who neither enjoyed the benefits of, nor had the opportunity to get disillusioned by, the so-called 'sexual revolution': for them, it has not gone too far, it never really started. We seem to find it necessary either to elevate the sexual to a pinnacle, or to cast it down into the pit. In the process the difficult, ambiguous, complex and subtle problems of sexual choice are ignored, and the genuine victims of sexual unfreedom pursue their lives in continuing anxiety and fear, untouched by any fashionable recantation of youthful foolishness.

We live in a world of contending truths, many of whose advocates are only too prepared to enforce *their* (changing) truth on others. Some years ago Edmund Leach warned us that 'all moral rules are conservative', while 'A zeal to do right leads to the segregation of saints from sinners.'[10] Surely as we approach the end of the second Christian millennium we can devise better ways of regulating things than to impose arbitrary distinctions between ourselves and others; between those of us who believe ourselves 'saved' and those we believe to be beyond 'salvation'.

I suggest, in contrast, that what is needed today is a politics around desire which is a politics of choice, which clarifies the criteria by which as sexual subjects we can *choose* our social

and sexual commitments. This is not, as I show, an easy ambition. 'Sexuality' does not readily provide its own answers.
But it is a crucial task, and this book is a contribution to the
setting of an agenda for that necessary process.

CHAPTER 2

The 'sexual revolution' revisited

Sex in the twentieth century is a consciously,
anxiously reinterpreted mystery ... a dirty,
secret.

ANN BARR SNITOW, in *Signs* 1980

In contrast to the politics of class, race,
ethnicity and gender, the politics of sex are
relatively under-developed. Sexual liberals
are defensive and sexual radicals almost non-
existent.

GAYLE RUBIN, *Coming to Power*

The current crisis

Despite the sustained efforts of generations of moralists there
has rarely been a time of consensus in the West on moral and
sexual standards. Even during the periods of greatest ecclesiastical control, formal and informal standards diverged spectacularly, while that renowned period of moral certainties and
fixed standards, the 'Victorian age', was characterised less by
an easy acceptance of 'traditional values' than by a battle over
conflicting beliefs and behaviours. Sexual standards varied
then, as they do now, between different classes and regions,
religious, racial and ethnic groups. The dominant moral values
which twentieth-century radicals have inveighed against and
social puritans have mourned—the marital ethic, the taboos on
non-genital sexuality, the stigma against non-marital relations
and illegitimacy, the privileging of heterosexuality and the
ostracisation of homosexuality—were only ever precariously
hegemonic (though their victims might have wished they were
more precarious), sustained by varying social, medical and

15

legal forces, constantly challenged, and frequently ignored. There was no Golden Age of sexual propriety, and the search for it in a mythologised past tells us more about present confusions than past glories.[1]

The belief in a Golden Age can, however, have real effects, particularly when we try to come to terms with important shifts in sexual attitudes and behaviours. Over the past generation, many of the old organising patterns and controls have been challenged, and often undermined, and sexuality has come closer than ever before to the centre of public debate. This has produced a crisis over sexuality: a crisis in the relations of sex, especially in the relations betweer. men and women, but also, perhaps more fundamentally, a crisis around the meaning of sexuality in our society. In the resulting confusion there has been an unprecedented mobilisation of political forces around sexual issues. A hundred years ago the possibility of a sexual politics was virtually unthinkable. Today it is commonplace on Right and Left, with the Right taking the initiative more eagerly than the Left. Sex has become a potent political issue because of a perplexing and seemingly endless conflict of beliefs as to the appropriate ways of living our sexualities. In recent years we have witnessed a faltering, and retreat, of 'sexual liberation', a resurgence of a political movement in defence of traditional norms, a wave of moral panics around sex, of which the recent crisis over AIDS is an example, and finally a deadlock over the appropriate forms of regulating sex. Their combination provides a witches' brew of problems.

Sex has conventionally been seen as the most intractable of natural energies, rebellious against the efforts at repression, resistant to the modifications of climate and culture. Protein levels (if we are to believe some writers) might regulate potency, work patterns, might modify will or desire, but sex as a power and potentiality seemed natural and inevitable. Against the dogmatisms of this tradition I want to suggest that sex—far from being the most recalcitrant of forces—has long been a transmission belt for wider social anxieties, and a focus of struggles over power, one of the prime sites in truth where domination and subordination are defined and expressed. On its terrain not surprisingly symbolic battles have been fought out—and countless 'deviants' have consequently suffered—

because of the importance attributed to this particular moral position, or that. The changes in behaviour that have indeed taken place in recent years have become a particularly vivid *casus belli*. By the standards of the sex radicals the changes may have been modest. By the guide lights of conservatives (of all political colours) the changes have seemed disruptive and destructive. They have come to represent all other things that have changed.

In the nineteenth century crises as varied as the French revolution, industrial reorganisation, urban development and local political controversies found a powerful—if rarely material—resolution through struggles over sexual mores. The seismic sensitivity of sexuality to wider social currents has meant that more recently a series of complex social anxieties, products in part of a developing siege mentality among significant sectors of the American and European populations, have similarly been displaced on to the issue of sex. It has come to seem a frontline in the battle for the future of western society. At stake is the legacy of the so-called 'sexual revolution' of the past generation. For many—though not all—progressives during the first two-thirds of the present century the call for 'sexual freedom' has been one of the touchstones of radical intent. *That* was always an ambiguous ambition—freedom from whom, by what means, at whose expense?—and its achievement today seems even more ambivalent. Terms like the 'sexual revolution' and 'permissiveness' have been jumbled together as loose descriptions of the changes that have occurred—but their meaning is opaque. This has not stopped the sceptics, doubters and plain opportunists from rallying against them. The rise of 'permissiveness' has been much heralded and much reviled. Its fall now appears imminent.

The myth of 'permissiveness'

Politics operate through metaphors. They condense anxieties and aspirations and they mobilise energies and will. Few political metaphors in recent times have been as powerful as that of 'permissiveness'. Disowned as a useful term by those who have been claimed as its main proponents, it has become in the hands of its enemies a vigorous cutting weapon.[2] And if 'permissiveness' evokes a trail of expectations and hopes, and of fears and anxiety, the 1960s becomes its singular moment of promise and success. The British Conservative Prime Minister, Margaret Thatcher, gave vent to a representative diatribe of the 1980s:

> We are reaping what was sown in the sixties. The fashionable theories and permissive claptrap set the scene for a society in which the old virtues of discipline and self-restraint were denigrated.[3]

In the struggle between old and new, tradition and the modern, virtue and vice, the 1960s appear as the key moment of transition, the decisive meeting place of conflicting values. In the writings of neo-Conservatives, New Rightists, and moral puritans alike 'the sixties' stand for all that has gone wrong. This was the key moment of 'moral collapse' for the proponents of the new morality, and the source of the detritus that marks and mars our contemporary world.[4]

If it were only explicitly conservative forces that revelled in attacking the supposed 'excesses' of the 1960s then we might acknowledge its organising force, but perhaps reject its representative nature. The peculiarity is that the reaction against that dramatic but historically heterogeneous decade has a wider resonance in at least two other quarters. In the ranks of those we might call 'disillusioned liberals' (many of whom, of course, gravitate fairly easily to the growing ranks of the new conservatism) there is a developing argument also that in the 1960s 'things went radically astray'. For them the sexual legacy of the 1960s is seen in an epidemic of venereal disease as much as in greater sexual choice, in the rise of an aggressive language of sexual abuse as much as in greater verbal freedom, in the worship of quantitative sex as much as a qualitative change in human relations. In a book significantly called *The Limits of Sex* the British journalist Celia Haddon confesses that:

> In some ways, the sexual revolution had freed me from guilt and anxiety; in other ways it had enslaved me anew, with different fetters.[5]

The real 'prisoners of sex' in this argument are the persons who believed too ardently in the claims of the pioneers of permissiveness—amongst whom 'the sexologists' are prominent—and who found in their pursuit of sexual achievement and success a new penance. They are experiencing, in well advertised anguish and guilt, a revenge from the swinging sixties.[6]

Curiously, this critique has parallels with a second one, whose origins are elsewhere, in the 'radical' (as opposed to 'liberal' or 'socialist') feminist attacks on male domination. Where the old liberal sought individual fulfilment in sex and found disillusion (and disease), radical feminism seeks escape, through *collective* endeavour, from the trammels of male power, only to find that male power operates insidiously through the dominant definitions of sex and especially in the rhetoric of 'sexual liberation'. The 'sexual revolution' that supposedly took place in the 1960s is therefore, by definition, a male-oriented one which subordinated women ever more tightly to the heterosexist norm. From this belief stems a strong, often violently worded, rejection of that decade, and all its works. In this view, the real enemies of women become the old sexual radicals.[7]

By a curious twist, radical feminism finds a common target with its ostensible ideological enemies in feeding the new puritanism of our time.[8]

The fact that such disparate streams of thought and political action cohere on a single symbolic period should give us pause for thought. There are two possibilities. Either the 1960s was a pretty awful decade, the source and origin of our present discontents. Or, the various proponents find in the period a convenient scapegoat for changes whose sources are actually diverse and often lie elsewhere. I prefer the latter explanation.

What all seem to agree on is that the past generation saw radical changes in attitudes to sex and in sexual behaviour. A more measured view would query even this.[9] Certainly there were vivid eruptions of sexual display in the 1960s—from the erotic posturings of rock stars to the growth of usually sleazy areas of commercialised sex in many major cities of the metropolitan west. There is evidence that attitudes more or less gradually relaxed, towards birth control, abortion, divorce, pre-marital and extra-marital sex, cohabitation and homosexuality—and this slow change in attitudes has continued into the 1980s despite an increasingly conservative political climate in the United States and Europe.[10] Western Europe saw a wave of reforms in the laws relating to sexuality, and the United States in particular played host to a spectacular growth of new subcultures of sex, and especially of homosexuality. As Dennis Altman suggested, the love that once dared not speak its name had become extremely voluble.[11] This was important in itself, but it also represented a wider shift. If the history of recent sexuality can be seen as an explosion of speech around sex then the 1960s experienced a decisive, qualitative escalation of the volume. Sex today is spoken about, written about and visually represented as never before. Many, especially the sexually oppressed and exploited, have gained a precious breathing space from this. Others have been wearied by its insistent discourse.

Against this we must place the strong persistence of what we still call 'traditional' attitudes (although their history is actually fairly recent) which provided a reservoir of support for the emergence of a new moral right; limited legal changes which ensured continuing controls on sexual free speech; the continuance of police and popular harassment of sexual 'deviants'; and the persistence—indeed growth—of the popularity of marriage. Of the generations of women born since the 1930s in the United States more are married than ever before and the same is broadly true of Britain. Only in the 1970s and early 1980s did the marriage rate show signs of dropping slightly.[12] Many of the changes that did occur had origins in the early years of this century. Some of the changes attributed symbolically to 'the sixties' actually happened later. Moreover, the mood of the period was never unified, and its transformations were unevenly experienced. Nor were these changes unproblematic. What for the Radical Right now appear as the worst examples of 1960s excess—feminist and militant gay movements—grew explicitly *in opposition to* the dominant tendencies of the decade. Yet the 1960s still have a symbolic resonance as the age of cutting change.

So what did happen in that much heralded 'sexual revolution'? Before we can answer that we need to escape from the imprisoning categorisation of a calendar decade, and to redefine our concern. The real object of interest is a particular unstable conjuncture of social and political elements which we can best characterise as the 'permissive moment'.[13] It covers a period roughly from the mid-1950s to the mid-1970s, though its parameters vary from country to country, and its character is defined as much by national peculiarities as by international trends. There was no single social imperative that controlled its emergence, no inherent tendency within capitalism to produce what Herbert Marcuse designated as 'repressive desublimation', the controlled engineering of consent to an illegitimate social order via a mis-recognised 'sexual freedom',[14] no single political strategy that organised and underpinned relevant legal and political adjustments. Yet there are common features, structuring elements, which make 'permissiveness' a recognisable phenomenon in many, if not all, advanced capitalist societies.

If we look at the period fairly schematically four sets of changes seem particularly important in shaping the current situation: the continuing, even accentuating, commercialisation and commodification of sex; the shift in relations between men and women; changes in the mode of regulation of sexuality; and the emergence of new, or the re-ordering of old, social antagonisms and the appearance of new political movements. These provide the framework for the contemporary sexual crisis.

The commercialisation and commodification of sex

'Capitalism', by its anarchic nature, has no controlling will. Its central imperatives—expansion, realisation of surplus value, profit—ensure a certain indifference to the terrain it is working on and through. The expansive energy of capitalism has certainly changed the world, but it has not changed it according to any masterplan. It has inflected a huge variety of social relations, but it has not done so in any unilinear fashion. If we look at a key moment in the establishment of a bourgeois moral hegemony, England in the early decades of the nineteenth century, we will seek in vain for any easy articulation between the interests of factory owners and the chief proponents of a new morality. Entrepreneurs were indifferent to the moral impact of employing women and children as well as men in the textile mills and the coal mines. Bourgeois ideologists, whose social location lay in finance capital, land, or the ancient professions, did care, and mounted evangelical campaigns in the working class to prevent the promiscuous coupling of the sexes in overcrowded, overheated, foetid places of work. The purposes of 'business' and 'morality' often clashed—and the latter frequently lost. By the end of the nineteenth century sections of the English working class had established an intricate evangelical type moralism of its own, but had created it out of its own experience rather than from simple acceptance of 'respectability'. If we look at attitudes to prostitution, birth control and abortion, marriage and divorce, even homosexuality, we find different class standards, the coexistence of different standards within the same class—and of course a constant gap between belief and behaviour. Capitalism did not create a personality type to fit its needs, let alone a sexual morality that was essential to the success of capital accumulation.[15]

It is important to state this. But having done so we are still left with the question of what was the relationship between capitalism and sexuality. Theoretical attempts to explain this have shown a notable paucity of insight, while descriptive accounts have offered the gory detail but little explanation. The best we can do at this stage is to suggest that the articulation between sexual mores and capitalism occurs through complex mediations—through moral agencies, political interventions, diverse social practices—whose histories still need to be uncovered.

But if we take a central strand of capitalist expansionism—its tendency to penetrate and colonise ever-increasing areas through its commoditisation and commercialisation of social life—then we can discern certain key points of articulation between changes in the structure of capitalism and changes in sexual life—the unintended consequences of capitalist growth.[16]

The major relevant shift during this century has been from capitalist accumulation to capitalist distribution, from production to consumption. The latter decades of the nineteenth century saw the inception of this tendency in North America and Europe. But its triumph came with the great post-war boom, the most sustained period of expansion in capitalist history, from the late 1940s to the early 1970s. Much of this boom was predicated upon the huge expansion of the domestic market, especially in the United States. In a country like Britain, whose growth to affluence was less rapid and more shaky than others, and whose international competitiveness decreased, the growth of its own domestic market was the *sina qua non* of economic growth. This new age of affluence with its rising standard of living for most, even as it failed to eliminate poverty for the substantial few, had its echo in changes in sexual mores. Sex had for long been something you were. By the 1950s it was also something you could buy, not just in the traditional form (for men) of prostitution, but in the form of glossily marketed fantasy. As Cohen and Taylor put it in their book *Escape Attempts* (and sex was becoming one of the great escapes) the commonest bookstall proclaimed the popularity of one of the west's major cultural forms, masturbation.[17] The public transformation in the status of what used to be called the 'solitary vice' or self-abuse is surely one of the great achievements of the post-war world. From being one of the great sexual taboos from the mid eighteenth century to the early twentieth, the gateway to nameless horrors, by the 1960s, in the work of Masters and Johnson, it had been elevated to the most efficient means of attaining sexual release.[18] The advantage of masturbation, as Quentin Crisp inimitably put it, is that you don't have to dress up for it. It is also the way in which the individual can bridge the gap, via fantasy, between mundane existence and the plurality of desires. The recognition of this in the early 1950s by a man like Hugh Hefner, founder of *Playboy*, scion of a religiously conventional and sexually inhibited mid Western family and 'the first man to become rich by openly mass marketing masturbatory love',[19] paved the way for a revolution in public discourse, if not in individual behaviour. As Barbara Ehrenreich noted, '*Playboy* charged into the battle of the sexes with a dollar sign on its banner.' *Playboy* and the like were the respectable side of a sexual coin that went into ever more dizzying circulation by the 1960s and 1970s, producing on its offside the multi-billion growth industry of the post-war world, pornography.[20]

The growth of a pornocracy was based on tendencies implicit within capitalism from at least the turn of the century—the expansion of perceived sexual needs, particularly among men.

Not only was sex an area that could be colonised by capitalism; it was also one that could expand ever more exotically. The increasing separation of eroticism from procreation, itself in part a product of technological developments within capitalism with the development of efficient means of birth control, opened up the way for the proliferation of new desires as the pursuit of pleasure became an end in itself. Much of this was potentially liberating, as the sex-procreation nexus was definitively broken up. But at the same time it provided the possibility for the commoditisation of pleasure.[21] The range of what could be bought had expanded dramatically by the 1980s—from sex aids to recreational drugs, from dating services to telephone sex-calls, from erotic clothes and fetishisms to away from it all sexual holidays. If you wanted sexual information and advice—and many did, as sexual misery and oppression continued to plague society—then the torrent of sex manuals could help you. If you needed more personalised or 'expert' assistance, then sex therapy, which by the 1970s had become a highly profitable industry in the wake of Masters and Johnson's pioneering success, was available. If you wanted casual sex (as a man) then the oldest profession was being modernised to adapt to your individual needs. Or if you wanted a more relaxed casual partnership among equals, then the growth of explicitly sexual pleasure palaces such as Plato's Retreat and the Sandstone sex commune in the mountains of California awaited you.[22] New ways of establishing contact and sexual initiation developed with the commercialisation of courtship—in cinemas, dance halls and discos—and greater geographical mobility associated with the motor car. Sex became an aid to sell everything from the automobile to soap flakes as images of female sexuality proliferated in ever more explicit forms. At the same time, new markets for sexual products were constantly being discovered or created—amongst adolescents in the 1950s, women in the 1960s, gays in the 1970s. The growth of the gay community, itself a triumph of political activity and subcultural organisation over continuing social oppression, produced its own explosion of new personal possibilities and commercial opportunities.[23]

Only rarely in history has sex really been a pre-eminently private concern. As early as the 1940s Alfred Kinsey was able to observe the practical breakdown of the private-public distinction even within the heartlands of respectable America. The social acceptance of petting, he observed, allowed public displays of sex which were acceptable simply because they fell short of the formal definition of sex, intercourse. Already he is suggesting the shaping importance of social definitions of what is allowable or not.[24] By the 1970s explicit sexuality (or at least of a heterosexual sort) pervaded the social consciousness from newsstands to televisions, from private clubs to theatres and cinemas, from advertising billboards to street life. A new community of knowledge projected sex into all corners of social life. And America led the way. A British feminist visiting New York in the early 1980s wrote of:

> a society in which sex, the body beautiful, homosexuality—everything—is commercialised to a degree as yet unknown in Europe ... the Manhattan streets where vividly dressed women and men dramatize their sexual identities in fashion codes and consciously stalk an individualistic ideal of self-fulfilment—across an urban landscape of futuristic beauty and immense squalor, where success and despair jostle on every block.[25]

The old bourgeois values of thrift and self-restraint, 'saving' rather than 'spending', the work ethic and standing on your own two feet, which Mrs Thatcher lamented, may have never been more than a minority practice. Their validity was radically challenged by the new consumerised sexuality.

Shifts in sexual relations

The chief proponents—and beneficiaries—of the sexual changes of the post-war world were undoubtedly men: as entrepreneurs of the new sexual opportunities, as laid-back indulgees in the liberated lifestyle promised by the likes of *Playboy*, or simply as voyeurs. But the targets of their interest—and of the new consumerism as well—were women.[26] Out of the complexities of the changes in the infrastructure of sex came an abundance of often contradictory discursive constructions of womanhood: women as mothers and consumers, as domestic companions and sexual partners. But lurking behind these forms of representation was another, a less high-profile one, of woman as worker, whose income in many advanced capitalist countries was the indispensable prerequisite of continuing domestic economic expansion. It was woman as worker and consumer in chief who guaranteed post-war expansion. The sexualisation of the female body was thus a problematic phenomenon, for it was not an autonomous development.

There is plentiful evidence for such a sexualisation. In much of the advanced industrialised world there has been a progressive increase in female pre-marital sex, so that today the majority of women do experience sex before marriage. In Sweden some 99 per cent of women as well as men have sexual experience before establishing permanent unions. In the United States something like 50 per cent of women do. There is a similar increase in the incidence of extra-marital sex. Kinsey's figures in the early 1950s suggested that around 26 per cent of women had adulterous relations. In more recent surveys this has risen to between 30 and 36 per cent amongst women compared to some 50 per cent of men.[27] Given the fact that more women marry than at almost any previous time, and the increased emphasis on the importance of sex in marriage, it is likely that more women have regular sexual relations than at any earlier period. There has been a major transformation in female sexual patterns, or at least there has been a major incitement to female sexual fulfilment.

It would be wrong to see these changes as straightforwardly negative. As Deirdre English has affirmed, the 1960s sex revolution was not an unmitigated disaster: 'The sexism was there, but women were actually having more sexual experience of different kinds and enjoying it.'[28] But the reality and significance of the changes that did occur were tempered by other realities, of women's continued familial dependence, of their recurrent exploitation as low paid workers in factories and offices, and of a new regime of female attractiveness which sexualised the female body while continuing to subordinate women to male definitions of desire. To put it more precisely the 'sexual liberation' of women was developing in a dual context: of male definitions of sexual need and pleasure, and of capitalist organisation of the labour market and of consumption. The junction of the two came through the material reality of family life. The economic position of most women—lower pay, fewer job opportunities—still ensures that marriage is seen as a gateway to financial as well as social security and position. And increasingly during this century sex, or at least sexual allure, has emerged as a guarantee for attaining status and security. We pay homage to an ideology of voluntarism in relation to marriage; the reality is often of an iron determinism, especially for women: economic, cultural, moral—and sexual.

The importance of the stress on sex as a key to marital harmony is not, of course, new. The idea of sex as a marital obligation is deeply rooted in the Christian west (and not just there), while a tradition of evangelical Christianity has since the seventeenth century emphasised the sacramental and binding quality of married love.[29] But the idea that choice of marriage partner—and the very nature of marriage—should be dictated by sexual attraction and compatibility is relatively new. Randolph Trumbach and others have argued that the 'rise of the egalitarian family' since the eighteenth century is dependent upon free choice of marriage partners. Nevertheless, despite the new domestic ideology, most people throughout the nineteenth century did not experience an easy union of domesticity, love and intimacy. Many sought friendships and warmth through kinspeople, neighbours and work companions of the same sex rather than their marriage partners.[30] It was not until the 1910s and 1920s that 'sexologists' expanded the concept of couple rapport to include sexual intimacy. The writings of such 'experts' as Havelock Ellis, Bertrand Russell, Marie Stopes, Van de Velde, Ben Lindsay and many others popularised the idea of a passionate union whose success could be judged largely by the degree of sexual harmony. By the outbreak of the Second World War this was already a dominant model in the United States, and by the early 1950s the idea of the 'democratic' family was widespread in Britain. Today the primarily sexual nature of conjugality seems to be universally accepted, whatever the reality.

This is not as a result of ideological manipulation. It is grounded in wider social changes. North America and Europe have witnessed, since the Second World War, a breakdown in many of the old forms of non-marital conviviality. The increased separation of work and leisure has fractured ties with workmates. Urban renewal has broken up well-established neighbourhoods, and with them well-established links of female and ethnic solidarity. Ties with kin are weakened by suburbanisation and upward and outward mobility. Marriage—or at least surrogate marriage partnerships—increasingly assume the responsibility for personal fulfilment.

The divorce figures reinforce this view. For American women born in the 1940s, 38 per cent of first marriages and 44 per cent of second will probably end in divorce. Most remarry, ever in search of the elusive fulfilment. Marriage carries with it high ideological burdens, not least of which is the burden of sexual skill. Most people seem willing to bear it. There have been shifts. In her investigation of late 1970s marriage-advice books Ellen Ross found an overwhelming emphasis on the importance of the heterosexual couple.[31] As divorce rates rise, fertility declines, and the distinction between married and unmarried tends to blur, 'the couple' rather than marriage emerges as the one seeming constant of western life. But sex becomes even more central to its success. Asked for an explanation for the growth of clinics for sex therapy, William Masters gave as one reason:

> A man and a woman need each other more now than ever before. People need someone to hold on to. Once they had the clan but now they only have each other.[32]

There is an unconscious slippage from the need for personal relations to the success of sexual performance. Sex has become the cement that binds people together.

The problem is that sexual ties are notoriously fragile. The heterosexual couple is still seen as the building block of our society, the forum of ambition, achievement and happiness. Its ideological hold on the population is immense. Yet the forces holding it together are tenuous. Here is fertile ground for social anxiety.

The regulation of sexuality

A repertoire of possible responses was available for coping with the sexual situation as it developed. The actual responses were shaped by particular social conditions and traditions, although a common feature was the struggle over forms of legal control, which, as Edwin Schur has pointed out, 'are likely to be specifically consequential, ... because of the great symbolic significance that attaches to such "authoritative or semi-authoritative" symbols'.[33]

There were, however, telling differences. Countries like Holland, West Germany, Sweden and Denmark saw a number of successful attempts to liberalise the laws governing homosexuality, abortion and pornography. Britain (or rather England and Wales) in the 1960s had an impressive set of legal changes, the most significant since the 1880s, justified by a coherent legal and political position—the 'Wolfenden strategy'. The changes in these countries represented a clear shift from laws rooted in religious moralism or even deriving from ecclesiastical precedents, to new forms of regulation dependent upon more utilitarian calculations. The secularisation of the law was perhaps the most significant feature. As early as 1958 the Lambeth Conference of the Anglican Churches saw in the new freedom of sexuality a 'gate to a new depth and joy in personal relationships between husband and wife'. A move in the position of the major establishment churches was an essential precondition for wider changes in the law. In Britain, a partial shift in the established church in attitudes to divorce, abortion and homosexuality meant that it met up with more radical sects, such as the Quakers, to support a less moralistic legal code.[34]

The United States, on the other hand, already had an official secular ideology embodied in its constitution. Here the struggle was not to change the law nationally (though many states did enjoy legal changes) but to campaign around the Constitution either by securing the Equal Rights Amendment, which until it failed in 1982 was a major focus of feminist campaigning; or by working in the courts against certain laws on the grounds that they were abridgements of guaranteed Constitutional rights. The campaign against the anti-abortion laws in Western countries are a good example of the differences. The 1967 Abortion Act in England was passed by a coalition of forces whose unifying desire was to break with the moralism of the old enactments and replace it with an act whose concern was

with health and welfare. Abortion was not freed of control—
there was no abortion on demand—but a shift in the mode of
regulation did take place, with medicine replacing the law as
the chief means of policing abortion. Two doctors were given
the responsibility of deciding whether an abortion was war-
ranted to prevent unnecessary harm to the patient. The United
States witnessed a more vigorous campaign through the courts
to get the Supreme Court to declare anti-abortion laws uncon-
stitutional—which it eventually did, in 1973.[35]

Most Western countries, then, saw a shift away from legal
moralism to a more liberal legal regime in the 1960s and 1970s,
and this was reflected in a crop of reforms especially concerned
with sexuality. The struggle for liberalisation had, however, a
different meaning in each country. In the United States the
campaign rhetoric was couched in the terminology of *rights*.
In Great Britain the struggle was conducted in terms of the
appropriate jurisdiction of the law in relation to private and
public behaviour. As a result the British legal changes—on
Prostitution (1958), on Obscenity (1959 and 1964), Male
Homosexuality and Abortion (1967), Theatre censorship
(1968) and Divorce (1969)—were preoccupied with subtle distinctions, more refined means of control, welfare and health,
but never with right or justice. The American case demanded
drama and national campaigns, and these were genuinely concerned with expanding the definition of autonomy. The British
case depended on delicate manoeuvring, parliamentary persua-
sion and political stealth—and produced 'piecemeal moral engineering'. Neither achieved a full liberalisation of the legal
controls on sexuality—or even properly mounted the foothills.
In the various states of the USA draconian laws on sexuality
remain on the statute books, and are selectively and randomly
invoked. In Britain the limitations of the 1960s reforms have
been well advertised, and in some cases (such as male homosexuality) police prosecutions actually increased after the new
acts were passed.[36] Yet in both countries, the legal changes
that did occur became symbolic of all the other changes that
had taken place. This was where the most visible changes had
occurred. In the United States the Supreme Court decision on
abortion became a *cause célèbre* amongst moralists fearing a
descent into immorality; and produced, as a counter-move,

an attempt to write into the American Constitution an
anti-abortion amendment, which fed into the politics of the
developing New Right. In Britain too the legal changes of the
1960s, modest as they appeared to those who had campaigned
for them, and limited for those whose lives were still controlled
by them, were deeply representative for conservatives of the
moral bankruptcy facing the nation.

Social antagonisms and political movements

None of these changes were uniform or universal in their impact; nor have they gone unchallenged. The social transformations of the post-war world, and especially the expansion
of capitalist relations into most spheres of social life, has produced new forms of social domination—and new forms of
resistance and politics. The widening definition of politics in
recent years is more than an arbitrary extension of a term: it
reflects a changing social reality. New 'social antagonisms'
have appeared, in opposition to new configurations of power.[37]
These do not displace old antagonisms such as those of class
or race or ethnicity. Indeed some traditional forms of conflict,
such as those between the sexes, have been reinvigorated by
the changes. But at stake is the issue of social—and hence
political—complexity. The bureaucratisation of the state which
accompanied its expansion during the great boom has produced oppositions to the excesses of paternalism: in welfare
provision, housing and health and many other spheres.
Changes in the ordering of gender relations and sex have produced, more dramatically, the feminist and sex radical movements of recent years. Following in many ways the organisational form of the black movements of the 1960s these new
social movements have constructed within them new political
subjects now prominent on the political stage—especially in
the United States. In the immensely complex tangle of social
relations produced by advanced capitalist societies, the claim
to priority of one form of struggle over another seems to have
no final status. This has profound implications for the future
of democratic politics, for the new movements are placing on
the agenda the question of the expansion of the term to include
a *sexual* democracy. A slogan like 'our bodies are our own'

has major implications for the current forms of social regulation of sex. It proposes the justice of sexual self-determination against the law and existing moral positions (including the
'reformed' law of the 1960s and 1970s); but by the very organisational form of its supporters in the women's and gay movements it proclaims the collective nature of the work necessary
to realise it. Its major achievement so far has been to bring
within the sphere of politics issues that have previously been
regarded as scarcely political at all: the questions of identity,
pleasure, consent and choice.

This broadening of the political process began amongst progressives and the general alignment was firmly with the radical
left. The new sexual movements were, however, clearly
attempting to expand the definition of politics against two
forces at once; firstly, of course, against the upholders of sexual
authoritarianism, whether political or religious; but secondly,
against an older progressive tradition which gave priority to
largely economic and class issues. At stake was not the relevance of those conventional struggles; but the equal relevance,
to those engaged in them, of the new agenda. The political
paradox of the late 1970s and early 1980s is that it has been
the traditional moralists—or at least their latter-day progeny—
who have recognised the opportunity provided by the new
political complexity and the growth of sexual politics; and the
old left which has signally failed to respond to the new politics.
Increasingly, therefore, the contemporary political agenda on
sexual issues is being written not by the libertarian left but by
the moral right. And in reconstituting the domain of sexual
politics it has been able to draw on a host of assumptions
embedded in the 'sexual tradition': of sex as danger and threat
rather than opportunity, demanding not the extension of
democracy but the reimposition of control.

CHAPTER 3

The new moralism

'The Bible on the table and the flag upon the wall'
may be the signs of secret deviance more than of
'right thinking'.

LAUD HUMPHREYS, *Tearoom Trade*

The Moral Majority is Neither.

Popular wisdom, early 1980s.

The new moralism and the New Right

There is a curious feature of the rise of the new moral Right.
Its success since the mid-1970s, in the United States and to a
lesser extent Britain, in capturing the political initiative on
sexual policy has been at a time when popular support for
liberal attitudes continues to grow. On issues such as homosexuality there is evidence in both countries of a continuation
of that slow shift in attitudes that had been going on since the
1960s. This did not herald full acceptance, more a 'toleration'
whose limits have been well rehearsed by gay activists. But at
least there appeared to be no mass base for the triumph of
anti-homosexual hysteria, as the failure of such reactionary
interventions as the Briggs initiative in California in 1978 illustrates.[1] Similarly with abortion: despite abortion becoming one
of the key issues in New Right mobilisation during the 1970s,
popular support for abortion continued to grow. One survey
in the United States suggested that apart from a sharp dip in
support in 1978, support for abortion increased steadily from
1965 to 1980. A *Newsday* poll in February 1981 showed that
72 per cent of those questioned rejected the anti-abortion position. In Great Britain at the same time conservative efforts to
limit the (unexpectedly wide) effects of the 1967 reform proved
repeatedly unsuccessful, largely because of popular mobilisation against restrictive changes.[2]

33

Yet contemporaneously social purity movements in both countries were able to mobilise sizeable constituencies and obtain some legislative purchase—with America proving the most successful testing bed. The juncture in the United States in 1979 of New Right political forces and Jerry Falwell's evangelical Moral Majority movement provided a strong cadre of footsoldiers in many parts of the country to ensure Ronald Reagan's Presidential election victories in 1980 and 1984. In Britain the union of evangelical Christian and right-wing political forces was less obvious in the Conservative election victories of 1979 and 1983, though strong personal and ideological links did exist.[3]

The *Conservative Digest* in 1979 stated that

> The New Right is looking for issues that people care
> about, and social issues, at least for the present, fit the
> bill.[4]

The American New Right had a political agenda—on the economy, race, law and order, defence, and the family—whose origins go well back into the 1960s and before. The usefulness of the so-called 'social issues'—a pleasant euphemism generally for matters concerning the family and sexuality—was that they provided an ideological framework through which to construct and organise a potentially powerful mass base, to articulate genuine social anxiety through a referential system in which 'sexual anarchy' became the explanation of social ill. Sexual anarchy, wrote Mrs Mary Whitehouse, 'is the forerunner of political anarchy. Political anarchy is the precursor of either dictatorship or destruction'.[5]

Two elements have been absolutely central in building mass support for this position: a constituency of embattled Christians, and a constituency of largely middle class, morally concerned women (not that the two are exclusive). The unifying motif was defence of 'the family', a metaphor as powerful as that of 'permissiveness' (and its polar opposite) to condense a number of hopes and fears, anxieties and possibilities around the social and the sexual. In the United States, much more than in Britain, this combination tapped a huge reservoir of strong moral belief, and dissatisfaction with all the changes that had occurred, which promised to make for a potent political force.

Increasingly in American society, Gusfield suggests, 'ceremonial and symbolic issues begin to pre-empt space customarily reserved for a more instrumental politics'.

The decline of the organising force of political parties, the increased role of government, a new style of conservative politics combined with new political technology, has made the western political system more vulnerable to the mobilisation of interest-group power. Simultaneously, the social definition of the family as a problem area in the 1970s offered a powerful totem around which this new fluid type of politics could mobilise.

In countries like Britain where class and basic economic issues were still of fundamental moment, this was less the case; but in the United States defence of the family effectively unifies the particularist concerns of various groups into a graspable political project, especially when linked to religious preoccupations.[6]

Religion has been vitally important in the articulation of moral positions and the regulation of sexual practices. Just as the move towards a more liberal interpretation of religious attitudes in the more influential British churches was a decisive precondition for the sex reforms of the 1960s, so opposition to the effects of these reforms was, contrariwise, predicated upon a largely religious world outlook. Mrs Mary Whitehouse, as the leading British social purity campaigner, adopted explicitly religious criteria to excoriate the secular influences of the 1960s—'South Bank (i.e. liberal) Theology', sex writer Alex Comfort, and the BBC, particularly its liberal Director General Sir Hugh Greene. These, and particularly the latter, were held responsible, in the court of moral absolutism, for the 'moral striptease' that had devastated the country.[7] By the 1970s secularisation had gone very far in Britain. But in the United States there remained a vast religious constituency whose values, and continuing way of life, seemed threatened by the transformations of the post-war world. Richard Viguerie, the chief fundraiser of the New Right, estimated there were some 85 million Americans with which to build a 'pro-family' coalition: 50 million born-again Protestants, 30 million morally conservative Catholics, 3 million Mormons, and 2 million orthodox and conservative Jews. Jerry Falwell's broadcast 'Old

Time Gospel Hour' had a regular weekly audience of 50 million, producing contributions of $1 million per week.[8] Here was a gigantic resource of money, moral commitment and political energy to support conservative and moral purity causes.

At the same time mobilisation in defence of 'the family' and its values could become a supremely emotive rallying-point. The family, as Lynne Segal has written, 'symbolises our deepest dreams and fears ... dreams of love, intimacy, stability, safety, security, privacy; fears of abandonment, chaos and failure.'[9] For many fundamentalist Christians the family and religion were intimately interwoven. Religion—and especially the authority of the Bible—provided a cement for personal relations and a resolution of a sense of social displacement. The family, on the other hand, was often the basis of the local religious grouping and certainly the fundamentalist churches saw themselves as extensions of kin—in rhetoric and organisation. For these and for many others 'the family' represented an image of certainty, stability and social position, whose foundations had nevertheless been fundamentally undermined.

An emphasis on family life as the fount of social and moral security is a major source of the joint appeal of moral purity and the New Right to many women. The Right in the United States, the radical feminist Andrea Dworkin has written, 'is a social and political movement controlled almost totally by men but built largely on the fear and ignorance of women'.[10] Women have been active, especially at local level, in all the major single-issue campaigns that have fed the currents of the moral Right, from groupings such as Phyllis Schlafly's campaign against ERA, and the 'pro-life', anti-abortion campaigns in America to Mary Whitehouse's campaign to 'clean up television' in Britain. In both countries this female constituency seems largely to be made up of economically dependent, middle-aged, middle-class, deeply religious women, living in rural areas and on the fringes of large cities, offering a classic sociological fit between social location and the retention of religious belief.[11] There is also a clear articulation between this sort of social background and concern with protecting the 'family'. At the simplest level the social purity campaigns represent an obvious extension of traditional women's work around the family, children, church and morality. But stronger forces are at work than this simple voluntaristic relationship might suggest. For women, 'sex spells potential danger as well as pleasure'.[12] The bitter anti-feminism of many women can be traced in part to the threat that the feminist break with traditional domestic forms seems to represent in sexual terms. Right-wing women live in the same world as feminist women, and experience the same threats (of male sexual violence) and the same possibilities of sexual objectification. In the case of right-wing women this is not countered by any sense of feminist solidarity though other forms of female community may be asserted. On the contrary feminism may be seen as precisely a force that is undermining women's basic hold on social, economic and sexual stability—marriage, family life and protection by men. In a culture where it is still relatively difficult for many women to become economically independent, and where status depends on the position of the male, women may see their very survival as dependent upon family life.[13]

There appears to be a complex knot of feelings at play here. The most obvious enemies are the social movements that explicitly threaten the old values—feminism and gay liberation particularly. Behind this is perhaps a more pervasive fear: that the changes of the past generation have served to undermine the ties that bind men to women. A powerful force in the anti-ERA campaign, was a fear of the sexes mingling, of a breakdown of the traditional boundaries between the sexes, and of women losing traditional male support as a result. The male 'flight from commitment' that Ehrenreich has traced, through easy sexual consumerism and the relaxing of marriage loyalties, has undermined marital trust. Here is one source for the fervour of the opposition to abortion. Abortion on demand, far from being an extension of women's freedom, can be seen as a further undercutting of male responsibility towards women and children by seeming to make pregnancy entirely a woman's choice.[14]

None of these fears are new. Similar feelings can be traced in the women's and social purity campaigns of the late nineteenth and early twentieth centuries. Then *feminist* opposition to mechanical birth control was based on a fear that this might weaken male ties with women. A dislike of sexual exploitation of women by men sometimes slid unconsciously into an anti-sex moralism in which the sexuality of women as well as men was to be ever more tightly controlled. And then, as today, the family, demarcated sex roles and religion were promiscuously evoked as a necessary antidote to sexual chaos. The male adoption of female standards of morality through acceptance of family responsibility and sexual restraint was seen then, as it is still apparently seen now, as an essential counter to social disruption.[15] The difference between the two periods is that today these familial and social purity positions have been welded into partnership with a political movement, in a period of heightened sexual antagonisms, to produce an effective, though far from triumphant, social and political grouping—on the right.

The experience of conservative governments in the United States and Britain which were elected with New Right support suggests that there is no automatic relationship between popular constituency and legislative action. But what has been clearly demonstrated is the potentially *political* nature of sexual issues. The idea 'that the personal is political' was a discovery of the left—but the traditional left generally fumbled the challenge. Feminism became an issue on the left only when its own effectiveness was demonstrated, and more delicate issues of sexuality, especially gay rights, were frequently shunned. As a result whole areas of social life, defined as outside real, material politics, have been evacuated for colonisation by the right. What Linda Gordon has described as 'The left's inability to articulate and unify around a progressive response, at least to the sex—and—family part of the current crisis'[16] has allowed many otherwise non-conservatives to be swayed by an ostensibly humanitarian rhetoric. The real triumph of the right has been its recognition that ideological interventions on traditionally personal or private issues can capture significant support for a wide-ranging social and political agenda. It can constitute and unify political forces on the right in a way that older conservative interventions were unable to do.

The American New Right has various organisational sources. Firstly there were (largely negative) single-issue campaigns, developing from the mid-1960s onwards, against compulsory bussing (with a barely concealed racist agenda), sex education, abortion, ERA, pornography and gay rights. Secondly a new political right has emerged as a strong political force from 1974 onwards, concerned with fundraising, elections and legislation, and drawing on diverse sources of support, from products of the new sunbelt industries to ex-Democratic neo-conservatives, alarmed by the 1960s drift to lawlessness. Finally a religiously based evangelical right has publicly emerged, of which Falwell's Moral Majority is the best publicised example.[17] Each of these have their own histories, different intellectual lineages and have constructed their own constituencies. Moreover, two distinct political priorities have emerged: the one stressing economic liberalism, the other social and moral order. The two strands are not necessarily incompatible. The economic changes promised by the New Right (lower taxes, economic freedom, reduction of bureaucracy and the cutting back of welfare) can be seen as removing the factors which are believed to have undermined the family; while the agenda of the moral right has the potential, as Jim O'Brien has argued, 'to help grease the skids for the economic changes', by providing the moral framework and ideological legitimation for greater social discipline.[18] In practice the two priorities have often clashed as the realities of government have promoted a degree of compromise (with the early lack of support from the first Reagan administration for the moral right's Family Protection Bill as a good example of cautious pragmatism triumphing over election winning ideology).

The central ideological deployment of 'the family' magically resolves some of these inevitable conflicts. *The* family as conjured up in social purity rhetoric rarely exists—and perhaps never did. The blasé pluralism of a *Readers' Digest* advertisement for a new magazine, *Families*, captures a little more of the current reality

Today's family is:
Mom, dad and 2.4 kids
A couple with 3 kids—his, hers, theirs
A 26-year-old secretary and her adopted son
A couple sharing everything but a marriage licence
A divorced woman and her stepdaughter
A retired couple raising their grandson.[19]

But the very diversity of these forms (and they are of course even more diverse if we include alternative forms, which are striking by their omission from this list) becomes the source of anxiety. Against this apparently amoral liberalism a hypothetical or mythological 'family' serves as a strong metaphor of order and harmony.

This is an hypothesised family with its own romantic history: deeply rooted in the realities of English individualism or of the American frontier, subversive site of individual freedom or of good Christian values.[20] There is no necessary adherence to religious values. Ferdinand Mount's conservative defence of the 'subversive family' is partly on the grounds that it is a bastion against religious dogmatism. But whatever the starting position, the organising centrality of the family for social policy is affirmed. A more sensitive reading of the past would show a more complex history than is allowed in these polemics: of diverse sets of relations, of fracturing of kin ties by economic and social necessity, of survival against the tyranny of patriarchal authority, of women's equal, or greater, participation in productive activity, and of sexual repression.[21] But the mythologised family enables the combination of various social issues, and acts as a standard by which to judge them.

Not all of these issues relate primarily or at all to sexual matters. There is a strong case for arguing that an implicit racism is as powerful a force as an explicit anti-feminism—though the two can easily become intertwined. The influential neo-conservative, D.P. Moynihan, made the relevant connections in his famous report on the 'Negro Family' in the 1960s, when he argued that the deterioration of Negro family life was due in large part to the emasculation of the black male by the working female. Sometimes the racist implications become less subtle. Pat Robertson, a fundamentalist television preacher, explicitly compared the home, as the basic unit of the fabric of society, with 'the flotsam and jetsam of the ghetto where young people don't know who their parents are'. Hunter has rightly remarked that

> In juxtaposing the family to the sexual promiscuity of the (black) ghetto, he has used non-racial criteria for writing

blacks out of the moral middle strata and into a place beyond.[22]

Similarly, the rhetoric of Christianity, or of economic self-reliance, or of denunciations of reliance on welfare, or of 'law and order', are ways of invalidating all but a narrow social experience without the words black or white passing the lips. In political terms they encode and call up racist feelings.[23] The complex linkages between white racism and fear of black sexuality have long been a subject of controversy. In the rhetorical evocation of the family by the New Right we can find an intricate marriage of race, gender, sex and class, in which all but the 'traditional values' are denigrated and devalued, and which effectively construct a white, largely male and middle-class view of what constitutes appropriate sexual behaviour. The campaigns against feminism or permissiveness thus have more than a negative agenda. They have a vision of a new order. In the homely rhetoric of the pro-family coalition lies the promise—or threat—of a new absolutism, an authoritarian populist project which nudges us gently to what has been called an 'apple-pie authoritarianism' in the United States,[24] and which in Britain urges a return to the security of 'Victorian values'.

The historical irony of this is that it often takes place on the territory marked out by radical sexual politics, and this has heavily shaped the right response. Even Mary Whitehouse in Britain has found it necessary to call for a sexual ethic that is 'neither reactionary nor libertarian', and in support of this she draws on the writings of the American New Rightist George Gilder (whose *Wealth and Poverty* was distributed to his Cabinet by President Reagan in 1981).[25] For Gilder, as for many radical feminists, it is men who are the problem, and wives who are the solution. There has been a major shift in the conservative interpretation of the heterosexual bond. The typical nineteenth-century view saw male sexuality as rampant, and the woman as little more than a passive receptacle. Today, fed by the dulcet appeal of sociobiology (the new morality is not averse to this branch of the sexual science), women's nature-endowed role as nurturer (and hence embodiment of women's particular strengths) is more assertively stressed. So Roger Scruton, the English New Right philosopher, can obscurely counterpose the 'unbridled ambition of the phallus' to the (presumably nature-given) task of women to 'quieten what is most vagrant'.[26] A fundamental difference and divide between male and female sexuality is reasserted against those who would deny distinctions; but the hazardous complementarity of the sexes is affirmed. Male desire contains a 'vector which negates obligation', as Scruton puts it. At the same time, as Phyllis Schlafly suggests in *The Power of the Positive Woman* (and how evocative that title is!), this strength of desire conceals a passivity in men, a need to be appreciated, admired and loved. Positive womanhood can supply this need, to the benefit of society. The essential conduit is the family. For Gilder:

> A married man . . . is spurred by the claims of family to channel his otherwise disruptive male aggressions into his performance as a provider for wife and children.[27]

By a skilful theoretical manoeuvre, the feminist case against male violence is turned into a defence of conservative social forms.

Few people today would fully embrace the libertarian attack on the family of the 1960s. The 'narrow privacy and tawdry secrets' of the family might be recognised, but we seek the source of our discontents far wider than 'the family'.[28] But there is a case still to be made against the elevation of *the* family as the necessary form of domestic organisation and the focus of all social policy. It is a common New Right argument that the obvious personal discontent and anxiety that exists is a product of the weakening of traditional bonds. It can equally well be argued, as Barrett and McIntosh suggest, that the over-emphasis on the family drains all other social relations of meaning.[29] There are both individual needs and collective needs that cannot be satisfied through a single 'traditional' form—and one moreover that in practice few of us live in at any particular time. The fundamental weakness of the New Right case is that despite its emotive appeal, only a minority of the electorate, to judge by their preferences shown in life-styles and opinion sampling, seem to want it enforced on them. But the success of the New Right's hegemonising of family politics means this case cannot easily be made. Many on the left have attempted to recuperate the family for a progressive politics by adapting to this new mood. The famous jeremiad of Christopher Lasch (wittily described by Ellen Ross as the Edmund Burke of this crisis)[30] against contemporary narcissism, and call for a return to the safe haven of the frontier family, explicitly rejects the claims of feminism and is implicitly anti-homosexual. Others (including feminists) have attempted to redefine feminism as being essentially about struggle in the family, or have attempted to construct pro-family socialist organisations (such as Friends of the Family). Even among feminists the increased emphasis on the threats posed by sexual freedom as opposed to its promise can be seen as one veiled response to this ideological offensive.[31]

The victims of this effort are all those who live outside the family form—and who are likely to continue to do so: the single person, the divorced, the unattached parent, the independent old, the collective-household dweller, the lesbian, the male gay. Few would argue against the nuclear unit as one road of choice. A strong case can be made against elevating the family into the fundamental norm of our variegated society.

In the New Right vision of social order the family has a policing role. It ensures carefully demarcated spheres between men and women, adults and children. It regulates sexual relations and sexual knowledge. It enforces discipline and proper respect for authority. It is a harbour of moral responsibility and the work ethic. This is contrasted to the ostensible moral chaos that exists outside.

Given this set of beliefs, it is not surprising that the New Right is so vehemently opposed to the sex radical movements. Gusfield has distinguished between 'gestures of cohesion' and 'gestures of differentiation'. If wrapping around you the flag of the family is a powerful symbol of cohesion, strong antipathy to women and gays is a source of differentiation, suggesting 'that some people have a legitimate claim to greater respect, importance, or worth in the society than have some others'.[32] Feminists challenge the old ways of relating between men and women. Lesbians and gay men offer a coherent alternative to conventional ways of living. More fringe sexual groupings threaten orthodox differentiations between generations, or be-

tween accepted and unacceptable types of activity. All tend to
affirm the significance of individual autonomy and needs, the
importance of choice, and the merits of sexual pleasure. A
clear line runs between the two types of sexual politics, that of
the right and that of the left. In the current climate it is the
right who have the political initiative. As Gayle Rubin has
said, 'the right has been spectacularly successful in tapping
(the) pools of erotophobia in its accession to state power.'[33]
The effect is to close the space that seemed to be opening up
in the 1960s and 1970s for experiment and change. The victims,
inevitably, are those on the margins of acceptability.

Sex as fear and loathing: the example of AIDS

Sexuality is a fertile source of moral panic, arousing intimate
questions about personal identity, and touching on crucial
social boundaries. The erotic acts as a crossover point for a
number of tensions whose origins are elsewhere: of class, gender, and racial location, of intergenerational conflict, moral
acceptability and medical definition. This is what makes sex a
particular site of ethical and political concern—and of fear and
loathing.

The history of the last two hundred years or so has been
punctuated by a series of panics around sexuality—over childhood sexuality, prostitution, homosexuality, public decency,
venereal diseases, genital herpes, pornography—which have
often grown out of or merged into a generalised social
anxiety.[34] Over time there have been shifts in the focus of those
events. Today the public indecencies of pornography have replaced the nineteenth-century preoccupation with the 'fallen
sisterhood' of prostitution, and the homosexual as folk devil
has been dislodged by the child molester (though the two are
often willy-nilly moulded into one). More crucially, over the
past hundred years the language of condemnation has changed:
from the anathemas of received morality to the rhetoric of
hygiene and medicine. The transition between the two
modes—a long revolution in sexual regulation—has never been
easy, nor finally realised. Like poor Oscar Wilde in the 1890s,
you might be denounced in the public press as wicked, found
guilty in the courts as a criminal, and subjected to medical and

psychiatric investigation as some species of 'erotomaniac'. Certain forms of sexuality, socially deviant forms—homosexuality especially—have long been promiscuously classified as 'sins' *and* 'diseases', so that you can be born with them, seduced into them and catch them, all at the same time. But today you are less likely to be condemned as immoral and more likely to be labelled sick. Disease sanctions govern and encode many of our responses to sex. It is this which makes the moral panic around AIDS (acquired immune-deficiency syndrome) so important. It condenses a number of social stresses and throws unprecedented light on them. What is so very striking about the moral panic around AIDS is that its victims are often being blamed for the illness. And as most people with AIDS to date (at least in Western industrial countries) have been male homosexuals, this must surely tell us something about the current sexual climate.

The mechanisms of a moral panic are well known:[35] the definition of a threat in a particular event (a youthful 'riot', a sexual scandal); the stereotyping of the main characters in the mass media as particular species of monsters (the prostitute as 'fallen woman', the paedophile as 'child molester'); a spiralling escalation of the perceived threat, leading to the taking up of absolutist positions and the manning of the moral barricades; the emergence of an imaginary solution—in tougher laws, moral isolation, a symbolic court action; followed by the subsidence of the anxiety, with its victims left to endure the new proscriptions, social climate or legal penalties. In sexual matters the effects of such a flurry can be devastating, especially when it touches, as it does in the case of homosexuality, on public fears, and on an unfinished revolution in the gay world itself. As Dennis Altman has remarked, in America today the homosexual is partially accepted but homosexuality is not.[36] Despite (or perhaps because of) the huge expansion of the gay communities since the 1960s, there is a large residue of anxiety and social hostility and a continuing social marginality. There is also, in the New Right and its evangelical and social purity affiliates, a political force able to capitalise on this social climate to propagate its own moral agenda. The eruption of AIDS since 1979 on to this fertile ground was fortuitous, but the social reaction it engendered was not.

Susan Sontag has observed the importance of illness—especially cancer—as metaphors, with illness given a particular moral stigma when related to an activity or a group of people otherwise disapproved of.

As if to confirm these arguments the *New Republic* made an explicit linkage. AIDS is a metaphor that 'has come to symbolize ... the identity between contagion and a kind of desire'.[37] In the fear and loathing that AIDS evokes there is a resulting conflation between two plausible, if unproven theories—that there is an elective affinity between disease and certain sexual practices, and that certain sexual practices cause disease—and a third, that certain types of sex *are* diseases. In the climate produced by such assumptions rational thought is very near impossible.

From the first AIDS was identified as a peculiarly homosexual affliction. The first major newspaper breaking of the story was in the *New York Times*, 3 July 1981, which headlined its story 'Rare cancer seen in 41 homosexuals'.[38] Kaposi's Sarcoma quickly became known as the 'gay cancer', though as it became clearer that this was only a symptom of a wider problem, a new term was adopted: GRID, 'Gay-related immunodeficiency'. Soon it became apparent that this rubric also was inadequate, for though male homosexuals amounted to threequarters of the reported cases, other groups of people were vulnerable: intravenous drug users, haemophiliacs, and significantly for the heated speculation about causes, Haitian immigrants into the USA'. From 1982 'AIDS' was generally accepted as the more accurate term. This did not stop the media recurrently referring in these early days to the 'gay plague'. The *New York* magazine spoke of a 'plague' spreading like wildfire—and in media shorthand this term became a common signifier of AIDS.[39]

By mid-1983 a generalised panic was in full swing, not only in the USA but elsewhere. The London *Sunday Times* reported in August 1983 that 'Fear of catching the mysterious killer disease, AIDS, is causing more harm in Britain than the disease itself', with one London hospital reporting 'hundreds of patients suffering from AIDS-related anxiety—some to the point of considering suicide'.[40] The United States first saw the grim appearance (soon echoed elsewhere) of what Sontag has called 'practices of decontamination': medics refused to treat AIDS patients, trash collectors wore masks when collecting garbage from suspected victims, undertakers refused to bury the dead. In Britain prison officers refused to move prisoners and the fire brigade worried about mouth to mouth resuscitation. Most of these practices were directed at homosexuals, though a hidden agenda of racism also had its corrupting impact: Haitian immigrants were initially targeted as a reservoir of disease, just as in the 1950s, when they first arrived in the USA, they had been branded as syphyllitics and TB carriers. Disease, deviant sex and race were intricately interwoven.[41]

There was in fact a dual crisis: one in the response to the disease itself; and one in the gay community. Both revolved essentially around the question of homosexuality and the gay lifestyle. The difficulty for both lay in deciding what the source and meaning of 'the plague' was. Two theories at first vied for supremacy. One stressed that it was the gay lifestyle that was the cause of infection; the other that it was a viral infection, probably transmitted through close contact and blood, which turned out to be the real situation. The 'bad blood' motif was a powerful and emotive one, and it served to unite the environmentalist and viral theories.

In his autobiographical work, *Breaking Ranks* (1979), Norman Podhoretz, a leading Neo-Conservative author and editor of *Commentary*, expressed his distaste for gays. Homosexuality, he wrote, was a plague that attacks 'the vital organs of the entire species, preventing men from fathering children and women from mothering them'.[42] In such a view (ironically coming from a prominent member of the Jewish community which itself had suffered for ostensibly having it too) homosexuals were displayed as having bad blood (homosexuality itself was the plague) and spreading it (weakening the vital fibres of others). The magical link was through a key term. 'One word', the gay writer Nathan Fain has written, 'is like a hand grenade in the whole affair: promiscuity.'[43] Although promiscuity has long been seen as a characteristic of male homosexuals, there is little doubt that the 1970s saw a quantitative jump in its incidence as establishments such as gay bath-houses and back-room bars, existing specifically for the purposes of casual sex, spread in all the major cities of the

United States and elsewhere, from Toronto to Paris, Amsterdam to Sydney (though London remained more or less aloof, largely due to the effects of the 1967 reform). Michel Foucault has written characteristically of the growth of 'laboratories of sexual experimentation' in cities such as San Francisco and New York, 'the counterpart of the medieval courts where strict rules of proprietary courtship were defined'.[44] For the first time for most male homosexuals, sex became easily available. With it came the chance not only to have frequent partners but also to explore the varieties of sex. Where sex becomes too available, Foucault suggests, constant variations are necessary to enhance the pleasure of the act. For many gays coming out in the 1970s the gay world was a paradise of sexual opportunity and of sensual exploration.

But these developments had scarcely gone unremarked. Delicate and not so delicate warnings about the dangerous connection between outrageous sexual indulgence and growing political power had for several years past been broadcast in the media. The CBS television documentary 'Gay Power/Gay Politics', in 1978, had contained explicit condemnation of gay sado-masochistic practices as a way, so it seemed to many in the gay community, of weakening the respectability and political pull of that community.[45] Moreover, it had become the object for numerous conservative offensives during the 1970s of which Anita Bryant's crusade in Florida and the Briggs initiative in California were only the public tips. San Francisco, Babylon by the Bay, was already targeted by the late 1970s for Moral Majority inspired evangelical assaults—and physical attacks inevitably followed in their wake. Midge Decter (Podhoretz's wife) has spoken scathingly of 'the homosexual's flight from normality'.[46] This was precisely the point: the developing gay way of life ran radically counter to the received sexual norms which the New Right was busy mobilising behind in the 1970s. AIDS provided proof positive that the fault was in the essence of homosexuality, of which promiscuity and disease was the inevitable product. It was blood which caused it and blood that revealed it. 'The poor homosexuals', Patrick J. Buchanan, later an assistant to President Reagan, wrote in the *New York Post* (24 May 1983), 'they have declared war upon nature, and now nature is exacting an awful retribution.'[47] By the summer of 1983 the Reverend Jerry Falwell was suggesting that gays be rounded up and quarantined like sick animals.[48]

The parallel that immediately comes to mind is with the association made in the nineteenth century between female prostitution and the incidence of venereal disease. One response in England in the 1860s was the passing of the Contagious Diseases Acts, which enforced compulsory inspections in certain garrison towns of women suspected of being carriers.[49] A similar chain of association existed by the early 1980s—promiscuity, VD, the undermining of the innocent nation's health. And there was a similar sort of response in what Schur describes as the call for 'social-psychological and moral containment'. As one gay activist put it,

> no one blamed war veterans for Legionnaire's Disease, no one attacked women over Toxic Shock Syndrome. But right-wing publicists are having a field day spreading panic and hatred against us over AIDS.[50]

AIDS produced, or accentuated, a crisis in societal responses to homosexuality. But the media-medical panic was paralleled by a moral crisis in the gay subculture itself. Beyond the medical sandstorm, one ring-side commentator said, 'lies a truly awesome hurricane of feeling within the gay male neighbourhoods of large United States cities'.[51] A large part of this was obviously due to the ghastly nature of the disease itself. Beyond this, the form of the reaction is illustrative of real strains within the gay world. For AIDS focused attention on just those practices and beliefs which have been central to the emergence of a coherent gay identity since the 1960s, but which simultaneously have been major sources of tension, both within the gay community and with the outside world.

The incidence of promiscuity and casual sex, the use of stimulants such as amyl nitrite ('poppers') and the extension of accepted sexual practices to include sado-masochism and fist fucking, have all been explored as aetiological factors of AIDS, and have all been the subject of heated controversy both within and outside the gay subcultures. Even more crucially, a large part of the male gay revolution of the 1970s lay in the celebration of the body. The 'machoisation' of the male gay world in those years was in part at least a product not of a simple aping of traditional male values but of an attempt to break away from the easy assumption that male homosexuality represented an effeminisation of men. It was a demonstration that you could be male *and* gay. The cultivation of the body beautiful was a vital part of that. But AIDS is a disease of the body, it wrecks and destroys what was once glorified. As Sontag has written (of cancer), 'Far from revealing anything spiritual, it reveals that the body is, all too woefully, just the body.'[52]

Transcending all these issues of lifestyle was the potent question of the gay identity itself. The gay identity is no more a product of nature than any other sexual identity. It has developed through a complex history of definition and self-definition, and what recent histories of homosexuality have revealed clearly is that there is no necessary connection between sexual practices and sexual identity. But since the late 1960s, with the emergence of a gay movement and the huge expansion of the gay subcultures, coming out as homosexual, that is openly assuming a gay identity, has been crucial to the public affirmation of homosexuality. Homosexual desire was no longer an unfortunate contingency of nature or fate; it was the positive basis of a sexual and, increasingly, social, identity. AIDS implicitly threatened that, firstly by offering fearful consequences for being actively gay, but secondly, more subtly, by undermining the assumption that homosexuality in itself is valid.

AIDS, like nineteenth-century cancer, is seen as the disease of the sexually excessive just as 'the homosexual' is seen as the social embodiment of a particular sexual constitution. The association of AIDS with homosexuality thus serves to critically undermine the basis of the gay identity. AIDS is the punishment for the forthright expression of certain sexual desires.

Given this background it is not surprising that AIDS produced several different responses amongst gay activists. The first may be described as one of controlled hysteria. Its authentic note was struck by the novelist Larry Kramer in an article in *New York Native* emotively entitled '1, 112 AND COUNTING'.

> If this article doesn't scare the shit out of you we're in real trouble. If this article doesn't rouse you to anger, fury,

rage and action, gay men may have no future on this earth. Our continued existence depends on just how angry you can get.[53]

Kramer was the author of a novel, *Faggots*, in 1977 which rather suggested that the gay world was ripe for retribution. His contribution to the AIDS debate was widely echoed, suggesting that there were indeed deep reservoirs of guilt to be mined. One AIDS person, understandably upset at attempts to minimize the illness, wrote to the Toronto gay paper, *Body Politic*:

There is no mutant virus; there will be no vaccine ... Denying that promiscuity is the cause of AIDS related death is going to decimate the gay male community. By refusing to see that the promiscuous lifestyle is potentially fatal, one may permit the ultimate triumph of the Moral Majority: we will kill ourselves.[54]

Here promiscuity was both cause and symptom of disaster. A second position comes from the opposite end of the spectrum. 'Promiscuity', the gay journalist Ken Popert has written, 'knits together the social fabric of the gay male community.'[55] From this position the AIDS panic is seen as an attempt by the medical definers of deviance to recuperate their loss of control over the gay community:

Like helpless mice we have peremptorily, almost inexplicably, relinquished the one power we so long fought for in constructing our modern gay community: the power to determine our own identity. And to whom have we relinquished it? The very authority we wrested it from in a struggle that occupied us for more than a hundred years: the medical profession.[56]

AIDS in this view is a tragic reality, but it is being used to reaffirm social marginalisation and control.

A third position lies somewhere in between these two. It calls for a cool response to the crisis, but recommends a pragmatic adaptation to the perceived dangers. Arnie Kantrowitz struck a representative note:

> As a member of the 'most-likely-to-contract-Kaposi's'
> crowd I knew I had to change my ways. They weren't
> wicked ways, I knew. My experiment in sexual anarchy
> was a rare delight, a laboratory lesson in license, an
> opportunity to see both flesh and spirit gloriously naked. I
> will never apologise to anyone for my promiscuity. I
> practised it with high ideals. But if I endanger my own
> mental or physical health, then I am myself an apology.[57]

All three positions are understandable responses to a genuine
crisis or combination of crises: a crisis of individual lives, a
crisis of the hopes that have directed the often painful shaping
of a public gay identity, and a crisis in the politics of sexuality
as the forces hostile to homosexuality have seized on a human
tragedy for their own moralistic ends. But it seems to me that
in an unstable situation the two extreme positions tend to
cancel each other out. Fervent denunciations of the past cannot
bring back the dead, while celebration of its pleasures does not
give much comfort to the fearful living. As Kantrowitz has
written:

> What is the bad news? Is sex dead? No. Is God wreaking
> cosmic vengeance on us? No. The bad news is simply that
> we have to take responsibility for our actions.[58]

Paradoxically, the very divisions within the gay community's
responses to AIDS have been a sign of that community's potential strengths. The debate has been passionate and polemical
because much seems at stake. But even those most critical of
gay lifestyles have continued their campaigns *within* the gay
movements (Kramer was one of the founders of the Gay Men's
Health Crisis organisation). Those movements themselves
have proved far from helpless as they used their growing political clout in the USA to put pressure on representatives for
funds and assistance. Within the gay subcultures themselves,
gay men appeared to be cautiously adapting to new sexual
circumstances—certainly suggested by a possible reduction in
the incidence of sexually transmitted diseases. In the columns
of the gay press there was a new emphasis on what constitutes
a healthy lifestyle and it has often been openly gay doctors

who have monitored the progress of the disease and the fight against it. As an AIDS person, Bobbi Campbell, said on the 1983 Gay Pride Parade in San Francisco:

> We are not victims, we are fighters ... It is not important
> to worry about when we will die; rather we should be
> more concerned about how we live.[59]

It would be a nice irony of history if a moral panic directed largely at homosexuals were to end up by strengthening the ties of solidarity of the gay community. It will not be the first time this has happened. No doubt it will not be the last.

Strategies

The example of AIDS illustrates the density of organising beliefs that shape sexuality. Each episode in its history is constructed from a myriad human interventions, guided by diverse concepts of what amounts to appropriate behaviour. Unfortunately, we all too often confront this complexity with moral and political positions that assume we *know* what constitutes correct sexual behaviour, and with powerful interests which seek to enforce them. When faced with sex we readily abandon respect for diversity and choice, we neglect any duty to understand human motivation and potentialities, and fall back on received pieties, and authoritarian methods. The result can be devastating for those who are forced to live on the margins of social acceptability—and inhibitive for those who do not.

Historically, the Christian west has offered three conflicting strategies for the regulation and control of sexuality, which I shall call the absolutist, the liberal, and the libertarian approaches.[60] Each of these evokes differing assumptions about the true meaning of sex. The absolutist position is the most clear-cut and familiar. It is not so much a coherent set of beliefs as a conviction that there is a clear morality (usually a strongly familial and monogamous one) which must guide personal and social life. In the west this morality has been generally rooted in Christianity—though this is not inevitable. The forms of regulation have changed, of course, over the centuries, and most of the surviving sexually conservative legislation in Britain and the USA derives from the social purity legislation passed between the 1880s and the 1920s rather than from medieval canon law (though sometimes you would not think so). But absolutist or fundamentalist positions are still firmly dominant in the Roman Catholic Church—indeed Pope John Paul II has ostentatiously reaffirmed them—and the evangelical Protestant churches, who as we know have powerful sociopolitical lobbies especially on the New Right. For these, sex clearly represents disruption and danger.

Against this we may set a second tradition, the liberal or liberal-pluralist position, which despite challenges has become highly influential over the last generation. As we have seen the liberal traditions differ in North America and Europe (and also differ incidentally between different European countries). In America the organising idea is that of 'rights'—and it is significant that in the abortion campaigns each side speaks in the language of rights, the rights of the unborn child versus the right of a woman to her own body. The result can be a dissolution back into the language of moral absolutes in which both sides simply proclaim different truths. In Britain, on the other hand, civil rights have always been a residual category though this has to some extent been balanced by a certain restraint in direct state intervention.[61] Where both positions meet is in a concern in defining the limits of public intervention into private behaviour.

Rooted in the debates of nineteenth-century liberalism, and in particular the work of J.S. Mill, this issue has been most clearly debated in England. Its classical statement is the 'Wolfenden Report' on homosexuality and prostitution published in 1957.[62] The focus of its argument is the distinctions it draws between morality and law. The duty of law is to regulate public order and to maintain acceptable (though by implication changing) standards of public decency, not to patrol personal life. From this distinction flowed most of the 'permissive legislation' of the 1960s, and the inspiration for the officially sponsored investigations of sexual matters since. It has been an important strategy in undermining the absolutist approach, and in creating certain spaces for greater individual freedom. But it is explicitly not a libertarian approach.

The Wolfenden strategy deliberately avoids speaking of the merits of particular forms of sexuality, and relies instead on shifting appraisals of what is socially acceptable. This in turn is based on a wholly artificial distinction between the personal and public, treating them as if they were natural and eternal categories, while actually constituting and delimiting them through legislative proposals. The result has been confusion over the definition of 'private' (especially with regard to homosexuality and pornography, where the definition constantly seems to shift) and over 'consent', which is crucial to the liberal approach. In Britain girls can consent to sex at 16, male homosexuals at 21, while rape in marriage is impossible, which by implication denies wives the right to refuse consent. Perhaps more significantly, the Wolfenden strategy provides a framework for potentially extending rather than reducing the detailed regulation of sexual behaviour either by new forms of legal surveillance of the public sphere, or by refined modes of intervention (medical, social work) into the private. The imagined public opinion of the average sensual man can become a tyrannous master when applied to sexual diversity.

The libertarian approach also has a substantial history, in this case extending from the radical pioneers of the late eighteenth century (if not earlier) to the sexual politics of today. In its most characteristic form it speaks of a sexuality that has been denied, to the detriment of individual freedom and social health. Its naturalistic approach to sexuality mirrors that of the major tradition of sexual thought for the past century, but it has been given an intellectual cutting edge through the work of the left Freudians, Wilhelm Reich and Herbert Marcuse especially; and a social grounding and political coherence through the counter-culture of the 1960s and the sex radical movements of the 1970s. At the heart of this approach is the belief that sexual repression is essential to social oppression; and that the moment of sexual liberation should necessarily coincide with the moment of social revolution. It is a utopian and millenarian project, and that has been its major source of energy. Rejecting the narrow certainties of conservative absolutism and the cautious and subtle distinctions of liberalism, it has offered a critique of contemporary sexual chaos from the viewpoint of an unalienated sexuality in the future. Its weakness is that, like the other approaches, it relies entirely on a fundamentalist view of sexuality whose truth it seeks to express. As a result its celebration of sex can easily become a glorification of all manifestations of desire. The effect of this, as feminists have pointed out, can be to impose a view that sexual expression is not only pleasurable, but necessary—often at the expense of women. The real problems, of defining alternatives and constructing new forms of relating, are ignored. The difficulty, and the danger, of simple libertarianism is that unfortunately sex does not unproblematically speak its own truth.

Against the certainties of these positions I want to canvass the merits of a fourth—what I shall call the 'radical pluralist' position. Like the liberal position at its best, it speaks out for individual needs. Like the libertarian approach it embraces the legitimacy of many hitherto execrated and denied sexual practices. Unlike the absolutist approaches, whether the old absolutism of religious dogmatism or the new, born of political certainties, it speaks out for the acceptance of diversity. It is, as yet, a position in the making rather than a fixed set of ethical or political practices. But it is apparent that two related aims need to be pursued.

The first involves a challenge to the idea that sexuality embodies the working out of an immanent truth. It is not a true and final nature which our sexual behaviour expresses but the intimate (and barely understandable, as yet) elaboration of a complexity of biological, psychic and social influences, all of which are deeply embodied in relations of domination and subordination. We need, therefore, to tear open the assumptions which lock us into conflicting views about what is natural or unnatural, true or false, right or wrong. We should begin to understand the hidden assumptions which organise the sexual tradition.

If the first task is to question the absolutism of 'Nature', the second is to explore the possibilities of an approach which is sensitive to what I believe to be the really fundamental issues around sexuality today: the social nature of identity, the criteria for sexual choice, the meaning of pleasure and consent, and the relations between sexuality and power.

All these issues pose major difficulties and problems. But a radical pluralist position is peculiarly concerned with the contradictory nature of sexual experience and the hazard-strewn path of sexual politics. It does not seek a sexual utopia outside history, because of its belief that it is only in and through history that sexuality has any meaning. We have recently been warned of the danger of seeing a future, socialist, polity as a completely homogeneous society in which all antagonisms will have disappeared. Instead, it is argued, we should begin to see socialism as the organising belief of 'a society in which antagonisms will be settled in a truly democratic fashion'.[63] Sexual antagonisms and contradictions probably cannot be entirely eliminated either, but we can find more democratic ways of handling them, to eliminate arbitrary exclusions and to maximise the possibilities of a non-exploitative freedom of choice. This is not an easy agenda. Only when we begin to shape it will we finally have escaped from the seductive embrace and certainties of the sexual tradition, with its claim to provide a privileged access to the absolute truths of Nature.

PART TWO

The sexual tradition

... myth has the task of giving an historical
invention a natural justification,
and making contingency appear eternal.

ROLAND BARTHES, 'Myth Today' in *Mythologies*

CHAPTER 4

'Nature had nothing to do with it': the role of sexology

The great fundamental impulses in human
life, as among animals generally, are
those of nutrition and of sex, of hunger
and of love. They are the two original
sources of dynamic energy which brings
into existence the machinery of living in
lowlier organisms, and in ourselves
constitute the most elaborate social
superstructures.

HAVELOCK ELLIS, *The Psychology of Sex*

Sexology is very much concerned, in the
final analysis, with the interconnected-
ness of what goes on between the groins
and between the ears relative to procreation
of the species.

JOHN MONEY, *Love and Love Sickness*

The invention of a creature whose feelings
were legitimately 'hetero' and 'sexual' was
something new in the late Victorian night,
a creature quite as unique as the 'homosexual'
under the late Victorian moon. .... That
newly invented 'heterosexual' was no more
'natural' than the 'homosexual' was
'unnatural'. To paraphrase Mae West, nature
had nothing to do with it.

JONATHAN KATZ, *Gay/Lesbian Almanac*

Science of desire or technology of control?

Appeals to 'Nature', to the claims of the 'natural', are amongst
the most potent we can make. They fix us in a world of

apparent solidity and truth, offering an affirmation of our real selves, and providing the benchmark for our resistance to what is corrupting, 'unnatural'. Unfortunately, the meaning of 'Nature' is not transparent. Its truth has been used to justify our innate violence and aggression and our fundamental sociability. It has been deployed to legitimise our basic evil, and to celebrate our fundamental goodness. There are, it often seems, as many natures as there are conflicting values.

Nowhere is this more true than in relation to our sex. It *appears* to be the most basic fact about us. We are, as Havelock Ellis suggested, defined by it:

> Sex penetrates the whole person; a man's sexual
> constitution is a part of his general constitution. There is
> considerable truth in the dictum: 'A man is what his sex is'.

Sex has become, as Michel Foucault has famously polemicised, the 'truth of our being'.[1] Our essence and our ultimate identity is somehow an effect of what our sexual nature dictates: we are constructed upon a bedrock of natural impulses.

Yet when we try to explore this realm of truth we find ourselves in a corridor of mirrors. The images, real and distorted, are powerful enough. But there are so many of them! And which is the real one? Where lies the truth of this truth? This has been the question which has dominated sexual theorising and sex research during the past century and despite many challenges it is a question whose time is not yet exhausted. From the dissection of rats to explain homosexual behaviour to the DNA determinism of contemporary sociobiology the search for the natural roots of our being goes on. What if, as now seems very likely, it is this constant seeking for truth that is the problem? We would be forced then, to look again at the role and function of those earnest proclaimers of the truth of sexuality, those would-be scientists of desire, the sexologists and their camp followers.

In the Preface to the first edition of his vastly influential compendium of sexual case studies and speculations, *Psychopathia Sexualis*, Richard von Krafft-Ebing wrote in 1887 that:

> Few people are conscious of the deep influence exerted by
> sexual life upon the sentiment, thought and action of man
> in his social relations to others.

Little more than half a century later, Alfred Kinsey could comment that:

> there is no aspect of human behaviour about which there has been more thought, more talk, and more books written.[2]

Few now, it seemed, doubted that 'deep influence'. Leaving aside for the moment the issue of whether Krafft-Ebing's statement was itself an accurate account of the nineteenth century, it is clear that the period between the two comments saw an extraordinary efflorescence of writing about, thinking about, talking about, sexuality; and a no less ardent effort to live it. 'King Sex' has reigned over the twentieth century: Krafft-Ebing and Alfred Kinsey have been two of his most famous and assiduous courtiers. The question that inevitably arises is: how important were these writers and researchers, this apostolic succession from Krafft-Ebing to Masters and Johnson, from Havelock Ellis and Freud to Kinsey and beyond, in shaping the way we think—and hence experience—our sexualities? They themselves had no doubt of their pioneering role in discovering the significance of the sexual. But as the mists clear, and as sexuality becomes increasingly an area of contestation, we can see that they actually played a more positive role in constructing that significance. 'Modern sexuality' is in part at least an invention of sexological pens, and like all such inventions its effects have been contradictory. These self-proclaimed pioneers, those avatars of sexual enlightenment, worked to build a science of desire, a new continent of knowledge that would reveal the hidden keys to our nature. In so doing they also lent support to other, more dubious activities, from the pathologising of 'perverse' sexual practices to the construction of racist eugenics, from the celebration of sexual antagonisms to the institutionalisation of dubious 'treatments'. They contributed, in diverse ways in the twentieth century, to the shaping and maintenance of an elaborate technology of control. The more we delve into this complex, sometimes noble, sometimes murky, history, the more we can perceive that 'Nature', pure human nature, had very little to do with it.

Pioneers

The last decades of the nineteenth century saw a spectacular new preoccupation with the scientific study of sexuality, giving rise to this new subdiscipline, 'sexology'. The Founding Fathers of sexology (and for once the patriarchal metaphor is an appropriate one; few women participated in this first wave of sexual theorising) had a clear vision of their task. There was, it is true, an often tentative note in their apologias, not surprising given their sense of the opposition. Krafft-Ebing modestly suggests in a preface to *Psychopathia Sexualis* that 'The object of this treatise is *merely* [my emphasis] to record the various psychopathological manifestations of sexual life in man ...' But the addendum was more profoundly ambitious: '... and to reduce them to their lawful condition'. The task of these early sexologists was no less than the discovery, description and analysis of 'the laws of Nature': to harmonise, as August Forel wrote in *The Sexual Question*:

> the aspiration of human nature and the data of the
> sociology of the different human races and the different
> epochs of history, with the results of natural science and
> the laws of mental and sexual evolution which these have
> revealed to us.[3]

Just as the founding moment of sociology in this very period sought, through the writings of Auguste Comte, Karl Marx, Herbert Spencer, Emile Durkheim, Max Weber and many others, to find the 'laws of society', so, in a complementary and equally influential fashion, the early sexual theorists attempted to uncover the silent whisperings, the hidden imperatives, of our animal nature—'on account of its ... deep influence upon the common weal'.[4] The science of sex was a necessary adjunct to the science of society; each came to rely, implicitly but absolutely, on the other. A dichotomy between 'sex' and 'society' was written into the very terms of the debate.

A preoccupation with the source, manifestation and effects of the bodily pleasures was not, of course, new to the late nineteenth century. Great swathes of the non-Christian world had long practised the erotic arts, where pleasures were pre-

cisely graded and gained through access to erotic techniques.[5]
By the nineteenth century the finest products of oriental sexual
wisdom and techniques were circulating amongst the know-
ledgeable, imported by travellers and pioneering anthropologists, destined to be essential partners in the sexological ven-
ture. Sir Richard Burton's translation of *The Kama Sutra*
appeared in a small edition in 1883 dedicated to 'that small
portion of the British public which takes enlightened interest
in studying the manners and customs of the older East'. (The
enlightened did not include Lady Burton, who burned Sir
Richard's more dubious manuscripts on his death.)[6]

Far more significant for the ideological formation of the
West was the tortuous history of Judaeo-Christian disquisi-
tions on the sins of the flesh (contrasted with the spiritual joys
of salvation). These had been elaborated since the earliest times
of the Christian era in treatises, canon law, bulls and peniten-
tials, and codified since the seventeenth century in the procedures of the Confessional (in Southern Europe) and the conscience of puritanism (in the North of Europe and America).
Twentieth-century sexologists, from Ellis to Kinsey, were
rightly to stress the formative role of Christian categories in
shaping our response to the body.[7]

By the eighteenth century, however, a more ostensibly secular literary concern with the erotic was in the ascendance.
Alongside the first appearance of tracts warning of the dangers
of masturbation (Samuel Tissot's famous essay *On Onania*
appeared in 1758), there developed a burgeoning literature of
bawdy novels, moral tracts, and even popular self-help sex
advice manuals presaging the torrents of the present century.[8]
By the end of the eighteenth century the Marquis de Sade had
already detailed the thousand sins (and pleasures) of sodom,
providing a benchmark by which the discourse of sexology
was to measure the range of the perverse. Nothing the sexologists could write would compete with the vividness—or amor-
ality—of the divine Marquis's imagination. It was to be the
late twentieth century before it became possible again to celebrate his utopia of polyvocal desire.

What *was*, however, new to the nineteenth century was the
sustained effort to put all this on to a new, 'scientific' footing:
to isolate, and individualise, the specific characteristics of sex-

uality, to detail its normal paths and morbid variations, to emphasise its power and to speculate on its effects. Samuel Tissot's fulminations against the all-pervasive and disastrous effects of masturbation had already marked a crucial transition: what you did was now more than an infringement of divine law; it determined what sort of person you were. Desire was a dangerous force which pre-existed the individual, wracking his feeble body with fantasies and distractions which threatened his individuality and sanity. From this stemmed a powerful tradition of seeing in the gentle joys of masturbation the cause of character defects ranging from feeble-mindedness and homosexuality to laziness and financial incompetence, and hence social disaster. Nineteenth-century sexologists were to refine this insight (though they differed about, and then came to dismiss, the aetiological role of 'self-abuse'—curiously, to be reinstated by devotees of that most modern of sciences, sociobiology).[9] In so doing there was often a tendency, as Alfred Kinsey bitingly noted, to produce 'scientific classifications ... nearly identical with theologic classifications and with moral pronouncements of the English common law of the fifteenth century'.[10] But the aspiration to fully scientific status gave the embryonic sexology a prestige—and more important, a new object of concern and intervention in the instinct and its vicissitudes—that has carried its influence, definitions, classifications and norms into the twentieth century.

The decisive stage was the individualising of sex, the search for the primeval urge in the subject itself. Already by the 1840s Henricus Kaan was writing (in Latin) about the modifications of the 'nisus sexualis' (the sexual instinct) in individuals, and other formative works followed: on the presence and dangers of childhood sexuality, the sexual aetiology of hysteria and on the sexual aberrations.[11] Karl Heinrich Ulrichs (1825–1895), himself homosexually inclined, published twelve volumes on homosexuality (given its name by Benkert in 1869) between 1864 and 1879, an achievement that was greatly to influence Carl Westphal's 'discovery' of the 'contrary sexual impulse' by 1870, and Krafft-Ebing's wider speculations on sexual aberrations thereafter.[12] Two moments are particularly important in this emergent discourse, importing elements which were to profoundly inflect its course. The first was the impact of Darwinism. Charles Darwin's *Origin of Species* had already hinted at the applicability of the theory of natural selection to man. With his publication of *The Descent of Man, and Selection in Relation to Sex* (1871) another element was added: the claim that sexual selection (the struggle for partners) acted independently of natural selection (the struggle for existence) so that survival depended upon sexual selection, and the ultimate test of biological success lay in reproduction. This allowed a legitimate revival of interest in the sexual aetiologies ('origins') of individual behaviour and a sustained effort to delineate the dynamics of sexual selection, the sexual impulse, and the differences between the sexes.[13] Biology became the avenue into the mysteries of Nature, and its findings were legitimised by the evidence of natural history. What existed 'in Nature' provided evidence for what was human.

The second decisive moment was the appearance of *Psychopathia Sexualis*: it was the eruption into print of the speaking pervert, the individual marked, or marred, by his (or her) sexual impulses. The case studies were a model of what was to follow, the analyses were the rehearsal for a century of theorising. It was Krafft-Ebing who began to bring together the scattered trails to forge them into a new approach. As Professor of Psychiatry at the University of Vienna, his earliest concern was with finding proofs of morbidity for those sexual offenders dragged before the courts, to satisfy the late nineteenth century's intensification of legal concern with sexual pecadillos. The first edition of his *Psychopathia Sexualis* was seen by him as a modest intervention. But it immediately evoked both professional approval and a popular response. Like many writers on sex since, he found himself deluged with letters and information from the sufferers of sexual misery and the targets of sexual oppression. *Psychopathia Sexualis* grew, as a result, from 45 case histories and 110 pages in 1886 to 238 histories and 437 pages by the 12th edition of 1903. His success encouraged many others: between 1898 and 1908 there were over a thousand publications on homosexuality alone.[14] In his *Three Essays on the Theory of Sexuality*, published in 1905, and itself a major stimulus to the growth of sexual theory, Freud acknowledged the contribution of nine writers: Krafft-Ebing, Albert Moll, P. J. Möbius, Havelock Ellis, Albert

Schrenck-Notzing, Leopold Lowenfeld, Albert Eulenburg, Iwan Bloch, and Magnus Hirschfeld.[15] To these could be added a host of other names, from J.L. Casper and J.J. Moreau, to Cesare Lombroso and August Forel, to Valentin Magnan and Benjamin Tarnorwsky, names scarcely remembered today, some even mercifully forgotten during their lifetimes, but significant shapers of the modern discourse of sexology.

Central to their work was the notion that underlying the diversity of individual experiences and social effects was a complex natural process which needed to be understood in all its forms. This endeavour demanded in the first place a major effort at the classification and definition of sexual pathologies, giving rise to the dazzling array of minute descriptions and taxonomic labelling so characteristic of the late nineteenth century. Krafft-Ebing's *Psychopathia Sexualis* announced itself as a 'medico-forensic study' of the 'abnormal' (its subtitle noted its 'especial reference to the Antipathic Sexual Instinct') and offered a catalogue of perversities from acquired sexual inversion to zoophilia. Urolagnia and coprolagnia, fetishism and kleptomania, exhibitionism and sado-masochism, frottage and chronic satyriasis and nymphomania, and many, many more, made their clinical appearance via or in the wake of his pioneering cataloguing. Meanwhile, Iwan Bloch set out to delineate the strange sexual practices of all races in all ages. Charles Fréré intrepidly explored sexual degeneration in man and animals. Albert Moll described the perversions of the sex instinct. Hirschfeld wrote voluminously on homosexuality and in a path-breaking way on transvestism, while Havelock Ellis's *Studies in the Psychology of Sex* was a vast and eloquent encyclopaedia of the variations of sexual expression.[16]

Secondly, this concentration on the 'perverse', the 'abnormal', threw light on the 'normal', discreetly shrouded in respectable ideology but scientifically reaffirmed in clinical textbooks. Ellis began his life's work on the 'psychology of sex' by writing *Man and Woman*, a detailed study, first published in 1894, and subsequently reissued in much revised versions, of the secondary, tertiary and other characteristics of, and differences between, men and women. The study of the sexual instinct in the writings of others became an exploration both of the source of sexuality and of the relations between men and

women.[17] Krafft-Ebing's 'natural instinct' which 'with all con-
quering force and might demands fulfilment'[18] is an image of
male sexuality whose natural object was the opposite sex. Just
as homosexuality was defined as a sexual condition in this
period, so the concept of heterosexuality was invented (*after*
the former) to describe, apparently, what we now call bisexuality, and then 'normality'.[19] Sexology came to mean therefore
both the study of the sexual impulse and of relations between
the sexes, for ultimately they were seen as the same: sex, gender, sexuality were locked together as the biological imperative.

Not surprisingly, the generation that followed the pioneers
had little doubt of their significance. Alfred Kinsey, the initia-
tor of the second wave of sexual writing, just as Krafft-Ebing
was of the first, was never over-generous in his assessment of
the contribution of either his contemporaries or his precursors.
He found Krafft-Ebing's work 'unscientific', G. Stanley Hall,
the American author of the pioneering study of adolescence,
was judged 'moralistic', as was Freud for his attitudes to masturbation. Ellis was dismissed as 'too timid', while Hirschfeld
offended Kinsey by his political openness. He was disdainful
of the great anthropologist Bronislaw Malinowski and quar-
relled with Margaret Mead. He was, as his biographer Claude
Pomeroy has written, intolerant of every other approach but
his own. But despite this elaborate disdain of their scientific
and political qualities, even Kinsey in the end expressed his
admiration of the pioneers, 'because they broke new ground'
and 'They made our job possible'. Echoing Freud's own esti-
mate, he compared them to Galileo and Copernicus.[20] This
was the authentic tone, which sustained the sexologists' own
perception of their role. They sundered, as Krafft-Ebing put it
in the Preface to *Psychopathia Sexualis*, the 'conspiracy of
silence' on sex in the nineteenth century. They saw themselves
as in the vanguard of the struggle for modernity, and in this
two strands were interwoven: their commitment to the protocols of science; and their devotion to the sexual enlightenment
of the twentieth century.

The early sexologists perceived themselves as engaged in a
symbolic struggle between darkness and light, ignorance and
enlightenment, and in this 'science' was their surest weapon.

Krafft-Ebing had from the first asserted that the importance
of the subject 'demands scientific research'. Havelock Ellis, as
an isolated man teaching in the Australian bush in the early
1880s, looked forward to a new Renaissance where reason and
emotion combined, and dedicated himself to the scientific
understanding of sexuality. Freud was the model of 'the great
scientist' and was outraged when Ellis preferred to see *his*
work as that of a poet rather than of a man of science.[21] The
criticisms that came from subsequent generations were not
because of this concern with science but over its inadequate
development. Kinsey upbraided his predecessors because they
were not scientific enough, not true to the demands of the age.
'Twelve thousand people', he wrote in *Sexual Behavior in the
Human Male*, 'have helped in this research primarily because
they have faith in scientific research projects.'[22] That was the
true spirit of the age.

A similar faith pervades the work of his successors, even as
they dismantle his conclusions. The critical issue has been, as
Kenneth Plummer has argued, the 'scientific integrity'[23] of the
work—whatever the effects. The old faith lives on; the belief
in science has captured the whole debate on sexuality.

Sexology is, then, in an important sense, an heir to the
post-enlightenment faith in scientific progress. But, as Plummer
has also observed, 'all good scientific work is difficult', and the
sense of the difficulty of the battle against unreason gives a
peculiar missionary tone to much of sexological writing—
what Jonathan Katz has called its 'sombre seriousness'.[24] In
the hands of an Ellis or Freud this could give rise to an elegant
lucidity of expression which succeeded in presenting as convincing fact what was often inspired speculation; from the pen
of a Krafft-Ebing or William Masters could flow a prose of
gloomy turgidity that faithfully reproduces the search for a
scientific earnestness.

Whatever their literary merits, these ambitiously scientific
efforts simultaneously had a social and political purpose: to
bring sexual enlightenment to a variety of social practices.
There was, in the first place, a sense that the law was deeply
ignorant of sexual realities. Krafft-Ebing took up the work
of Ulrichs, himself homosexual and a pioneering advocate of
the rights of 'Urnings' or the 'third sex', because of the inad-

equacy of medico-forensic views of homosexuality. Most of these early writers on sexuality endorsed the removal of penal laws against homosexuality—from Lombroso in Italy, to Ellis in England, Hirschfeld in Germany, Krafft-Ebing and Freud in Austria—because they conflicted with the insights of the new sexual science. They embraced a form of political rationalism, for, as Krafft-Ebing put it, 'erroneous ideas' prevail. Magnus Hirschfeld founded in 1898 the Scientific Humanitarian Committee (a characteristic title) to promote the cause of sex reform generally and homosexual reform in particular. He later became the founder of the Institute for Sexual Science in Berlin and the leader of the World League for Sexual Reform and the promoter of the World Congresses for Sexual Reform. His watchword was 'Per scientiam ad justitiam', and on the eve of his death, in exile, and with the fruits of his life's work destroyed by the Nazis in Germany, he could still affirm his faith:

> I believe in Science, and I am convinced that Science, and above all the natural Sciences, must bring to mankind, not only truth, but with truth, Justice, Liberty and Peace.[25]

By the late 1920s the World Conferences brought together the leading scientific sexologists of the world to debate the iniquities of censorship, the marriage and divorce laws, lack of birth control, penal sanctions against abortionists and homosexuals and others as well as the more dubious merits of eugenics.

Havelock Ellis, more timid publicly, nevertheless was rooted in the ethical and socialist revival of the 1880s and later sponsored the British Society for the Study of Sex Psychology and, with Forel and Hirschfeld, became an honorary President of the World League. Ellis, indeed, went further than anyone in asserting the significance of struggles over sex. What debates over religion and work had been to the nineteenth century, so would, he believed, the sexual question, by which he meant relations between the sexes, be for the twentieth. Nineteenth-century progressive thought had worried about the point of production; the twentieth should worry about the 'point of procreation'.[26]

Kinsey for a later generation as passionately as the pioneers invoked 'scientific fact' to demonstrate the gap between sexual activity as revealed in his studies and moral codes:

> at least 85 per cent of the younger male population could be convicted as sex offenders if law enforcement officials were as efficient as most people expect them to be.[27]

Sexual science was to be the handmaiden of sexual reform, the harbinger of a new sexual order built on a rational understanding of our true sexual nature. The fact that they frequently disagreed on the empirical evidence, the theoretical underpinnings and the social implications of their science scarcely mattered. Their commitment was absolute. Krafft-Ebing representatively hoped that his work might 'prove of utility in the service of science, justice and humanity'. So said all of them.

What remains of this aspiration is more contentious. In recent years a serried army of protesters have advanced on the structures that the pioneering sexual theorists so assiduously constructed. Historians have challenged their claims to modernity. Philosophers of science have queried their scientificity. Feminists have attacked their patriarchal values. Homosexuals have resisted their medicalising and pathologising tendencies. The walls of the citadel are still standing; but their foundations are beginning to crumble under the challenge. Each science attempts to rework its history as a history of progress, as a constant refinement of what has gone before.[28] This was always a dubious endeavour, for scientific breakthroughs come more often from breaks with the past, from a re-ordering of their mode of enquiry and object of concern as from the inheritance of received wisdom, and today few of us have undiluted faith in the inevitably progressive nature or inevitability of science. Such doubts must be redoubled when we approach the inexact human sciences, and the even less precise domain of sex. The object of sexological study is notoriously shifting and unstable, and sexology is bound, by countless delicate strands, to the preoccupations of its age. It is impossible to understand the impact of sexology if we simply accept its own evaluation of its history. Sexology emerged from, and contributed to, a dense web of social practices. This should propel us at least to look again at its claims to enlightenment, and scientific neutrality.

The social relations of sexology

Sexology did not appear spontaneously at the end of the nine-teenth century. It was constructed upon a host of pre-existing writings and social endeavours. This alone must force us to reconsider at least some of its claim to oppositional status. In many ways, far from being at odds with nineteenth-century trends it was peculiarly complicit with them. As much recent historical work has shown, our image of the nineteenth century as a uniquely sexually repressive period must be challenged.[29] There were indeed draconian penal measures—against so-domites, prostitutes, pornography, birth control, abortion—which often increased in personal effectivity, though changing and often liberalising their forms, in countries such as Ger-many, Britain and the United States as the century wore on. And there was a reign of euphemism and elaborate delicacy, which strictly delineated what could be said and written. But even the refusal to talk about it, as Michel Foucault has sug-gested, marks sex as *the* secret, and puts it at the heart of discourse.[30] For the nineteenth century saw an explosion of debate around sexuality. From the end of the eighteenth cen-tury, with Malthusian debates in England about the overbreed-ing of the poor and about the sexual excesses of the aristocracy contributing to revolutionary collapse, sexuality pervades the social consciousness: through the widespread discussions of working-class morality, birth rates, life expectancy and fertility in the early part of the century, to urgent controversies over public health and hygiene, working conditions, prostitution, public and private morality, divorce, and education from mid-century, to the panics over population, race and incest at the end. No final consensus emerges. The Victorian period sees a battle over appropriate sexual values in a rapidly changing world. Precisely for this reason sexuality comes to be seen as so important. It is the subject that is not publicly discussed as such, but traverses, and intersects, a vast array of debates.

Foucault has suggested that sexuality becomes central to the operation of power in the nineteenth century because it is the focus of a two-pronged shift in the productive operations of power. This leads, firstly, to a new preoccupation with policing of the population as a whole, the maximisation of its health, productivity and wealth; and secondly to a new tehnology of control over the body. Sex 'was a means of access both to the life of the body and the life of the species'.[31] This somewhat abstract formulation is useful in pinpointing the emergence of a new positive form of power (what Foucault calls 'biopower'), concerned with spreading its tentacles of regulation and control ever-more thoroughly into the nooks and crannies of social life, and in suggesting the centrality of sex to its operation. But talking about sex is not the same as living it or controlling it. And it is not the case that subjection and subjectification through sex is the only mode of control, either in the nineteenth century or today. It is nonetheless true that sexuality becomes a terrain of contestation in the nineteenth century as it emerges as an area central to the operations of the body politic.

What we see in the nineteenth century is a 'grappling for control' in the light of rapidly changing social and economic conditions. All these produced major shifts in relations between the genders, and in the relationship between behaviour and moral codes. Sexuality becomes a symbolic battleground both because it was the focus of many of these changes, and because it was a surrogate medium through which other intractable battles could be fought. Anxieties produced in the bourgeois mind through large gatherings of workers, men *and* women, in factories, could be emotionally discharged through a campaign to moralise the female operatives, and exclude them from the factories. Worries over housing and overcrowding might be lanced through campaigns about the threat of incest. Fear of imperial decay could be allayed by moralising campaigns against prostitution, the supposed festering carrier of venereal infection, and hence of the weakening of the health of soldiers. Concern with the nature of childhood could be re-directed through a new preoccupation with masturbation and sex segregation in schools and dormitories. A fear of the effects of feminism in relations between the sexes could be channelled into social purity crusades to expunge immorality. In a significant array of social practices the sexual is discovered as a key to the social. Through these concerns, worries, campaigns (and the resistances they evoked), sexuality is being constituted as a key area of social relations. Far from being the area most resistant to the operations of power, it is the medium most susceptible to the various struggles for power. Sexology emerges out of these struggles and social practices; it begins the task of analysing them, codifying them, and hence constituting on a theoretical level what is already emerging on the level of social practice as a unified domain of sexuality, sexuality as an autonomous force and realm.

The sexologists translate into theoretical terms what are increasingly being perceived as concrete social problems. Anxieties over the social categorisation of childhood are transformed into a prolonged debate over the existence, or not, of childhood and adolescent sexuality.[32] The question of female sexuality becomes focused on discussions about the aetiology of hysteria, the relation of the maternal to the sex instinct, and the social consequences of female periodicity.[33] A concern with the changing relations between the genders produces a crop of speculations about bisexuality, transvestism, intersexuality, and the reproductive instinct.[34] The growing refinement in the legal pursuit of the perverse, with the abandonment of old ecclesiastical for new secular offences, leads to a controversy over the cause of homosexuality (hereditary taint, degeneration, seduction or congenital) and consequently over the efficacy of legal control. As Krafft-Ebing noted, the medical barrister:

> finds out how sad the lack of our knowledge is in the
> domain of sexuality when he is called upon to express an
> opinion as to the responsibility of the accused whose life,
> liberty and honour are at stake.[35]

It is also significant that sexology emerges, in the 1880s and 1890s, at the very period when in countries like Germany, Britain and the United States a social purity consensus achieves a precarious dominance, reflected in a consolidation of legal codes, a refined concern with private morality as opposed to public vice, a desire to reform and remoralise the public domain through campaigns against alcohol and prostitution, and when imperialist rivalries are giving rise to a new preoccupation with race and reproduction. Sexology, like the sex reform movements which in many ways parallel it, develops not against a pre-existing monolithism of sexual repression, but

alongside an emergent social hygiene and moral reform hegemony with which in many ways sexology and sex reform are
implicated. Havelock Ellis, like many other of his contemporaries, was not only a pioneering advocate of the removal of
legal penalties against homosexuals, but also a supporter of
eugenics, the technology of selective breeding of the best, with
all its racist and Eurocentric implications, and sat on the committee of the British National Council for Public Morality.
There was no clear-cut divide between the eugenicist, the social
moralist and the reforming sexual theorist: they inhabited the
same world of values and concepts. As Ellis wrote as late as
the 1930s:

> At the present time it is among the upholders of personal
> and public morality that the workers in sexual psychology
> and the advocates of sexual hygiene find the warmest
> support.[36]

It is clear from this that sexology to a large extent moved
with, not against, the grain of nineteenth-century preoccupations. The question that arises is why then the early sexologists
saw themselves as so embattled, so much in the vanguard of
progress? We must be careful here to distinguish on what terms
the sexological writings were accepted. There was certainly a
general absence of barriers to publication of sex works on the
European continent,[37] and someone like Magnus Hirschfeld
was able to publish various volumes and even a yearbook on
homosexuality in Germany in ways which Havelock Ellis in
England was not: the German version of his *Sexual Inversion*
was published in, 1896; his English version was effectively
banned in 1897 and published thereafter only in the United
States. There were cultural and moral differences between
countries, and different rhythms in the acceptance of sexual
literature. Conjunctural factors, the balance of forces between
social purity advocates, social reformers and political constituencies, were as crucial in dictating the pace of acceptance of
new material then as now, and in England, notoriously, the censorship was more severe than in Germany, Austria or France.[38]
    On the other hand, even in the apparently more relaxed
mores of central Europe the regulation of what and how things
could be said was precise. Krafft-Ebing was a physician who

wrote for others of the same profession; hence, as he put it, 'technical terms are used throughout the book in order to exclude the lay reader', and the more graphic sexual descriptions were rendered in Latin. In the 12th edition, after, and *because of*, its great commercial success, the number of technical terms and the use of Latin increased.[39] (Even this was not satisfactory to the more moralistic British: the *British Medical Journal* complained in 1893 that the whole book should have been written in Latin, hence veiling it 'in the decent obscurity of a dead language'.) Books on sexuality won acceptance when addressed precisely to the medical and medico-forensic professions. Ellis lost the support of his peers in Britain largely because it was felt his *Sexual Inversion* was too popular in tone, published as it happened, by a spurious and crooked publisher.[40] Ironically, the refuge he sought for the subsequent volumes of his *Studies in the Psychology of Sex*, F.A. Davis of Philadelphia, was very strict about selling only to the profession.[41] Not until Random House took over the series in 1936 was there a general sale. The medical press was surprisingly explicit compared to the delicacy and innuendo of the popular and middle class press,[42] but its circulation was limited.

These parameters, moreover, were not peculiar to the nineteenth century or the earlier part of this century. Kinsey was urged strongly to publish his findings with a medical publisher. The Indiana University President thought that the book would then:

> go into the hands of the most reputable people, those who needed it for scientific purposes, and consequently would have little other circulation and so not be misinterpreted.[43]

(He also urged Kinsey not to publish during the 61 days of the Indiana Legislative Session, underlining the political parameters; the first volume, *with* a medical publisher, nevertheless sold 200,000 in the first two months, illustrating another point: the institutions of regulation might prescribe and proscribe but people respond in their own often subversive ways.)

William Masters, anxious to follow the work that Kinsey had begun on observing physiological processes, was advised by *his* mentor to wait till he was 40 before beginning, to establish a reputation elsewhere first, and then to be sponsored by a major medical school,[44] injunctions he followed almost to the letter. Clearly, for most of this century it has not been what you have published but with whom and for whom you have published that has been most crucial.

In brief, the findings of sex research and theorising have been allowable when they have been compatible with an acceptable discourse, usually that of medicine. When sexual theorists were, on the other hand, explicitly political in their commitments they became vulnerable to challenge and attack. They were especially vulnerable when they took the side of sexual deviants. An Ulrichs, a lawyer rather than a doctor, and a propagandist (even if, as Numa Numantus, pseudonymously) for homosexuality, was less likely to be taken seriously than a Krafft-Ebing, who could transmute his thoughts into a suitably medical language. In Britain, Havelock Ellis, as a more or less respectable scientist, could expect a generally more respectful audience than his compatriot, the socialist and homosexual writer, Edward Carpenter. Ellis had recognised from the early 1880s that in order to be listened to he had to train as a doctor. The early sense of embattlement that Freud expressed may well have stemmed from his slight disdain for the medical profession: medical jurisprudence was the only examination in his life that he failed.[45]

It was through its symbiosis with the medical profession that sexology became respectable. It was indeed the new 'medical gaze' of the nineteenth century, the new concept of a systematic exploration and understanding of the body, that also, in a very important sense, made sexology possible by reshaping the questions that could be asked about the human (sexed) body and its internal processes.[46] But the other side of this was that sexological insight could easily become subordinated to a medical norm. Many commentators in the nineteenth century, especially feminists, were noting the elevation of the medical profession into a new priestly caste, as the profession itself sought to consolidate itself, and as its principles and practices were utilised in social intervention, especially in relation to women.[47] At best doctors, with few exceptions, generally acquiesced in stereotyped ideas of womanhood even if they were not militant in shaping them. At worst doctors intervened to actually shape female sexuality, through case work, organising against women's access to higher education because of their incapacity for intellectual work, supporting new forms of legal intervention and evidence, campaigning against abortion and birth control. Commentators observed that nineteenth-century medicine created women as no more than wombs on legs, as little more than the mechanism by which life was transmitted. Ellis's comment that women's brains were in some sense 'in their wombs' or Otto Weininger's that 'Man possesses sexual organs; her sexual organs possess women' called upon, reaffirmed, and recirculated such assumptions of medical discourse.[48]

Early sexology, then, drew much of its claim to legitimacy from its association with more acceptable institutions of power, especially medicine and the law, and this is a tendency that has continued. Sex research, Plummer has observed, makes its practitioners (even in the 1980s) 'morally suspect',[49] and in the rush to protect themselves many sexologists have become little more than propagandists of the sexual norm, whatever it is at any particular time. The call upon science then becomes little more than a gesture to legitimise interventions governed largely by specific relations of power. The production in sexological discourse of a body of knowledge that is apparently scientifically neutral (about women, about sexual variants, delinquents or offenders) can become a resource for utilisation in the production of normative definitions that limit and demarcate erotic behaviour. By the 1920s the traditional social purity organisations, deeply rooted as they were in evangelical Christian traditions, were prepared to embrace a cocktail of insights from Ellis and Freud.[50] Today the moral right finds it opportune to legitimise its purity crusades by reference to (selected) sexological findings. Sexology has never been straightforwardly outside or against relations of power; it has frequently been deeply implicated in them.

The biological imperative

Masters and Johnson at one point genuflect to the power of 'Authority'.[51] The sex researchers have made themselves authorities who have the power to legitimise or deny. This, not their personal predilections or beliefs, is what makes them signifi-

cant in our century, and in this lies their power for good or ill.
Many sexologists have recognised this and have carefully
explored the ethical and political difficulties of sex research:
the effects the research might have on the subject, the biases of
the findings, the impact that any changes in sexual attitudes
might have, the difficulties of establishing guidelines.[52] These
are all areas of legitimate and proper debate. But even more
significant, and less discussed, has been the impact of the sexologists' demarcating their own domain of knowledge, the
body and its sexuality, in conditions where they have the
power to adjudicate on normality and abnormality. For it is in
their claim to specialised knowledge of the sexual origins of
behaviour that the real power of sexology has lain. And stemming from this their achievement has been to *naturalise* sexual
patterns and identities and thus obscure their historical genealogy. The results have been profound in shaping our concepts of sex and sexual subjectivities.

There are three closely related areas where the power to
naturalise has been particularly strong: in relation to the characteristics of sex itself, in the theoretical and social privileging
of heterosexuality, and in the description and categorisation of
sexual variations, particularly homosexuality. I want to look
at each of these in turn.

I

The emphasis on the significance of sex to the individual has
been central to the sexual theorists of the twentieth century. It
has been seen as the source of our personal sense of self and
potentially of our social identity. It is according to Ellis both
'all-pervading, deep-rooted, permanent', and the last resort of
our individuality and humanity.[53] It is the most private thing
about us, and the factor that has most profound social significance. And yet, when they came to define the nature of this pervasive force, sexual theorists were on less safe ground. The best
authorities, suggested Havelock Ellis, 'hesitate to define exactly
what "sex" is',[54] and certainly, despite much endeavour before
and since, we are no more able than those 'best authorities'
were to define its ultimate essence. But this has not stopped
sexual theorists adopting a firmly essentialist idea of sexuality.
Sex has been defined as an overpowering urge in the individual,

a 'physiological law', 'a force generated by powerful ferments',[55] which is the guarantor of our deepest sense of self. The image of male sex as an unbridled almost uncontrollable force (a 'volcano', as Krafft-Ebing graphically put it, that 'burns down and lays waste all around it; ... an abyss that devours all honour, substance and health'[56]) is one that has dominated our response to the subject. We perceive what has been called a 'basic biological mandate', a powerful energy that presses on, and so must be controlled by the cultural matrix. Sex is a force outside, and set against society. It is part of the eternal battle of individual and society.

This view has the merits of appearing commonsensical, closest to our (or at least male) perceptions of our sexual impulses. It is moreover a view endorsed by a long tradition. Thus St Augustine in the early Christian era sees the sexual act as a kind of spasm:

> This sexual act takes such a complete and passionate
> possession of the whole man, both physically and
> emotionally, that what results is the keenest of all
> pleasures on the level of sensations, and at the crisis of
> excitement it practically paralyses all power of deliberate
> thought.

Much later in the seventeenth century, one William Bradford, a member of the Plymouth colony in America, evoked this graphical traditional response; he likened sexual wickedness to water dammed up. When the dams break the waters 'flow with more violence and make more noise and disturbance than when they are suffered to run quietly on their own channels'.[57] Sex is an engulfing natural phenomenon.

Metaphors such as these—'spasms', 'water dammed up', or even later ones of 'saving' and 'spending', hydraulic images all—abound in the discourses on the sexual. They recur throughout the writings of the sexologists, from Krafft-Ebing to Kinsey. It is clear, wrote the latter,

> that there is a sexual drive which cannot be set aside for
> any large portion of the population by any sort of social
> convention ... For those who prefer to think in simpler
> terms of action and reaction, it is a picture of an animal

who, however civilised or cultured, continues to respond to the constantly present sexual stimuli, albeit with some social and physical restraints.[58]

Whether it's the elegant volumes of Ellis (who preferred the term 'impulse'), the essays and papers of Freud (whose concept of 'the drive' ambiguously relates to the tradition), the politically engaged writings and 'metatheoretical excursions' of the Freudian left, the ethnographic field work of social anthropologists, the statistical forays of a Kinsey, the laboratory work of Masters and Johnson (in their notion of 'physiological response') or in the genetic determinism of sociobiology, where the agency of the genes replaces the imperative of instincts; in all, there is an enduring commitment to what can best be called an essentialist model. Where the sexual theorists differed from their canonical precursors was in their effort to put this model on a scientific basis by attempting to define the ultimate nature of this instinct.

The general concept of the instincts had a long provenance, going back to Plato and Aristotle, reappearing in the Middle Ages in the concept of natural law, and present in the eighteenth century in notions of conscience, benevolence, sympathy and other 'moral sentiments'. But it was Darwin who provided the most important turning-point in the history of the subject: a chapter in *Origin of Species* was devoted to the subject and, though not in relation to humans, its extensions were obvious.[59] Its significance was that the instincts were put into an evolutionary context which stimulated biologists to speculate on their source, varieties and effects. This did not automatically imply a biological determinism. Darwinism inspired a revived interest in the inheritance of (environmentally) acquired characteristics as much as an interest in genetics. Haeckel's fundamental biogenetic law', which proposed culture as a flowering of monistic evolutionary tendencies, with individual development repeating the developing of the race[60] (which Freud was to adopt and adapt) was one child of Darwin's. Weismann's discovery of the continuity of the 'germ plasm', the unit of heredity, and the revived interest in the Abbé Mendel's experiments with sweet peas, which emphasised the independence of genetics from environmental influence, was another.[61]

Biological arguments were contested. But what Darwinism did do was to fuel speculation on the origins of phenomena, and hence stimulate the search for the prime motor of behaviour. The concept of 'the instinct' usefully filled the gap.

The dominant view of the instincts up to the 1920s argued that they laid down the basic and permanent ends of human activity, providing the fundamental 'cravings', the persistently recurring impulses, common to all members of the species, which were heritable and to which the different behaviour patterns were a response.[62] The early sexologists attempted to develop the idea of a *sexual* instinct in this context.[63] A traditional view (present, for instance, in the writings of Martin Luther) that was still utilised by Charles Féré as late as the 1890s was that the sex instinct was little more than the impulse of evacuation. The obvious deduction from this was that sexuality was essentially male, with the woman just a hallowed receptacle: 'the temple built over a sewer'. A more respectable view was that sexuality represented the 'instinct of reproduction', a more appealing theory in that it did reflect one result, at least, of heterosexual copulation, and could offer an explanation of women's sexuality as a product of the 'maternal instinct'. But it scarcely adequately explained sexual variations, except as a failure of heterosexuality. Nor, of course, did it explain most heterosexual relations, only a fraction of which are guided by reproductive or parental yearnings alone. Darwin, in *The Descent of Man*, had suggested that other complementary factors were at work, namely the processes of aesthetic and erotic responses which ensured sexual selection, and these inspired sexologists such as Moll and Ellis to theorise the sexual instinct as a complex process involving both biological and psychological factors. Amongst some writers this gave rise to a pansexualist vision where sex became the sole explanatory force for social phenomena. Amongst more sophisticated writers like Ellis and Freud the impulse of sex was theorised as only one of the great forces in contention which shaped civilisation, hunger and self-preservation, and love and sex.

The way was open for a theorisation of the process of sexual stimulation in a fashion which laid the groundwork for the later investigations of Masters and Johnson.[64] The rejection of pansexuality in its extreme form suggested that the sex instinct was always subject to restraint and modification. Krafft-Ebing noted, for instance, the modification of the instinct demanded by hereditarianism, moral, racial and climatic factors.[65] But this opened the way to problems. If the instincts were merely general sources of stimuli and not specifically object directed, then the naturalness of heterosexuality became questionable and the aberrations of the instincts could only be judged so on purely moral grounds. Yet simultaneously the pioneering sexologists were anxious to assert the absolute centrality of the heterosexual impulse, rooted as they saw it in natural processes. Men and women, it was agreed, had evolved differently in the interests of evolution. Herbert Spencer, the early English sociologist, believed that sex differences were a result of the earlier arrest in women of individual evolutions, necessitated by the reservation of vital powers to meet the cost of reproduction.[66] The subsequent break with Lamarckian concepts of the inheritance of acquired characteristics, via Weismann's discovery of the continuity of the germ plasm, accentuated rather than undermined this. Patrick Geddes and J. Arthur Thomson, in their influential work *The Evolution of Sex* (1889), found that the germ plasm, the fundamental unit of heredity, already displayed all the characteristics of sexual differentiation which could be seen as arising from a basic difference in all metabolism. At the level of the cell, maleness was characterised by the tendency to dissipate energy (katabolic) and femaleness by the tendency to store up energy (anabolic). By making sperm and ovum exhibit the qualities of katabolism and anabolism Geddes and Thomson were able to deduce a dichotomy between the sexes which, like Spencer's, could easily be assimilated to the conventional ideal of male rationality and female intuition, and which, laid down in nature, could not easily be overridden.[67]

And yet, as Geddes and Thomson put it in their textbook, *Sex*, instinct alone is not enough to guide us through the morass of danger and potential disaster. The sexual relationship of men and women, though biologically necessary and inevitable, is also beset by dangers which only social prescriptions —'self-control', 'healthy mindedness', 'clean living' and sex education—can help us control.[68] Hence the enduring paradox:

heterosexuality is natural yet has to be attained, inevitable but constantly threatened, spontaneous yet in effect to be learnt. It is this paradox that necessitated the investigation of the true natures of men and women, and of the sexual variations which in all their perverse splendour testified to the instability of instinct alone.

II

Two grand polarities, between men and women, and between normal sexuality and abnormal, have dominated sexual thinking. The definition of normality has usually been in terms of sexual practices which bear some relation to reproduction, but it has also been recognised that there are a host of sexual practices, falling short of reproductively successful coition, that while incurring ecclesiastical or legal injunctions, are still regarded as 'normal' in heterosexual relations: fellatio, cunnilingus, buggery, biting and so on. They only become 'abnormal', when they substitute themselves for reproductive sexuality, when they become ends in themselves rather than 'fore pleasures'. It was not a great leap from this (though one that many sexual theorists have found virtually impossible to make) to see a continuum between heterosexual practices and other 'abnormal', 'perverse' or later, 'deviant' practices. The idea of a continuum of sexuality was born. Latent in Ellis, manifest in Freud, it becomes the basis for Kinsey's radical refusal of moral judgment on sexuality. Nothing, it seemed, that was biologically possible was *in itself* intrinsically harmful. This view was never unchallenged, but it constitutes the core contribution of Kinsey to a radical evaluation of sex. But the first polarity, between men and women, has been taken much more as given, irreducible. So Kinsey even when challenging absolute distinctions noted that, 'It takes two sexes to carry on the business of our human social organisation.'[69] Notice the jump from bodily difference to social division.

Few indeed have sought to challenge such statements; and defining the division—and hence the *true* natures of men and women—has been a central imperative of sexual theorists. What in Darwin's theory of sexual selection had been taken for granted, mere differences which favoured reproductive sex, became in the hands of his immediate successors fundamental dichotomies that demand explanation. As Geddes and Thomson saw it,

> The differences can be read in the proportions of the body;
> in the composition of the blood; in the number of red
> blood corpuscles; in the pulse; in the periodicity of growth;
> in the amount of salt in the composition of the body.[70]

The many breakthroughs that have occurred in the knowledge of internal processes—of ovulation, the chromosomes and hormones, the DNA—have invariably been deployed to back up this assumption. Ellis, and most of his contemporaries, with the major, if partial, exception of Freud, sought biological explanations for the differences. Where sophisticated environmental explanations are adduced to explain differences in sexual practices, differences in gender characteristics are still attributed to genetic factors (Masters and Johnson). Even when writers go out of their way to demonstrate affinities between the sexes (as in Kinsey or later Gagnon and Simon), psychological or social explanations are developed to explain differences. The point is not that there are no differences, but that real differences need not automatically account for antagonistic interests or identities, and yet in the overwhelming mass of sexology the differences in sexual equipment were taken to account for the world of social division between men and women and as the fundamental cause of our differentiated subjectivities.

This in turn provides the basis for definitions of normality and abnormality. To be a normal man is to be heterosexual (attracted to the opposite sex); to be a normal woman is to be a welcoming recipient of male wooing. Gender-appropriate behaviour is being defined in relation to appropriate sexual practices. This may seem so basically obvious as not to merit comment. But these sharp demarcations are, I would suggest, *historical*, not natural phenomena. It might well be that dichotomisation is a fundamental mental activity, and certainly gender has long been a fundamental conceptual divide. As Lynda Birke has put it, 'Viewing the world in terms of a gender dichotomy may be an old and nasty habit.' What seems to have changed is the significance we attach to it.[71] Other cultures have seen differences as fluid and complementary. We tend to see them as sharp and appositional. The centrality given to gender in distinguishing appropriate behaviours must therefore be seen as a social process that needs explanation rather than a natural fact that must be taken for granted.

Once entrenched, however, the association of gender and sexual behaviour became extremely difficult to challenge.

The early sexologists played the leading role in theorising these distinctions. The question we must ask is why they felt it to be so important a task. Ludmilla Jordanova has argued that debates about sex and sex roles, especially in the nineteenth century,

> hinged precisely on the ways in which sexual boundaries might become blurred. It is as if the social order depended on clarity with respect to certain distinctions whose symbolic meanings spread far beyond their explicit context.[72]

Many attacks on nineteenth-century feminists were precisely because they threatened to blur the distinctions between the sexes, and it is certainly the case that much sexological literature is a direct response to the changing position of women. Freud's plaintive question, 'What does woman want?', was not uniquely his. It is the common note of the Founding Fathers.

But this accentuation of sexual difference was not solely a response to women; others have noticed how important distinctions and dualities generally became in the definition of the sexual (or of other areas of the social) in the nineteenth century: vice/virtue, hygiene/disease, morality/depravity, civilisation/animality, nature/culture, mind/bodies, reason/instinct, responsibility/non-responsibility.[73] Each of these distinctions had its own separate history, feeding into the developing definitions of sexuality: women were closer to morality and animality, to body and instinct, to nature and non-responsibility. Men to the opposite. These become the basis for sharp divisions, contradictions, opposites.

These *theoretical* developments reinforced *social* tendencies which were working to redefine the relations between the sexes. These were class specific, geographically and nationally varied, and never unilinear in their impact. The patterns of female subordination were never uniform, nor unchallenged as

the existence of a large feminist movement in most major capitalist countries suggests. But what sexologists could provide
were apparently scientific definitions which could be used to
justify social differences and changing assumptions and needs.
These in turn locked into, and made theoretical sense of, a
morass of popular beliefs about the proper spheres of men and
women, and the demarcation of sexual normality. Such
elements in the culture were often contradictory in form and
effect, and sexology helped to transform them into 'scientific'
concepts, which could then be challenged and transformed by
empirical studies. But sexology was successful precisely to the
degree that it made sense of inchoate feelings and beliefs—
that its theories could be recognised as true by 'common sense'.

Perhaps the human mind needs boundaries. But what is
problematic about the boundaries drawn by the sexologists is
that they were static ones, conforming to pre-given assumptions. In constructing what are no more than categories of the
human mind, and then making these the basis for empirical
investigation, they are narrowly delineating human potentiality
and reifying human characteristics. The most extraordinary
example has been in the changing definitions of female sexuality. From the denials of the existence of female sexuality of a
William Acton (which Ellis acknowledged to be peculiar to the
nineteenth century) to the glorification of female sexual potential
in the writings of Masters and Johnson, the feminine has been
defined by male experts. The contradictory effects of this are
illustrated in the medicalising of clitoral sexuality. There has
been no absence in sexological literature of a recognition of
the importance of the clitoris for female sexuality. Even Freud's
account of the suppression of clitoral sexuality in the young
girl was an attempt, though an inevitably ambiguous and ten-
dentious one, to account for the perceived characteristics of
adult female sexuality. But his throwaway remarks about the
clitoris being a vestigial phallus immediately, in the hands of
his followers, became an empirical fact, while his descriptive
account of female sexuality became normative. The Freudian
theory was never unchallenged, and there were subtle shifts
even in the writings of his most ardent followers. But for some
it became absolute truth that brooked no empirical challenge.[74]
Bergler equated frigidity with a failure to achieve *vaginal* or-

gasm, and not surprisingly found that this was a failure concerning 70–80 per cent of all women. Clitoral orgasms were only partial orgasms, and signs of immaturity. He famously castigated Kinsey:

> One of the most fantastic tales the female volunteers told
> Kinsey (who believed it) was that of multiple orgasm.
> Allegedly 14 per cent of these women claimed to have
> experienced it ... Multiple orgasm is an exceptional
> experience. The 14 per cent of Kinsey's volunteers, all
> vaginally frigid, belonged obviously to the nymphomaniac
> type of frigidity where excitement mounts repeatedly
> *without* reaching a climax. Not being familiar with this
> medical fact ... Kinsey was taken in by the near misses
> which these women represented as multiple orgasms.[75]

The result of such comments was to pathologise not only some types of activity but the persons who expressed it. The frigid woman becomes a potent image in a world which is, by the 1940s, busy sexualising all forms of behaviour.

III

The object of Bergler's scorn, Alfred Kinsey had already clearly stated his position in 1948, even if he could not live up to it. 'Nothing has done more', he wrote in *Sexual Behavior in the Human Male*, to block the investigation of sexual behaviour than

> the almost universal acceptance, even among scientists, of
> certain aspects of that behaviour as normal and of other
> aspects of that behaviour as abnormal.[76]

The obsession with the norm inevitably produced a sustained effort at accounting for the abnormal, the perversions, of which homosexuality became the prime, if ambiguous, example.

Divisions between acceptable and unacceptable forms of sexual behaviour were transparently not new to the nineteenth century. But the early sexologists helped produce a major conceptual shift. The fundamental divide throughout much of the Christian era had been between reproductive and non-reproductive sexuality. These were closely related to biblical injunctions about marriage and propagation being the only moral justification for sexual indulgence, the road to salvation being through abjuring the sins of the flesh. This meant, quite logically, that a hierarchy of sins made sodomy (non-reproductive intercourse) worse than rape (which was potentially reproductive). Sodomy became a catch-all category, which included sexual contact, not necessarily anal, between men and men, men and animals and men and women. It was universally execrated, though the details of its horror remained decently vague. There was a yawning chasm between sexual act and social being. Practising sodomy did not, in any ontological sense, make you a different sort of being. A 'sodomite' was someone who practised sodomitical acts, and the law, though draconian, was selective and arbitrary in its impact. But the nineteenth century produced a new definition and a new meaning. The sodomite, as Foucault has put it, was a temporary aberration; but the homosexual belonged to a species.[77]

In the course of the late nineteenth century the homosexual emerged as a distinct type of person, the product of the new dichotomy of heterosexual/homosexual. Sexologists rapidly intervened to define him (and it was, at first, 'him'). Building on the pioneering work of writers such as Ulrichs, sexologists attempted to explain the aetiology of this creature: corruption or degeneration, congenital or transmission of childhood trauma. Was homosexuality natural or perverse, inherent or acquired, to be accepted as destiny or subjected to cure? Alongside such tortuous questions they produced elaborate typologies which distinguished different types of homosexuality in a classifying zeal which has not diminished. Ellis distinguished the invert and the pervert, Freud the absolute invert, the amphigenic and the contingent. Clifford Allen distinguished twelve types, from the compulsive, the nervous, the neurotic and the psychotic, to the psychopathic and the alcoholic. Richard Harvey found 46 types, including the 'demoralised young man', 'the religious', the 'body builder', the 'woman hater', the 'war queen' and the 'ship's queen'. Kinsey invented a seven-point rating for the spectrum of heterosexual/homosexual behaviour. This allowed others to distinguish 'a four' from 'a five' or 'a six' as if essential being depended upon it. Even researchers anxious to break with rigid categorisation (in favour of the dubious pluralism of 'homosexualities') managed to discover five types of homosexual experience which danced along the fine line between description and categorisation.[78]

Many of the sexologists realised the danger of over-rigid definitions, for they just did not fit the empirical evidence. By the 1930s Ellis was talking of the more neutral idea of 'sexual deviations' than the horror-evoking notion of perversions. The way was being prepared for Kinsey's rejection of 'all or none propositions'.[79] But once the notion of 'the homosexual' (or the sadist or masochist, transvestite or kleptomaniac, paedophile or coprophiliac) was born it proved impossible to escape its entrails. Sexual practices had become the yardstick for describing a person. And as the modes of social regulation of sexuality shifted during and after the nineteenth century, as the catch-all categories like sodomy went down before the more refined, and more effective, pursuit of petty sexual offences, so the new definitions were brought into play not only to describe but to account for the miserable offenders brought before the courts or the medical profession.

The concept of a biological imperative thus had consequences way beyond its overt claims. As an explanatory theory, it was vague in scientific terms and ambiguous in social explanation. But it filled a conceptual space that made it indispensable. Sexologists were not sure what sex was; but they *knew* that behind it lay a sexual force which explained both the nature of the individual subject and his or her object choice and sexual practices. Without its explanatory power sexology would have been a much weakened discipline.

The limits of sexology

The claim of sexology to scientific and political rationality has given it a privileged status, and its influence has spread through a host of social activities: to the law, medicine, social welfare agencies, and even the most bigoted of religious organisations. Its definitions have consequently had major effects in shaping our concepts of male and female sexuality, in demarcating the boundaries of the normal and abnormal, in defining the homosexual and other sexual 'deviants'. This is a powerful achievement for a discipline that was variegated in origins, fractious and disputatious in development, peripheral in terms of the great social transformations of the century.

The very marginality of sexology, however, has been its saving grace. When working with the grain of accepted orthodoxy it was a force that could lock people into pre-set positions —as degenerates, perverts, sex dysfunctionals or what you will. At critical times, nevertheless, the findings of sex research had an alternative, potentially liberalising effect. The writings of Havelock Ellis or Magnus Hirschfeld on homosexuality, of Freud on the normality of sexual fantasy, of Alfred Kinsey on the spectrum of sexualities: all these punctured the sexual tradition and opened the path to more sensitive ways of coping with sexual diversity. They were creatures of their time, and their time was not ours, but we must judge the interventions of the pioneering sexologists not simply vertically —how they speak to us—but also horizontally—how they spoke to their own time. Their insistent claim to scientific truth was a dangerous weapon, but it was a weapon that might be turned. Above all, the sexological discourse, because of its very ambivalences and contradictions, was a resource that could be utilised and deployed even by those apparently disqualified by it.

The example of homosexuality is a useful one again, both because it was so central to the sexological endeavour and because there is now a well-developed documentation of homosexual history.[80] From this it is clear that while erotic activity between men and men and between women and women has existed in all times and all cultures, only in a few societies does a distinctive homosexual categorisation and sense of self develop. Today we have very clear lesbian and gay identities: we are what we are, our own very special creations. In the eighteenth and early nineteenth centuries relations between women were not clearly demarcated as sexual or non-sexual, lesbian or heterosexual, and despite subcultural formations and relationships, meeting places, transvestite clubs and the like, there was little evidence of a male homosexual identity.[81] The sexological 'discovery' of the homosexual in the late nineteenth century is therefore obviously a crucial moment. It gave a name, an aetiology, and potentially the embryos of an identity. It marked off a special homosexual type of person, with a distinctive physiognomy, tastes and potentialities. Did, therefore, the sexologists create the homosexual? This certainly seems to be the position of some historians. Michel Foucault and Lillian Faderman appear at times to argue, in an unusual alliance, that it was the categorisation of the sexologists that made 'the homosexual' and 'the lesbian' possible.[82] Building on Ulrichs's belief that homosexuals were a third sex, a woman's soul in a man's body, Westphal was able to invent the 'contrary sexual feeling', Ellis the 'invert' defined by a congenital anomaly, and Hirschfeld the 'intermediate sex'; the sexological definitions, embodied in medical interventions, 'created' the homosexual. Until sexology gave them the label, there was only the half-life of an amorphous sense of self. The homosexual identity as we know it is therefore a production of social categorisation, whose fundamental aim and effect was regulation and control. To name was to imprison.

Tempting as this seems, the actual history appears more complex, and the role of sexology more subtle. There is plentiful evidence of at least a homosexual male subcultural formation long before the intervention of sexology—in England going back to the seventeenth century, in Italy and elsewhere in Europe going back to the Middle Ages. Its development was uneven as between different cultures, and often broken in continuity. The population who used the subcultures were often casual participants, and certainly few adopted homosexuality as a way of life before the nineteenth century. Even more crucially, there were fundamental differences between male homosexual activity and lesbian.[83] Male homosexual practices seem to have developed *against* the wider patterns of male sexuality, as the strong association of male homosexuality and effeminacy well into the current century suggests. To be 'a homosexual' was to be a failed man, that is a pseudo-woman. Lesbianism before the present century merged much more easily into the general patterns of female interaction: silent because unthinkable, but present as part of the ties bred by the common experience of womanhood.

At the same time, there is evidence that sexologists produced their definitions in order to understand a social phenomenon which was appearing before their eyes: before them as patients, before the courts, in front of them as public scandals, on the streets in a still small but growing network of meeting places, for women as well as for men. By the end of the nineteenth century press and police exposure of male haunts were common, and 'passing' lesbians had their own meeting places. The definitions were largely attempts to explain such manifestations, not create them. The sexologists were, in a word, responding to social developments which were occurring through a different, if related, history. The definitions, of course, had powerful effects. They led, as Katz has graphically suggested, to the 'medical colonisation' of a people.[84] They set the limits beyond which in this century it has been very difficult to think. The homosexual identities, gay male and lesbian, have been established within the parameters of sexological definition. But they have been established by living and breathing men and women, not by paper caricatures floating from the pens of the sexologists.

This is the real point. Sexology, in association with the law, medicine and psychiatry, might construct the definitions. But those thus defined have not passively accepted them. On the contrary, there is powerful evidence that the sexual subjects have taken and used the definitions for their own purposes. An Ulrichs invented the 'third sex' to free homosexuality from legal restraint. An Edward Carpenter campaigned for law reform because he was homosexual. Magnus Hirschfeld advanced the science of sex to achieve sexual justice. More important, the anonymous people whose sexual feelings were denied or defined out of existence were able to use sexological descriptions to achieve a sense of self, even of affirmation. Kinsey noted the way in which his respondents used his interviews with them to enquire about their own problems.[85] From Krafft-Ebing on this has been the common experience. Even the hysterically anti-female views of an Otto Weininger could be used to support a positive sense of identity. Margaret Anderson, a Chicago reformer and lesbian, enquired of Havelock Ellis's wife in 1915:

What does Mrs Ellis think about Weininger's statement that intermediate sexual forms are 'normal, not pathological phenomena, . . . and their appearance is no

proof of physical decadence'? Does she agree with him ...
that inversion is an acquired character ...?[86]

Apparently, what was objectionable—the violent misogyny—
could be jettisoned while the kernel of apparent relevance was
extracted, bounced around and put into effective operation.
For what sexology did was indeed to propose restrictive definitions, and to be regularly at one with the controlling ambition
of a variety of social practices; but it also put into language a
host of definitions and meanings which could be played with,
challenged, negated, and used. Against its intentions usually,
countering its expectations often, sexology did contribute to
the self-definition of those subjected to its power of definition.[87]

There is an important lesson in this. The sexologists sought
to find the truth of our individuality, and subjectivity, in our
sex. In doing so they opened the way to a potential subjection
of individuals within the confines of narrow definitions. But
these definitions could be challenged and transformed as much
as accepted and absorbed. This suggests that the forces of
regulation and control are never unified in their operations,
nor singular in their impact. We are subjected to a variety of
restrictive definitions, but this very variety opens the possibility
of resistance and change.

The emergence of modern feminism and gay politics, often
on the very terrain marked out by sexology, points to the truth
of this. Sexology as the domain of 'the expert' on sex, is being
challenged by the very sexual subjects whose identities it
helped to define. As Gayle Rubin has put it, 'a veritable parade
out of Krafft-Ebing has begun to lay claim to legitimacy, rights
and recognition'.[88] At the very least this has given rise to a
'grass roots' sexology where those historically defined and
examined strive to do so for themselves. At the most there is
a powerful critique emerging of the powerful institutions which
have embodied the received definitions of sexual truth. The
limits of sexology seem to have been reached; its claim to be
the only authorised channel into the wisdom of our sexual
nature has been challenged. The problem remains of transforming the critique into a coherent alternative theory and
practice around sexuality.

CHAPTER 5

'A never-ceasing duel'? 'Sex' in relation to 'society'

The sex impulse has been the source of
most troubles from Adam and Eve onwards.

BRONISLAW MALINOWSKI, *Sex and Repression
in Savage Society*

Native human nature supplies the raw material
but custom furnishes the machinery and the
design ... Man is a creature of habit, not
yet of reason nor yet of instinct.

JOHN DEWEY, *Human Nature and Conduct*

'Sex' versus 'society'

'Sexuality' is as much a product of history as of nature. Shaped
by human action it can be transformed by social and political
practice. I believe these statements to be true, and basic to any
political project around the erotic. Their apparent clarity conceals, however, a cluster of problems and difficulties, many of
which are now something like a century old.

Two sets of critical relationships are involved. In the first
place there is the elusive problem of the precise relationship
between the various constituents of sexuality, between biological sources, psychological disposition and social regulation
in the making of sexual behaviour and identities. This issue is
fundamental to any full understanding of human sexualities,
and is one that has taxed most writers on sexuality. Its answer
has been presented in terms, historically, of a second problem,
of what exactly is the relationship between on the one hand
'sex', and on the other hand 'society'. Havelock Ellis concluded
the main volumes of his *Studies in the Psychology of Sex* with
one entitled: 'Sex in Relation to Society'.[1] This formulation is
so taken for granted that its validity has scarcely been questioned. Yet, as becomes clear with a moment's pause, this prob-

lem already assumes a response in terms of the pre-existence of two given entities: 'sex', the arena of nature, individuality, and identity, and 'society', the domain of cultural norms, social laws and (sometimes) history. The sex/society divide evokes and replays all the other great distinctions which attempt to explain the boundaries of animality and humanity: nature/culture, individual/society, freedom/regulation. We are offered two rival absolutes, which demand rival disciplines (biology, psychology, sexology, as against anthropology, sociology, history) to penetrate to the truth. Above all, it presents us with an opposition, even antagonism, between two separate realms which has made it virtually impossible to understand sexuality as a historical presence.

The theorists of sexuality have always been aware, in some parts of their minds at least, of the dilemma. Even when the pioneers were at their most adamant in their attempt to explain the biological imperative of sex, they nonetheless recognised a domain of socio-sexuality, a social order of regulation, ordering and control, on the borderlines of nature and culture, which varied within and across different societies. They observed different rules of marriage, monogamy, taboos against incest and responses to non-procreative sex even as they sought to naturalise them, to root them in evolutionary necessity and project a gradual ladder of progress. And, on the other hand, early social scientists such as Herbert Spencer, Karl Marx, Friedrich Engels, and Emile Durkheim, saw in sex and sexual relations an area which was crucial to their understanding of society, the 'privileged site', as Rosalind Coward has put it, for speculations on the origins of society.[2] The important debates in the latter half of the nineteenth century on the evolution of fundamental social forms such as kinship and the family revived earlier speculation, but did so within a set of concepts shaped by, and in turn reshaping, the new preoccupation with sex. Between them, the sexologists and the social theorists created the terms, and set the limitations, for the way we now conceive of sexual relations.

This has posed major problems which the bulk of this chapter will try to explore. But the reasons they are important extend far beyond arcane debates, for sustaining the elegance of the theoretical constructions are implicit but powerful political positions. Theory, on the terrain of sexuality, has often been the bedraggled servant of politics. Within the general formulation 'sex' versus 'society' two responses have been possible—what we can best term the 'repression model' and the 'liberatory model'. If, as Krafft-Ebing believed, 'life is a never-ceasing duel between the animal instinct and morality', then an absolutist policy of sexual repression and control is seen as inevitable to guarantee civilisation: 'Only willpower and a strong character can emancipate man from the meanness of his corrupt nature.'[3] This has been a strong position, endorsed by a particular reading of the Freudian tradition, and one to which many social theorists have added their weight. If, on the other hand, sex is seen as a beneficent energy, distorted and perverted only by the corruptive efforts of a 'civilisation' gone wrong, for which there has long been strong, oppositional support, then the possibility arises of a new freedom where men and women walk in tune with their true nature. From Rousseau's *Social Contract*, through the socialist utopian writings of Charles Fourier and Edward Carpenter, the metaphysics of the Frankfurt School to the stream of consciousness of the contemporary feminist Susan Griffin, who 'can look at the whole history of civilisation as a struggle between the forces of eros in our lives and the mind's attempt to forget eros', people have pursued the will of the wisp of a liberation from 'civilisation', a new freedom in which a healthy, natural, sexuality would flourish as the realisation of our repressed true selves.[4]

The difficulty, inevitably, lies in deciding what is natural or unnatural, good or bad. Rousseau disapproved of masturbation, and of active female sexuality, Wilhelm Reich of all non-genital sexuality and Susan Griffin of pornography and sado-masochism—all in the name of Nature. Others have seen in these practices the very essence of 'sexual liberation'. This argument forces us back to an ever-receding research for the truth of nature, which only the initiates, the true believers, can reveal. And unfortunately, they never seem to agree.

This split between the sexual and the social, I want to suggest, inscribes us in a search for false universals, and structures political choice in terms of rival absolutisms, either much sex, or no sex, a celebration of hedonism or an urging of restraint.

The effect has been to weaken our understanding of the social dynamics that shape sexual patterns, and to obscure the real options that are available to us as political and sexual subjects.

So, is sex social in origins, or biological? If we reject the latter, are we forced simply to accept the former? When we look at the debates on this issue since the early part of the century we can see that two distinct approaches have emerged, one rooted in anthropology and sociology, the other in ethnology. Neither, I believe, is able ultimately to confront the complexities involved in the making of sexuality. Both have produced enthusiastic bands of acolytes whose influence has coloured the science of desire.

The cultural matrix

Since the eighteenth century, when, as Havelock Ellis put it, travellers discovered the 'strange manners and customs' of primitive man in the 'new and Paradisiacal world of America', anthropology has been a vital focus for debates about sex and sexual regulation, with other cultures providing laboratories 'in which we may study the diversity of human institutions'.[5] From Rousseau to the pioneers of sexology, from Freud to Kinsey and beyond, other cultures have provided a test-bed and a comparative standard for speculations about the nature of sex and the reasons for its variations. In the debates amongst anthropologists we may, therefore, find critical insights into the difficulties of social explanations of sex.

The existence of transparent differences between cultures had to be explained, and in the resulting speculations crucial questions were posed about the relationship between the sexual and the social. Two general models resulted. The first, which dominated all debates from the 1860s to the 1920s, was an evolutionary one. Existing 'primitive societies' were remnants of our own forefathers' stunted growths on the evolutionary ladder. They therefore provided abundant, if rather ambiguous evidence, for the cultural practices of the earliest progenitors of the human race. As such they offered fertile grounds for the argument that 'culture' was an evolutionary triumph over the 'natural' or semi-animalistic behaviour of early man: modern culture was shaped by the animal/natural behaviour of its inhabitants, but also represented a limitation on them. A single line of progress to modernity was proposed, though what evolution was built on, or had triumphed over (primitive promiscuity and matriarchy or natural monogamy and patriarchy) was disputed.[6] Freud's *Totem and Taboo* in 1912 represented a polemical culmination of such speculation, not so much for its originality as for its influence, building as it did on much contemporary (if perhaps already dated) anthropological writing. Through a reading of the totemistic practices of aboriginal tribes he was able to deduce (or so he believed) crucial evidence for the mechanisms of the transition from nature to culture—the taboo on incest, guilt at the primal murder and the invention of the paternal law which not only explained cultural forms but also individual development: ontogeny repeated phylogeny, so that individual and social evolution formed a seamless whole.

This model was enormously influential, not least on the anthropologist Bronislaw Malinowski, who saw in *Totem and Taboo* a powerful argument for the cultural significance of psychological and sexual matters. But while never fully abandoning an evolutionary perspective[7] Malinowski was to become the leading proponent of an alternative anthropological model: one which saw in different cultures evidence not for our own forefathers' behaviour but for the *variety* of social developments in which questions of the origins of behaviour were suspended. This relativist model posed in a new way the question of the relationship of the sexual and the social, this time privileging the cultural over the natural, for the co-existence of different types of society suggested that what was crucial was not natural but social differences built on a basic human nature.

Several theoretical consequences flowed from this partial break with evolutionism in the 1920s. First of all, there was a perceived need to make sense of primitive societies in their own terms. Malinowski expressed a desire to break with the 'exoticism' of the past, to show that 'only a synthesis of facts concerning sex can give a correct idea of what sexual life means to a people'.[8]

This implied a rejection of arguments that practices such as promiscuity were mere 'survivals' of earlier stages of civilisation. Instead they were to be explained in terms of their function in particular societies. Culture was a self-contained reality which had to be understood in its own terms.[9]

This led, secondly, to the abandonment of speculative evolutionary or historical approaches in favour of ethnography, of empirical field work, of immersing oneself in a culture to imbibe all its inner meanings, subtle nuances and self-appraisals. Malinowski lived among the Trobriand Islanders whom he celebrated in *The Sexual Life of Savages*; Margaret Mead lived amongst others, with the Samoans (however briefly), the Arapesh, the Mundugumor and the Tchambuli, who provided the raw data for her cultural relativism.

But thirdly, the new approach led inevitably not only to the abandonment of any unitary model of human development but also of any attempt to explain different cultures. The result was a cultural relativism which deliberately avoided any theorisation of historical development. Culture becomes a series of inexplicable differences in which each society imposes itself on its inhabitants in a total way.

The curious effect of this privileging of culture in such a static and ahistorical way is that it does not challenge the status of the natural. The simultaneous recognition of cultural variations and the refusal to speculate on origins or development co-exists with a model of biological and psychological human needs as formed in the natural family.[10] What Malinowski sought in Freud was an explanation of psychic forms (shaped in the transition from nature to culture) which could exist with the sexual theories of Ellis and other sexologists. He praised Freud for offering 'the first concrete theory about the relation between instinctive life and social institution'.[11] With Ellis he went even further, celebrating his prophetic status, as the 'synthetic metaphysician of life', whose work was 'a lasting contribution to science'. Cultural anthropology, he believed, 'can and must' provide the basis of the social sciences by concentrating on 'the universally human and fundamental'. His eventual break with Freudianism came because he believed that psychoanalytic theories were too unrealistic, in specifying, for example, the transcultural form of the oedipal moment. He sought general characteristics of human nature which could take different cultural forms, for 'culture determines the situation, the place, and the time, for the physiological act'.[12] The science of society, reconstituted through the new methods of field research, would necessarily, therefore, co-exist with the science of sex, as set forth by the likes of Ellis and Freud.

'Sex', according to Malinowski, 'really is dangerous', a powerful and disruptive force which demands powerful means of regulating, suppressing and directing.[13] For the sex impulse, he argues in *Sex and Repression in Savage Society*, has to be experimental if it is to be selective, selective if it is to lead to the mating of the best with the best, a eugenic principle that governs human marriage as well as animal behaviour. Hence sexual jealousy and competition is human and natural, and this makes for serious social disruption. In animals oestrus allows some sort of limitation on this. But in man, for evolutionary reasons, sex is in a state of permanent readiness and tension. Cultural regulation, taboos and barriers therefore step in to fetter man, where natural endowment has left him freer than the beast.[14]

Instinct alone, then, does not dictate social forms. Rigid instincts which would prevent man's adaptation to any new set of conditions are useless to the human species, dysfunctional. So a 'plasticity' of instincts is the condition of cultural advance, and culture acts to positively promote social forms rather than simply negatively to control. Culture transforms instincts into habits which are learnt by tradition. On the other hand instinctual tendencies are there and cannot be arbitrarily developed or overridden. Cultural mechanisms must follow the general course imposed by nature on animal behaviour. Natural endowment provides the 'raw material' out of which custom is fashioned.

For Malinowski, as Kuper has noted, 'cultures were delicately attuned mechanisms for the satisfaction of men's needs.'[15] The problem was that these assumed needs were based on a model of instincts, derived from contemporary theory, which were never questioned. The result is that Malinowski reads into nature patterns of behaviour—monogamy, jealousy, the primacy of genital sexuality, and the inevitability of heterosexual pair bonding—which need to be explained rather than taken as given. Malinowski, for instance, recognises the existence of infantile sexuality, but evaluates it solely in terms of its relationship to adult genital sexuality, as a form of playing at genitality. In modern readings of Freud the transition from infantile polymorphous perversity to adult genital primacy is seen as an issue that has to be explained, and the attainment of heterosexuality (or indeed of homosexuality) is problematic, not pre-given. By ignoring, or rejecting, the radical questions posed by Freud and psychoanalysis in favour of a more generalised instinct model taken from social psychologists such as William McDougall and A. F. Shand, and sexologists such as Ellis, Malinowski is unable to transcend the sex/society dichotomy; indeed he contributed to its theoretical solidification. Sexual instincts become needs which society has to try to satisfy, or repress.

Contemporary critics of Malinowski recognised the problems in his position. Ruth Benedict, a leading proponent of a more culturalist anthropology, challenged Malinowski precisely for generalising from his study of the Trobrianders to all primitive societies. She, instead, stressed the importance of studying not 'primitive culture' but 'primitive cultures', thus extending the cultural relativism implicit in functionalist anthropology.[16] With it went an explicit rejection of apparently all non-cultural factors, and in particular once and for all rejection of the power of Weismann's germ-cell. The life history of the individual was shaped by the patterns and standards traditionally laid down in the community, and: 'not one item of his tribal social organisation, of his language, of his local religion, is carried in his germ cell.'[17] It was not biology that was important but the 'cultural configuration'. At the same time as this view endorsed an extreme cultural determinism, in which at best anthropology can only be descriptive of social forms, it paradoxically embraced in as passionate (if less open) a manner as Malinowski the idea of a universal human psychology, of general human characteristics upon which the social acted. But whereas Malinowski saw these characteristics as instinctual, with animal origins, the American 'culture and personality' school—Franz Boas, Margaret Mead and Ruth Benedict—stressed psychic characteristics, a concept dependent in large part on a particular appropriation of psychoanalysis married to the behaviourism of J.B. Watson and his school.[18] The key term was 'conditioning' which served to lay stress on the deliberate social moulding of psychological characteristics.

American culturalist anthropology had its origins in an explicit rejection of instinct theory. Like Malinowski's anthropology, it appropriated from the Durkheimian sociological discourse a concept of the autonomy of the social. But whereas Malinowski's borrowing stressed the functionalist aspects, Franz Boas emphasised the absolute division between social and biological, in an approach shaped within a specific set of political conditions. American culturalism was a conscious reaction to the racial and racist fantasies of eugenics, which in the United States and Britain as elsewhere was enormously influential in extinguishing the liberal emphasis on general *social* ameliorisation in favour of proposals for the planned breeding of the best. Both 'negative eugenics', the elimination of the unfit, and 'positive eugenics', the promotion of breeding in the best, claimed that the future of the race lay with selective propagation. The difficulty was that the criteria for who was judged fit or unfit corresponded closely with the characteristics of those who were already transparently socially privileged or unprivileged, and by the 1910s clear links were being made between colour and racial origins and mental capacities: blacks were consequently destined to their inferiority by reason of their inferior intellectual endowment, a position that many progressives, including sexologists like Havelock Ellis, endorsed.[19] Boas's adoption in the mid-1910s of an extreme form of cultural determinism was thus a political as well as theoretical rejection of such racist assumptions.

So when Boas enthused his most famous acolyte, Margaret Mead, in the mid-1920s he had a clear aim and ambition to transmit: to utilise anthropological field work to demonstrate the plasticity of human nature. Margaret Mead's famous (today perhaps even infamous) first field trip to Samoa had an explicit theoretical and political purpose: to study the patterns of adolescence, currently an issue of controversy. It was guided by the search for a 'negative instance', the exception to the supposed universal law of intergenerational conflict between adults and young people which would demonstrate that development patterns were culturally, not biologically, determined. One exception would prove that biology alone could

not explain individual characteristics. Her resulting lyrical por-
trait in *Coming of Age in Samoa*[20] of a very simple and 'un-
complex society', where a sense of sin and therefore of guilt
was absent, where oedipal conflicts were minimised, and where
the art of sex was highly developed in an easeful, Apollonian
state of bliss, became a powerful text for progressives in the
inter-war years. Its example suggested that new educational
attitudes could change behaviour, that sex reform could harmonise desire and necessity, that conflict need not be the hallmark of social life. What had been socially formed could be
socially transformed. The romantic vision that Mead constructed was no doubt influenced by the long tradition of ro-
manticising primitive cultures, serving subliminally, perhaps,
to suggest yet again that primitives are closer to nature, and
hence more joyously sexual. But it seemed a death blow to the
biologisms of her predecessors, a definitive proof for her contemporaries of the 'unbelievably malleable' nature of human
nature.

Today her legacy seems less assured. Her hurried and scanty
research in Samoa has been criticised, her image of an easeful
society without major conflict has been challenged, and her
ability to ignore or misunderstand counter-evidence to her conclusions has been excoriated.[21] All this is important, and
doubtless a proper subject for discussion. But to concentrate
on Mead's errors is to ignore the important contribution she
made to the discussion of sex. By describing in a vivid way the
different attitudes towards sex and gender behaviour in other
cultures, she helped put on the agenda the question of why
western cultures are as they are. Unlike the early anthropologists she refused to see contemporary mores as an evolutionary
necessity which transcended primitive ones; and unlike Malinowski she did not seek, though she may at times have assumed, cross-cultural evidence for common human characteristics. Her task was to throw into relief received beliefs, and
this has been of major significance in thinking about sexuality.

Her summing up in *Sex and Temperament in Three Primitive Societies* of the sex variations in New Guinea cultures
illustrates her strengths:

We found the Arapesh—both men and women—
displaying a personality that, out of our historically limited

preoccupations, we would call maternal in its parental aspects, and feminine in its sexual aspects. ... We found no idea that sex was a powerful driving force either for men or for women. In marked contrast to these attitudes, we found among the Mundugumor that both men and women developed as ruthless, aggressive, positively sexed individuals, with the maternal cherishing aspects of personality at a minimum. ... In the third tribe, the Tchambuli, we found a genuine reversal of the sex-attitudes of our own culture, with the woman the dominant, impersonal, managing partner, the man the less responsible and the emotionally dependent person.[22]

But to explain this powerful evocation of cultural diversity even within a small geographical area there is the ambiguous notion of 'social conditioning' which betrays the weakness of Mead's position. In *Male and Female* she suggests that

In every known society, mankind has elaborated the biological division of labour into forms often very remotely related to the original biological differences that provided the original clues.

But, she goes on, she knows of no society that has articulately argued that there is no distinction between the sexes, and concludes:

If any human society ... is to survive, it must have a pattern of social life that comes to terms with the differences between the sexes.[23]

In other words, even when the theory operates on the basis of the infinite malleability of human nature, there is a limit beyond which malleability does not go—the anatomical boundaries of the sexes. Although the content of the roles might vary, sexual division is unassailable. Mead rejects rigid sex dichotomisation as wasteful, but also rejects the standardisation of sex as a 'loss in complexity'.[24] She concludes *Male and Female* with a paean to the differences between, but complementarity of, the sexes: 'To both their own'. Mead advocates keeping the difference, but 'giving each sex its due', a position that became central to the rehabilitation and reconstitution of the family as a harmonious unit in the 1940s, when the book was written.[25] But there is no conception of why the difference is so necessary or how it has come about—except through, ironically, biological determination, a concept Mead had strenuously challenged from her earliest work. It is ultimately assumed as the irreducible pre-given norm of social relations. In this the nurturant family plays the major role: 'The family, a patterned arrangement of the two sexes in which men play a role in the nurturing of women and children . . .'[26]

For Mead no less than Malinowski is committed in the end to a taken-for-granted notion of the biological family as the basic natural as well as social unit, in which a division of labour between men and women is necessary and inevitable. Indeed, the break with evolutionism made it theoretically inevitable that this explanatory reliance on the family should actually increase.[27] Evolutionary theory had at least made it possible to interrogate certain forms of family arrangements and the position of women, for they could be seen as products of development and change. The critique of the manifest inadequacies of unilinear evolutionism, however,—its teleology and determinism in particular—and its replacement by a static functionalism or a descriptive anthropology, made it impossible to ask certain questions, about gender divisions, the origins of the family, about social determination or change, and created a theoretical vacuum which could only be filled from external sources. As a result biological or psychologistic theorists inevitably filled the gap, and anthropologists came to rely on the 'scientificity' of sexology for their explanations, just as sexologists relied absolutely on the science of society.

The lacunae in functionalist and culturalist theories in turn resulted, it may be suggested, from a totalistic theorisation of 'the social'. In the work both of Malinowski and his followers, no less than of Mead and hers, culture is taken to be a unified whole, expressing a common spirit, which moulds and organises the givens of human nature or the psyche. Readings both of the Marxist tradition, in which ideological and cultural forms were seen as the emanation of a determined social base, or of the sociological, in which 'society' was conceived of as a unified domain awaiting scientific investigation, served to further affirm the all-embracing power of cultural forms. As a result the complexity of the social, its ever-partial and provisional unifications of disparate social practices, relations and discourses, its contradictory effects in the constitution of individual subjectivities, is lost.[28]

This is not to deny the importance of the work of anthropologists such as Malinowski and Mead. They rightly pointed to the relevance of trying to understand each culture as a unique ensemble of phenomena, and of not judging them by an absolute standard. This approach in turn served to relativise assumptions about sexual behaviour and social norms, and thus to throw into stark relief the absolutisms and moralisms in our own culture—especially in relation to concepts of masculinity and femininity and the 'sexual perversions'. As a method, too, social anthropology encouraged the attempt to understand not only other cultures, but subcultures within our own society through grasping their inner dynamics and meanings. Here it met up with the sociological tradition deriving from George Mead and the 'Chicago School' of the 1920s which was to have an enormous influence on the understanding of the ecology of sexual life in the 1960s and 1970s.[29] But by avoiding attempts to understand the historical nature of sexual patterns, to explain their development and transformation, and to consider the range of their effects, anthropology failed to illuminate the social origins of sexuality. Ultimately, like the sexologists upon whom they often relied, they constructed their theories upon the basis of an assumed individual human nature which foreclosed further investigation.

The selfish gene

The impact of sociobiology stems in part from this crisis of social explanation. The social sciences despite, or perhaps because of, their overwhelming commitment to social determination, have left open a space into which it is easy to fit a deterministic explanation, a refurbished biological imperative under the protection of 'modern science'.[30]

This brings sociobiology surprisingly close at times to some of the writings of the social anthropologists. The fervent evangelical tone of sociobiology obscures its affinity to the Malinowskian desire to see every detail of human culture as a functional adaptation of the biological needs of the individual. But in sociobiology the anthropological concern with the forms of social regulation is displaced in favour of an intensified interest in the biological mechanisms that provide the bases of social phenomena. In doing this it offers more than an adjunct to the social sciences. It lays claim to displacing them.

Sociobiology, Janna L. Thompson has argued, 'is not so much a discipline as an undisciplined collection of theses and models for relating the biological and the social'.[31] But despite its lack of coherence and frequent contradictions its power lies in its belief that it is offering a new explanation of social life. E.O. Wilson, the Founding Father of sociobiology, defines it as 'the systematic study of the biological basis of all social behaviour'.[32] There is already here a claim to be offering a universal key for the understanding of human history. Sociobiology ambitiously proposes a resolution to longstanding deadlocks in social theory, by providing an explicit, unifying foundation for the sciences of man. Sociobiology, Barash has written, 'comes to upgrade social sciences, not to bury it'. It offers a 'breath of fresh air', and a new way of seeing things. E.O. Wilson concludes his founding text, *Sociobiology: the New Synthesis*, which is largely about insect behaviour, with a chapter entitled, 'Man: From Sociobiology to Sociology'. His next book on the theme, *On Human Nature*, goes much further in *its* last chapter. It is called 'Hope'.[33] The 'hope' of sociobiology is to provide solutions to intractable problems in social explanation.

It attempts to do this by claiming that any human behaviour that has a genetic component is adaptive: that is organisms survive, are selected and inherited, because they serve a function. So everything from jealousy and spite to tribalism, entrepreneurial skill, xenophobia, male domination and social stratification, from hair colour to sexual patterns, are dictated by the human genotype, the particular assemblage of genes selected and preserved in the course of evolution. Where early sexologists sought a proliferation of the instincts, sociobiologists seek a proliferation of genes, the basic 'unit of heredity'. A cosmic functionalism returns to haunt the social sciences, where nature, though blind in aim (for nothing is preordained), lurks behind the forms of social life. Nature in her wisdom wastes none of us—or any of our characteristics. They survive only in so far as they are useful. They serve a purpose, and have therefore an explanation.[34]

Sociobiology sprang ready-armed from the head of E.O. Wilson in 1975 with the publication of his first volume on the subject. But its ideological power is derived from its welding together of two intellectual strands: population genetics and animal ethology. The first is derived ultimately from Weismann's discovery of the continuity and 'immortality' of the germ plasm, with its concern with how species characteristics become established through the evolutionary selection of genetic material. The second is chiefly concerned with what animals do in their natural habitat, and had developed from the 1920s largely through the work of zoologists such as Konrad Lorenz and Niko Tinbergen.[35] Its aim had been to challenge the dominance of animal research in laboratory conditions (which behaviourism and Pavlovian experiments had encouraged) by offering comparative studies of animal behaviour in the wild.

Its effect was to reinstate notions of the *innate* in a climate in the interwar years which was challenging the simplicities of instinct theory.[36] Darwin, it could be said, had made possible a break with anthropocentrism, the belief that man was the measure of all existence, by placing humanity in an evolutionary process. Ethologists sought to go further, by breaking with *anthropomorphism*, the attribution to animals of human characteristics. By studying animals in their own terrain, they attempted to understand specifically animal behaviour. But the paradoxical result of this was an attempt, consequently, to understand the animal in man.

This gave rise in the 1960s particularly to an influential vogue for studies of the 'Naked Ape', in Desmond Morris's familiar phrase: Lorenz's own work *On Aggression*, Robert Ardrey's *The Social Contract* and *The Territorial Imperative*, Lionel Tiger and Robin Fox's *The Imperial Animal* and Lionel Tiger's *Men in Groups* amongst many others.[37] These had an enormous circulation (Morris's *The Naked Ape* sold over 8 million copies world wide), largely because they offered simple or comprehensible answers to complex and intractable problems (sexual antagonism, ceaseless warfare, competition for scarce resources). Even some of the progenitors of this approach felt the popularisation went too far: Lorenz suggested that Morris may have exaggerated the beastliness of man. But they were important forerunners of the sociobiological school, for, as Wilson saw it, they helped to break the 'stifling grip of the extreme behaviourists'.[38]

Where Wilson's sociobiology broke in turn with the ethologists was over the centrality of the individual. Ethologists made the assumption that the important factor in evolution was the survival of the species, or gene pool; that natural selection worked to maximise the chances of survival of particular groups. Sociobiology argued instead that natural selection worked to make the individual gene survive, and in this the individual was no more (though no less) than the vehicle for the transmission of the gene.

This was to lead to a fundamental ambiguity in sociobiology over whether the *capacity* for culture was genetically formed, or whether culture itself was genetically shaped. 'No human behaviour', Barash has written, 'comes entirely from our genes',[39] and this type of statement has allowed the acceptance of sociobiology into a variety of progressive discourses. If all we are talking about is the 'influence' of biology then few would dispute its relevance. But the claim of sociobiology to be offering a new type of general explanation suggests that the underlying ambition of sociobiology is much stronger. This is borne out by the fervour and generalising tone of its exponents. Biology *is* offered as the explanatory agent; a genetic determinism is the ultimate goal of sociobiology, for all social phenomena in the end are subordinated to its dictates, from petty inter-personal behaviour to the great edifices of art and culture. 'Beliefs', stated E.O. Wilson, 'are really enabling mechanisms for survival.'[40] It is difficult to read into such statements any scientific caution.

Charles Darwin wrote in *Origin of Species* of 'one general law, leading to the advancement of all organic beings—namely multiply, vary, let the strongest live and the weakest die.'[41] Sociobiology elevates this into the prime law for understanding social behaviour. The individual is the central focus of the resulting sociobiological theory but no longer formally as the unified, constitutive individual of classical liberal theory. The individual is seen now as simply the convenient means of re-producing genetic variations. Thus E.O. Wilson:

> Samuel Butler's famous aphorism, that the chicken is only an egg's way of making another egg, has been modernized: the organism is only DNA's way of making more DNA.[42]

Evolution, as Lecourt has aptly put it, is for sociobiology like a stock exchange transaction, the sole object of which is the eventual realisation of genetic dividends. Sociobiology gives central place to the 'natural fitness' not of the individual but of the gene, measured by the relative frequency of a specific gene in a population over the course of successive generations. In each generation the victorious genes, victorious by measure of their survival, separate and re-assemble to construct new organisms that on average contain a higher proportion of the more successful genes. The founding characteristic of these genes is their will to survive in the race for life, their selfish-ness. Dawkins argues for a 'fundamental law of gene selfish-ness', which in its most general form means the differential survival of entities. The law of natural selection is a law of competition and selfishness. The individual is programmed by genes to achieve their purposes so that: 'We are survival mach-ines—robot vehicles blindly programmed to preserve the selfish molecules known as genes.'[43] The individual can now be ex-plained as the product of genetic transmission, 'natural selec-tion has built us, and it is natural selection we must understand if we are to comprehend our own identities.'[44] Immediately there is a leap from biological elements to personal and social identities, as if there were an unproblematic link between the two. But the argument can go further, for if individual patterns can be explained by genes, then so can society, as 'a product' of individuals, be explained in terms of the imperatives of natural selection. A seamless web is constructed whereby the cultural becomes little more than an emanation of genetic char-acteristics. A new 'social contract' is discovered, which not only explains but justifies social phenomena. They are products of biological necessity, the exigencies of gene survival, with 'society and nature working in harmony'.[45]

It is, of course, obvious that not all behaviour is selfish, and altruism is common in all social groupings. How this is to be explained is a key problem in sociobiology, and leads directly to the question of sexuality. For in order for the selfish gene to survive individual selflessness may be necessary in the wider interests of the gene.

A selfish need for gene diversification demands a selfless choice of kin to further spread (kin-selection). By helping rather than competing with close relatives, by assisting them to survive and breed, the interests of the genes held in common are furthered. Altruism is thus functional to the diversification and survival of genes, their fundamental aim, and the sexual impulse is functional to both.

Sex, in sociobiological theory, serves a utilitarian purpose. Without it nothing is possible. But it is also problematic and dangerous. Sex, wrote E.O. Wilson in 1979, is 'an anti-social force in evolution', for it causes difficulties between people.[46] The male/female partnership is one of mutual mistrust and exploitation. Altruism is more likely when everyone is the same. So why does the organism not reproduce by partheno-genesis, and why have two sexes evolved, not one, or three, to engender sexed reproduction? Sex bonding and reproduction are necessary, it is argued, to achieve diversity, which is the surest way of genes surviving, 'the way a parent hedges its bets against an unpredictably changing environment'. Two genders, and heterosexual bonding between them, are 'adaptive', it is suggested, for 'two are enough to generate the maximum potential genetic recombination' to ensure reproductive success.[47] Courtship and formal sex bonding have evolved to override the antagonism which might prevent the necessary diversification. The forms of sexual life have emerged, there-fore, to ensure the survival of the gene. They might vary a little between different cultures, but the limits to those varia-tions, to those adaptations to the particular environment, are set by gene selfishness.

At the heart of sociobiological thinking about sex, then, is a basic acceptance of sexual division and antagonism, and conflicting interests, for, as H.J. Eysenck and Glenn Wilson have written, 'Men and women are fundamentally (i.e. psycho-logically and genetically) different in their sexual, as well as in their social attitudes and behaviour.'[48] These differences,

Steven Goldberg has suggested, have set 'immutable limits ...
on institutional possibility'. E.O. Wilson himself has tempered
such views by suggesting that differences between the sexes are
but cultural variations on a twig only slightly bent at birth.
But he goes on to suggest that the most socially useful thing to
do is not to eliminate differences, any more than one should
exaggerate them, but provide equal opportunity for each sex
in his/her sphere. This is the least costly of choices, and it
helps preserve the nuclear family, 'the building block of nearly
all human societies'.[49] By a familiar slide, relations between the
sexes are seen as problematic and troublesome, but necessary
and complementary. So a 'cosmic conservatism' is re-estab-
lished even as the way is opened to the consideration of alternatives.

This approach enables sociobiologists to derive social as well
as sexual differences from the differentiated roles that men and
women have evolved in reproduction. As Symons has written,

> with respect to sexuality, there is a female human nature
> and a male human nature, and these natures are
> extraordinarily different ... because throughout the
> immensely long hunting and gathering phase of human
> evolutionary history the sexual desires and dispositions
> that were adaptive for either sex were for the other tickets
> to reproductive oblivion.[50]

These differences begin and end, it sometimes seems, with the
evolutionary characteristics of the ova and testes. Because
males have an almost infinite number of sperm, while women
have a very restricted supply of ova, it is suggested that men
have an evolutionary propulsion towards spreading their seed
to ensure diversity and reproductive success, and hence towards promiscuity, while women have an equal interest in
reserving energy, towards conservation, and hence towards
monogamy. From this can be deduced the explanation of all
the other supposedly fundamental differences: greater intra-
sexual competition between men than between women, a
greater male tendency towards polygamy and jealousy whereas
women are 'more malleable' and amenable, and a greater sexual will and arousal potential in men than in women.

Symons, in what he obviously regards as conclusive proof,

adduces two pieces of evidence to substantiate the biological roots of these characteristics: the masculinisation of women that occurs when they are exposed to the male hormone, androgen; and the fact that male homosexuals tend to have more in common with male heterosexuals, and lesbians with heterosexual women than with each other.[51] Neither, it needs to be said, offer any proof whatsoever of any automatic relationship between biological capacities and social characteristics. There is a good deal of evidence for the separation between bodily and biochemical characteristics of the individual and gender and sexual identity. 'Nature' is less stern in creating sexual dimorphism than humans like to think.[52] The syllogism: all men want to be promiscuous, homosexual men are promiscuous, therefore homosexual men, free of the ties with womanhood, are the ultimate proof of masculinity, the living embodiment of male promiscuity, looks satisfying on the page, but scarcely lives up to examination. Some homosexual men are promiscuous, others are not; some are aggressive, others are not; some are hyper-masculine in style and appearance, others are not; some are misogynistic, others are not. The easy generalisation to back up a theoretical point is a characteristic of sociobiological writings on sex, but hardly one to inspire confidence in its 'scientific' quality.

The theoretical inadequacies of sociobiology have been thoroughly rehearsed elsewhere. The most effective arguments come from the three disciplines of biology, social anthropology, and history. Biologists have found in sociobiology a number of factual and methodological errors—Lewontin objects *inter alia* to the following typical procedures: reification, arbitrary agglomeration, false metaphors and conflation.[53] But the most fundamental criticism is that of 'reductionism', that sociobiology attempts to explain the property of complex wholes in terms of their constituent units. The result in sociobiology is the hypothesis of a gene to explain each type of behaviour, a hypothesis subject to the canons neither of proof nor of refutation.

Social anthropologists have gone further, in demonstrating that cross-cultural evidence is clearly at odds with sociobiological theory. Sociobiology assumes that human kinship can be understood in terms of genetically based behaviour. Yet as

Marshall Sahlins has argued, kin ties are not primarily ties of blood but social relations, often based on residential affinities and hostile to genetic affinities.[54] Similarly the sociobiological stress on the rituals of incest avoidance as a 'largely unconscious and irrational' 'gut feeling',[55] by emphasising the limitations of close biological ties ignores the social reasons for exogamy, marriage outside the kin (the circulation of people and the cementing of social ties) and conflates them with the biological.

The *historical* objections to sociobiology are to its static quality, to its inability to recognise variability and change. As Tiger and Fox saw it, 'nothing worth noting has happened in our evolutionary history since we left off hunting and took to the fields and the town ... we are still man the hunter, incarcerated, domesticated, polluted, crowded and bemused'.[56] The great waves of social transformation, it seems, are as nought compared to the fixed ideas of sociobiologists. 'Bemused', perhaps, is not the word.

But despite these objections, powerful and valid as they undoubtedly are, sociobiology has been influential, in a variety of social and political discourses, and this demands some interrogation. Sociobiologists themselves disclaim any political project. They insist on a rigid disjunction between *is* and *ought*. Sociobiology, they claim, is a neutral examination of what has happened and is happening in terms of evolution. It lays no claim to prescribing what should happen. Politics, Barash observes, is a 'tangled bank'. He rejects criticisms that it is racist, a genetic determination, that it abolishes free will, that it is sexist, that it provides a support for the status quo, that it offers an excuse or a rationale for social inaction. Sociobiology, he writes, 'has very few political, ethical or moral implications'.[57]

The problem is that it is the 'brute instincts', the natural limitations imposed by biology, rather than the ethical considerations, which are given most stress in sociobiological writings—and in the political appropriations of sociobiology. Barash is forced to make his list of disclaimers not because critics have viciously slandered sociobiology, but because it has been used to argue for these positions.[58]

One left response to this has been the suggestion that sociobiology is effective because it is simply a justification for the status quo, and Barash has agreed that 'sociobiology reads very much like laissez-faire capitalism operative in the realm of genes'.[59] Much of sociobiological terminology is derived from modern market and cybernetic systems, so the dynamic of human evolution is expressed in terms of genetic investment and accumulation and maximisation of genetic profit. The gene has all the apparel of the capitalist entrepreneur, and genetic determinism can easily be read as a justification for contemporary capitalist social relations.

But it would be limited to see sociobiology simply in these terms. Sociobiology has become popular in the last decade because it seems to explain the otherwise inexplicable, and because, as Joe Crocker has suggested, its explanations tally with people's lived experiences under capitalism.[60] Its theses correspond with common sense understandings of differences as inequalities; they draw on, and then lend theoretical sustenance to, elements which are common in the culture: about racial, gender, and intellectual differences. Sociobiology is influential and effective because of the paucity or ineffectiveness of alternative explanations.[61]

Sociobiology's naturalisation of certain issues has also ensured an audience for it among more progressive elements. Here it offers an ostensibly *material* explanation for what might otherwise seem merely ephemeral products of social determination: individuality, the impulse towards art, the recurring differences between the sexes, and the constant eruption of sexual variations. The Italian philosopher, Sebastian Timpanaro, while recognising the reactionary implications of a sociobiology detached from an understanding of the social relations of production, nevertheless insists on the refractoriness of biology as material priority and limit.[62] This *cri de coeur* has been very influential among left intellectuals disillusioned with arid sociologising theories, and is an appropriate one in so far as it reminds us of the biological sources of social behaviour. But such approaches all too easily become concerned with limits rather than possibilities, restraints rather than releases. Biology becomes meaningful through culture; the meaning of culture should not be searched for in biology. The result of an over-insistence on biological limits is that politics becomes trapped within categorisations and divisions whose historical genealogies and effects are once again ignored.[63] It prevents the asking of certain questions.

The sociobiological response to contemporary feminism is a good illustration of this. During the latter part of the 1970s a deadlock seemed to have been reached between the claims to equality of feminism and the forces that thwarted the achievement of that equality. This was a real political impasse which demanded a political understanding. The response of the *New York Times* amongst many others was to wonder whether *natural* limits did not exist to the achievement of full equality.[64] This in turn called upon deep-seated popular assumptions about sexual divisions, many of which were already gaining new credence through the dissemination of sociobiology. The effect was to evoke an apparently scientific explanation for a complex political situation. Such an explanation simultaneously explains and justifies existing difficulties, and prescribes limits to future programmes. It can do so because sociobiology seems to make sense.

Some feminists themselves have accepted the logic in this. Sociobiology addresses many of the issues—reproduction, kinship, sex roles—that feminism has traditionally been concerned with. And one strand of feminism in its reduction of all issues to the male/female divide, comes close to the essentialising of sexual differences that is one of the hallmarks of sociobiology. It is a straightforward move from that to support a feminism which argues for change within the constraints set down by nature.[65] This is what many of the early sexologists had advocated as feasible within the laws of nature. The idea of 'separate but equal' had in effect been the call of the first wave of feminism; in tandem with sociobiology it seems set to enjoy a modest revival.

The evocation of an earlier phase of feminism through sociobiology is paralleled in the revival of a 'natural rights' attitude towards sexual variations which recalls the work of Havelock Ellis, Edward Carpenter and Magnus Hirschfeld. Their concern had been to demonstrate that a 'perversion' such as homosexuality was little more than a harmless anomaly (Ellis) or evidence of an intermediate sex (Carpenter, Hirschfeld).[66] Nature in her wisdom had constructed sex variants, either by chance, or to fulfil a veiled purpose. Sociobiology has lent itself to similar explanations. E.O. Wilson has suggested that:

> All that we can surmise of humankind's genetic history argues for a more liberal sexual morality, in which sexual practices are to be regarded first as bonding devices and only second as means for procreation.[67]

With the removal of the centrality of the reproductive urge as the yardstick of normality, the way lies open to endorse tolerance of variations as 'natural' and 'eugenic'. What is remarkable about the resulting work is that, like the similar efforts of the sexological pioneers, it advocates tolerance within carefully demarcated limits. Ellis was able to combine a progressive response to homosexuality with an attitude to male–female relations which was, by our standards, extremely rigid and oppressive. Similarly, sociobiological writers are able to justify homosexuality, paedophilia and sado-masochism, while never questioning the differences between rather than across the genders. All of these are potentially functional.

In an argument that is curiously close to Edward Carpenter's at the beginning of the century, E.O. Wilson suggests that 'The homosexual members of primitive societies may have functioned as helpers ... (operating) ... with special efficiency in assisting close relatives.'[68] Homosexuality—like other variations—has survived because it aids the evolutionary process. What is obviously appealing is that a justification in nature can now be offered for the claim to 'rights' by the sexual minorities.[69]

My purpose here is not to denigrate biological evidence. Any theory of sexuality will need recourse to an understanding of bodily possibilities and limits. But the disturbing thing about the revived search for biological explanations of social behaviour is that the urge to fill a conceptual gap is stronger than an adherence to theoretical consistency and political judgment. A good example of the seductive temptations of an ostentatiously biological explanation is the Kinsey Institute's final publication on homosexuality, *Sexual Preferences*. The authors carefully explore the evidence (or lack of it) for the aetiology of homosexuality, and concludes that: 'What we seem to have identified is a pattern of feelings and reactions within the child that cannot be traced back to a single social or psychological root.'[70] But instead of then considering the possibility that homosexuality might not be a unitary phenomenon with a single causative explanation, as Kinsey himself had done, the authors resort to what is basically a rhetorical device: if a social or psychological explanation cannot be found, then a biological explanation must exist. 'Biology' fills a gap which social theorising has constructed. The result is an intellectual closure which obstructs further questioning.

It is this space in theorising about the sexual that sociobiology seems able to fill. Its own theoretical inadequacies are forgotten as the intellectual and political uses of it become apparent. But, I suggest, it takes us no further than the theories of the pioneering sexologists. Like them it claims validity from its employment of Darwinian insights. Like them it is trapped within categories it cannot either ignore or explore.

The web of sexuality

The overriding difficulty with all these theories is that they cannot function without some notion of 'natural man' (with woman as the natural other). With Malinowski and the sociobiologists this is explicit. But even when a liberal like Margaret Mead attempts to relativise social categories, she still assumes implicitly that there are previously ordered slots available for the roles and identities to fit into. The theoretical implications of this are important. But the political implications are even more significant, for if relations between the genders and the forms of sexual expression are in the last resort dictated by the laws of nature, by instinctual forces outside human control or by human needs practically outside human understanding, then forms of human action must be severely limited. It might be that this is the case, as sociobiologists in particular have proposed. There are, however alternative positions, which offer a more fruitful understanding of the social dynamics at work.

In recent years, from within radical sociology, structuralist anthropology, psychoanalysis and Marxist theory there has been a major challenge to the naturalness of 'natural man', the founding centrality of the 'unitary subject'. The declared aim is to understand 'the individual' as a product of social forces, 'an ensemble of the social relations', in Marx's famous (if contested) phrase, rather than as a simple natural unity, with a given identity.[71] The notion of the person, the concept of the self, the French anthropologist Marcel Mauss argued, is a 'category of the human mind'. In the same tradition, Michel Foucault has written that man 'is probably no more than a kind of rift in the order of things', a figure written in sand to be washed away by the tides of history.[72] All societies, of course, have ways of specifying individuals, through names, position or status, but they are not necessarily specified as *individual subjects*, unique entities with a distinct consciousness of self, who have the will and power to constitute social order and make moral judgment. Other societies have conceived of individuals through the dense network of obligations, duties and responsibility they owe: as lords and masters, priests and laymen and so on. Since at least the seventeenth century, however (and many argue that it occurred much earlier), the west has prioritised individual will and responsibility as the starting point of speculations on society. 'Man' exists prior to society. 'His' activity with others founds society. 'He' is the measure of all things.

So a challenge to the idea of this founding individuality has wide implications—not least to the idea of a pre-given essence of sexuality. The very concept of sexuality as biological necessity becomes possible, it has been argued, because of the new concept of man emerging by the eighteenth century, when human beings came to be interpreted as knowing subjects, and, at the same time, objects of their own knowledge.[73] The idea that 'man' was a coherent product of inner propulsions and drives, which biology since the eighteenth century sought to demonstrate, made it possible to specify sex as the most vital energetic force in the individual.

A rejection of the enticing model of the bourgeois individual in all 'his' world-making glory should not necessarily involve an abandonment of what we have come to regard as 'humanist values'. Love, solidarity, trust, warmth are not inconsequential qualities; they are fundamental to the 'good life' on any interpretation. But it is dangerous to base these on a supposedly fixed, continuous and eternal, human nature. Human beings are shaped by a flow of different forces and influences, swayed by contradictory appeals. Unification into a fixed identity is a hazard-strewn process. Who is to say what elements will predominate in the fixing of our allegiances: gender, sexual preference, race, creed or class? We become human in culture and cultures vary and change. So do the political priorities we assign to our various needs and desires.

This does not mean we can ignore the body. It is obvious that sex is something more than what society designates, or what naming makes it. We experience it in our bodies and live it out in our fantasies. It might be true that sex is not the truth of our bodies, nor need it be the relentless force that we often experience as unstoppable, beyond rational control. But it must be based on biological sources and bodily potentials.

The dilemma is that even for the biologists who reject the genetic determinism of sociobiology, the nature of the relationship between biology and social consciousness is far from clear. As Steven Rose has put it, in describing the workings of a group whose specific task is to generate an understanding of the 'Dialectics of Biology', our understanding is 'tentative'. He writes: 'Societies and organisms are composed of units whose interactions generate complexities qualitatively different from the component parts.'[74]

This is no doubt true, but the degree of interaction, the relative roles of each, and the efficacy of social intervention in changing behaviour, are less than clearly specified. All that can safely be said is that we are at the start of a project to promote a greater understanding of the relationship between the biological and the social; its outcome is far from obvious.

We can tentatively propose, however, that the body is a site for historical moulding and transformation because sex, far from being resistant to social ordering, seems peculiarly susceptible to it.[75] We know that sex is a vehicle for the expression of a variety of social experiences: of morality, duty, work, habit, tension release, friendship, romance, love, protection, pleasure, utility, power, and sexual difference. Its very plasticity is the source of its historical significance. Sexual behaviour would transparently not be possible without physiological sources, but physiology does not supply motives, passion, object choice or identity. These come from 'somewhere else', the domains of social relations and psychic conflict. If this is correct the body can no longer be seen as a biological given which emits its own meaning. It must be understood instead as an ensemble of potentialities which are given meaning only in society.

To leave it at that, however, would be unsatisfactory. We are certainly creatures of naming, of designation and of categorisation. But these definitions are multiple ones—our sense of self is a precarious unity of different, often conflicting definitions and meanings: as male or female, heterosexual or homosexual, working class or aristocrat, housewife or worker, black or white. How do we recognise ourselves in these namings? Which is, or should be, the dominant one? What is the nature of this 'desire' which is involved in speaking of pleasure and the body? Is there an intermediary stage between the biological possibility and social coding?

These happen to be the precise areas to which psychoanalysis has laid claim. So far I have deliberately deferred any detailed discussion of the Freudian tradition which haunted and taunted but still remained within the discourse of sexology. It is now appropriate to redress that omission: to explore the realm of the unconscious, and the challenge it poses to the orthodoxies of the sexual tradition.

PART THREE

The challenge of the unconscious

It is in his theory that he proved to be truly revolutionary.

OCTAVE MANNONI, *Freud: The Theory of the Unconscious*

CHAPTER 6

Sexuality and the unconscious

> I do not wish to arouse conviction. I wish to stimulate thought and to upset prejudices.
>
> SIGMUND FREUD, *Introductory Lectures*

> I am interested not in what Freud did but in what we can get from him, a political rather than an academic exploration.
>
> JULIET MITCHELL, *Psychoanalysis and Feminism*

Why psychoanalysis?

Words, Freud once remarked, were originally magic. Few utterances have had as magical an effect as Freud's, or as controversial and disputed a legacy. For our own study Freud's work is critical. He is as clearly of the sexual tradition as Krafft-Ebing or Ellis, Malinowski or Mead, and his work cannot be understood without reference to the history of sexology. But he was, too, a dissident within it, which has given psychoanalysis a persistently important role in the development of radical theories of sexuality, from the outpourings of Reich to the (quite different) critiques of modern feminism. Freud's work represents a high point of a would-be-scientific sexology—and a source of its potential distintegration.

There are many social psychologies which attempt to bridge the gap between the individual and society. The importance of psychoanalysis is that unlike most of these it directly challenges conventional concepts of sexuality and gender, and in particular it questions the centrality of sexual reproduction and the rigid distinction between men and women.[1] It does this because it is concerned with the unconscious and desire. Individuals are not determined products of biological imperatives, it argues, nor are they the effects simply of social relations: psychoanalysis proposes that there is a psychic realm with its own rules and history where the biological possibilities of the body acquire meaning. If true (and I believe that despite its problems it is 'truer' than any alternative approach), Freud's theory of the mind opens the way to a concept of sexuality and sexual difference which is alive to the body, aware of social relations, but sensitive to the importance of mental activities. As a result, psychoanalysis offers the possibility of seeing sexuality as more than the irrepressible instincts which wrack the body; it is a force that is actually constructed in the process of the entry into the domain of culture, language and meaning.

The early sexologists tended to see sexuality as a pool from which a number of distributaries flow: pre-eminently those of normal sexuality, but if blocked the stream of normality turns into the nightmare of perversity. Freud is preoccupied with the tributaries which in complex ways, over hazardous terrains, in never predetermined ways, go to make up the pool. The sources of this process lie in the possibilities of the body. Many of the constraints on these possibilities come from external necessity. Both these imperatives are mediated through the activities of the unconscious mind, which it has been the pre-eminent task of psychoanalysis to theorise.

It sometimes seems that there are as many Freuds as there are Freudians. Freud has become a resource from which we pick the bits we like and discard the rotten husks. I do not pretend here to recover or return to a 'real' Freud, nor at the other extreme do I want to embrace the whole of the legacy of psychoanalysis. But I am seeking in the theory of the unconscious insights which can challenge and disrupt the sexual tradition we have inherited. Buried in the corpus of Freud's work are elements which should be central to a radical theory of sexuality.

First of all there is the partial but critical displacement of biology. His earliest scientific interests were in the physiological structure of the mind, and he never abandoned a belief in the biological basis of mental activity. In two significant works of the 1890s Freud attempted to bridge the gap between neurology and psychology: in his paper *On Aphasia* in 1891, and in the so-called *Project for a Scientific Psychology*, written in 1895, sent to Freud's closest colleague of the time, Wilhelm Fliess, and then, it seems, totally forgotten.[2] But Freud never lost the hope that one day the two disciplines would be linked. There was a consistent thread of argument, and a structural continuity, throughout Freud's work, from the *Project* to his last text, *An Outline of Psychoanalysis*, written a year before he died.[3]

Nevertheless, the difficult but fundamental last chapter of *The Interpretation of Dreams* at the very end of the nineteenth century marks a decisive move to a new theory of the mind, conceived in the language of physiology perhaps, but showing the way to a concept of psychic reality as fundamentally different from biological and social reality.[4] Freud speaks of an 'aboriginal population of the mind' and vividly describes the id in a later work as 'the dark, inaccessible part of our personality ... a chaos, a cauldron of seething excitations'.[5] But despite this colourful language, Freud clearly distinguished the unconscious from any immediate relation to animal instincts, though these might provide a nucleus of some sort. What the unconscious 'contains' is not repressed instinct but ideas (instinctual representatives) attached to drives which seek to discharge their energy, wishful impulses which are denied access to consciousness. Some of these Freud came to believe were a result of the phylogenetic inheritance, the early experiences of the human race which are relived in the early stages of development of each human subject. But what fundamentally constitutes the unconscious are those wishes which are repressed in the face of the demands of reality and in particular the repressed (and incestuous) desires of infancy: 'What is unconscious in mental life is also what is infantile.'[6]

This was a key break. There were hesitations, particularly in relationship to sexuality, which were to delay the full emergence of a developed theory until quite late in his career. But there could be no real turning back.

The second major element is the centrality of language. *On Aphasia* and the *Project*, despite their physiological preoccupations, reveal a deep concern with the relationship between language and the mind. Already, in the *Project*, the psychical apparatus is defined as a succession of inscriptions of signs. Recent psychoanalysis, especially that derived from the followers of Jacques Lacan, has exclusively stressed the verbal contents of the unconscious.[7] It is a structure of representations, and this is clearly already implicit in Freud. With the *Studies in Hysteria*, his joint work with Joseph Breuer, (1895) and the *Interpretation of Dreams* symptoms come to be seen as meaningful, as representing repressed wishes and experience (particularly those relating to sexuality). The significance of this stress is that it precisely opens the way to a theory of the unconscious which removes it finally from physiology, and to an explanation of the structural significance of the unconscious as constituted in and through language. In this reading, the unconscious becomes the way in which we acquire the rules of culture through the acquisition of language. We become fully human through the entry into the order of language and meaning. Following the linguistic theories of Ferdinand de Saussure, for whom meaning is constructed not through inherent qualities but through the arbitrary relationship of signs, Lacanian and much feminist psychoanalysis has gone on to stress that growing awareness of separation and difference is the key element in the acquisition of self and subjectivity.[8]

This is crucial to the third major point: the displacement of the unitary human consciousness that Freud's work suggests. In his *Introductory Lectures* Freud talks of three great displacements in the field of human knowledge. The first came with the Copernican revolution, which demonstrated that the earth was not the centre of the universe. The second occurred with Darwin, who demonstrated the continuity of man with the animal world. The third was Freud's own 'Copernican revolution', with its demonstration that the ego was not even the master in its own domain, but the subject of unconscious urges and impulses over which it has little or no initial control.[9] The human animal is not born as a constituted human individual. It is more a 'blob of humanity', a bundle of impulses and potentialities, subject to conflicting desires and drives. The acquisition of culture is therefore constitutive of humanity, and hence, for Freud, the 'repression' necessitated by culture is not an imposition on our humanity but an essential stage in its emergence. It is through the repression of the contradictory play of our desires and drives, 'driven hither and thither by dynamic forces'[10] that we become human subjects in human culture. Inevitably, then, our humanity is achieved at a cost — a cost paid in neurosis, the originating object of psychoanalytic investigation. And 'identity' is as a result an ever-precarious achievement, for it is constantly undermined by the repressed wishes which constitute the unconscious. The first moment when a child realises (or imagines) the distinction between its own body and the outside, the 'other', is simultaneously the moment which announces the permanent alienation at the heart of identification.[11] The individual identifies with a wholeness or completeness which can never be attained, giving rise to a ceaseless desire for that which has been lost, and hence for an identity which can only be mythical. And the decisive moment for the acquisition of culture and our identity as male or female, the oedipal moment, signifies the smashing or repression of desires which cannot be activated or realised in civilisation, but which never disappear from the unconscious, can constantly re-erupt and displace identities. The significance of this is wide-ranging, for it involves a rejection of any theory reliant on the notion of a pre-given human wholeness or completeness. It differentiates the work of Freud from the efforts alike of Freudo-Marxists, such as Wilhelm Reich, and of American ego psychology, which seeks a normalising adjustment to a mythical healthy 'self'. For Freud, to be human is to be divided.

This leads to a fourth major element in psychoanalysis: the centrality of the wish or desire. Centrally for Freud desire relates to the experience of satisfaction. The experience of the satisfaction of a need gives rise to a memory trace in the form of a mental image. As a result of the link thus established, next time a similar need arises, it will give rise to a psychical impulse which will seek to recathect or re-energise the image to re-evoke the feeling of satisfaction. This is a wish or desire. A need arises from internal tension, and can be satisfied through a specific action. Hunger, for example, can be satisfied by the attainment of a particular object, by food. But wishes or desires are linked to memory traces of previous satisfaction and are fulfilled through hallucinatory reproductions of the perceptions, which have become signs of the satisfaction.[12] The search for the object of desire is not governed therefore by physiological need, but by the relationship to signs or representation. It is the organisation of these representations that constitutes fantasy, the correlate of desire and a principle of its organisation. Desire cannot therefore be a relationship to a real object, but is a relationship to fantasy. A child's fantasy of parental seduction is as real in its effects as an actual seduction. It is none the less potent for being imagined: what we believe to be true is a forceful shaper of our dreams and dilemmas.

For Freud the repression is particularly directed against sexual desires, and it is this (the fifth point) that accounts for the formative role of sexuality in psychical conflict. Freud was not, as he himself repeatedly stressed, a 'pansexualist': he did not argue that sex was the sole shaping force of human destiny. But he did believe that sexuality played a central role in the conflict at the heart of mental processes, and in particular in the aetiology of the neuroses.[13]

The centrality assigned to sexuality was a basic principle for Freud. It grew out of his earliest exploration of neuroses, where he became convinced that, as he put at the end of his life:

> The symptoms of neuroses are, it might be said, without exception either a substitutive satisfaction of some sexual urge or measures to prevent such a satisfaction; and as a rule they are compromises between the two.[14]

Freud had observed from the late 1880s the part played by simple sexual frustration among his patients in the causation of what came to be known as the anxiety neuroses, such as 'neurasthenia'. At the same time he was working on the much more complex psychoneuroses (or transference neuroses), especially hysteria, and soon became convinced here too of the aetiological significance of sexual repression, but now it was not a simple denial of sexuality in a physical sense, but a complex psychical process that he was perceiving. In particular he saw the traumatic effect of infantile experience. Working, with Breuer, on what became *Studies in Hysteria*, he reached the conclusion that at the root of hysteria and other neuroses was repression of sexual ideas associated with the experience of a trauma. By 1895 he was prepared to begin publishing his views, and to develop his first explanation of the trauma, which he saw at this stage as the delayed effect of actual infantile seduction by adults. What was repressed was the memory of a traumatic event connected with sexuality. It was the unlikelihood to his mind of the universality of such a causative fact

(though he never abandoned the perception of childhood seduction as a common fact) that propelled Freud's new theorisation.[15]

By 1897 Freud finally accepted the hypothesis of infantile
sexuality (which previously he had masked behind the seduction theory), the generality of perverse infantile desires, and
the fact that neuroses were the negative of perversion (that is
the symptoms replaced repressed perverse wishes)—and hence
he stepped boldly into the struggling-to-be-born discourse of
sexology.[16] From now on the prime aetiological significance of
sexuality was integral to psychoanalysis, one of its most pre-
ciously cherished tenets. Over it, Freud was prepared to break
with some of his most trusted colleagues, including his designated intellectual heir, Carl Jung. 'What is demanded of us',
Freud wrote to Jung in 1907, 'is after all that we deny the
sexual instinct, so let us proclaim it.'[17] Proclaim it he did.

The nature of sexuality

The claim of psychoanalysis that sexuality was central for the
mental life of individuals can only be fully understood if we
grasp the extension made by Freud of the concept of sexuality.
Freud consciously, deliberately, sought to sever the connection
conventionally made between the sexual instinct and heterosexual genitality:

> ... we have been in the habit of regarding the connection
> between the sexual instinct and the sexual object as more
> intimate than it in fact is. Experience of the cases that are
> considered abnormal has shown us that in them the
> sexual instinct and the sexual object are merely soldered
> together ...[18]

The very form of his first major statement on sexuality, *The
Three Essays*, deliberately emphasises his interest by beginning
with a discussion of homosexuality (thus severing the expected
connection between sexuality and heterosexual object choice)
and perversion (breaking the expected link between pleasure and
genitality). The accomplishment of heterosexual object choice
(if ever fully achieved) linked to the genital organisation of
sexuality has to be understood as the culmination of a process

of development not assumed as its starting point. Freud therefore warned of the need 'to loosen the bond that exists in our thoughts between instinct and object'.[19]

Freud's theory of 'the instinct' involved a major departure from conventional notions, with their usual implication of an unmediated biological force seeking a natural object. (The German word that Freud actually used was not *instinkt* with its connotation of animal instinct, but *triebe*, which is better translated as 'drive'; unfortunately the English *Standard Edition* of Freud's work translates both words as 'instinct'.[20]) The 'drive', for Freud, was:

> a concept on the frontier between the mental and the
> somatic, as the psychical representative of the stimuli
> originating from within the organism and reaching the
> mind, as a measure of the demand made upon the mind
> for work in consequence of its connection with the body.[21]

In the same way sexuality was a balance between biological source and stimuli and mental organisation of aim and object, a view which slowly emerged from Freud's researches and analyses.

There are at least three phases of Freud's theorisation of sexuality. The earliest was basically focused on the seduction theory—the traumatic effects at puberty, with the assumed birth of sexuality, of earlier assaults on the sexless infant. This collapsed by 1897 because of its apparent internal contradictions and led to his acceptance of infantile sexuality. This in turn opened the way to a transitional theory, culminating in the first version of the *Three Essays* in 1905, which stressed the endogenous nature of the sexual drive and its emergence through stages, and was the closest Freud ever approached to a straightforwardly biological theory of sexuality. A simple automaticity through oral, anal and genital phases is assumed in sexual development even though the inevitable achievement of the (heterosexual) goal is never simplistically assumed. Both fantasy and the Oedipus Complex are missing from the first published version of the *Three Essays* and are only included in later editions and footnotes. Moreover, it is the biological capacity for reproduction at puberty which is taken to be the real start of adult sexuality, playing upon infantile experiences which become meaningful because of the physiological changes. The reproductive imperative is still the lodestar of sexuality.

The final mature phase of Freud's theory opens with his exploration of children's theories of sexuality in 1907-8, and his case study of Little Hans,[22] and points the way more firmly to the significance, which formally at least he had recognised since 1897, of the psychic organisation of sexuality through fantasy (so it is a fantasy of seduction that from 1897 he believed to be operative in the aetiology of neurosis). The tangle of repressed wishes, layers of overlapping desires, elaborate edifices of unconscious and semiconscious dreams and hallucinations are ever at war with the simple urges of libidinal energy, moulding it into individuated and fantastic shapes. There is now no single 'reproductive instinct'; no pre-given aim; no predetermined object through which the instinct can be satisfied. Instead there is an initial variety of drives—'polymorphous perversity'; an openness concerning object choice —'bisexuality'; and a consequential struggle through which the potentially perverse, bisexual human animal infant is 'conscripted' into humanity, and into the rigid structures of normal genital (hetero-) sexuality which attempts to govern even those who ostensibly live outside its laws.

At the end of his life Freud summed up what he saw as the key elements in his broadening of the concept of sexuality:

a) Sexual life does not begin only at puberty, but starts with plain manifestations soon after birth.
b) It is necessary to distinguish sharply between the concepts of 'sexual' and 'genital'. The former is the wider concept and includes many activities that have nothing to do with the genitals.
c) Sexual life includes the function of obtaining pleasure from zones of the body—a function which is subsequently brought into the service of reproduction. The two functions often fail to coincide completely.[23]

The second and third points are in a real sense less challenging than the first (though still too challenging for most sexologists). The sexual impulses are, he observed, 'extraordinarily *plastic*'. Sexuality is manifested in neuroses where the symptoms constitute the sexual activity of the patient, or to put it another way, the symptoms represent a distorted wish-fulfilment. The sexual drives can be sublimated, diverted towards ostensibly non-sexual aims, to form the basis of civilisation and cultural achievement. Sexuality can take diverse and perverse forms, both in object choice such as homosexuality, and in aim (as in the aberrations described in Krafft-Ebing, Moll, Hirschfeld and others). The perversions are in fact keys to the understanding of sexuality in general, for they give insights into its nature that no others can. What a perversion and orthodox sexual activity have in common is a subordination of a component instinct to a dominant one, its governance he suggests in a significant phase by a 'well-organised tyranny'.[24]

The activities of perverts are unmistakably sexual because they usually (though not invariably, as in the case for example of voyeurism and transvestism) engage in activities which lead to orgasm. Such a criterion does not, however, apply to infantile sexuality, despite what Freud calls 'hints' of such proto orgasms in young people. It is this that makes the hypothesis of infantile sexuality so controversial. In his *Introductory Lectures* Freud, with his usual directness, sought to answer the standard objections:

> To suppose that children have no sexual life—sexual excitations and needs and a kind of satisfaction—but suddenly acquire it between the ages of twelve and fourteen would (quite apart from any observations) be as improbable, and indeed senseless, biologically as to suppose that they brought no genitals with them into the world and only grew them at the time of puberty.[25]

But it is not clear from this account why the activities of early childhood should be described as 'sexual' rather than, say, 'potentially sexual', for Freud admits that there is no generally recognised criteria of the sexual nature of a process; and what occurs in infancy cannot be either genital or orgasmic sexuality in any meaningful physiological sense. Freud realised he was on difficult theoretical ground and attempted two further justifications. Firstly, he suggests that infantile behaviour can justifiably be called 'sexual' because the analyst comes to an awareness of it through analysis of undoubtedly sexual elements in adulthood. It is the analysand who demonstrates the link, not the analyst. Secondly, he suggests that nothing is gained by *not* calling it sexual, or by trying to assert the purity of children. Moreover, by about the age of three undoubtedly sexual manifestations, such as masturbation, do appear, and this has been established independently of psychoanalysis.[26]

This ultimately begs the question, and it is difficult not to think that on this issue Freud's thinking is tautological. For he argues simultaneously that sexuality exists from the beginning, is a dynamic force through the development of the child, is detachable from all conventionally recognisable definitions of the sexual, while being unable to offer any criteria by which to define what *is* sexual.

Yet, despite the contradictions and problems in Freud's emphasis on infantile sexuality, psychoanalysis does offer a framework which allows us to describe childhood activity as 'sexual'. For as psychoanalysis pre-eminently demonstrates, the child does not develop in a vacuum, but in a world of unconscious desires amongst all around him or her. As Freud put it in the *Three Essays*,

> A child's intercourse with anyone responsible for his care affords him an unending source of sexual excitation and satisfaction from his erotogenic zones. This is especially so since the person in charge of him, who, after all, is as a rule his mother, herself regards him with feelings that are derived from her own sexual life: she strokes him, kisses him, rocks him and quite clearly treats him as a substitute for a complete sexual object.[27]

It is the pre-existence of adult sexual desires that ensures the sexuality of the child.

Not surprisingly, given this hothouse of unspoken (and unspeakable) desires, Freud suggests that infantile sexuality is 'distracted', composed of a host of desires, which the child displays 'without shame', and adult sexuality only emerges 'by a series of developments, combinations, divisions and suppressions, which are scarcely ever achieved with ideal perfection'.[28] The perfection is never really attained precisely because the advent of the rules of genital supremacy demand a complex process of recognition and renunciation, a hazardous journey which can rarely be negotiated 'successfully'. Every step on the path can become a point of fixation, or of dissociation, of the sexual drive. For Freud, a creature of his times, the goal was undoubtedly laid down by the laws of biology, history and culture, and he had no doubt that health depended on the completion of this hurdle race. But in the problematical evolution of each individual subject, success could never be guaranteed, and was rarely, if ever, fully achieved. 'Normal' sexuality was a brittle carapace constantly cracking from the strain of disciplining its discordant desires. Hence the vital importance of the oedipal moment, the most important stage on the road to sexed identity.

Oedipus and sexual identity

The Oedipus Complex, and its resolution, was for Freud the point of juncture between the individual and the social, but the difficult problem was how the social acted upon the individual —how the individual was inducted into the laws of culture. Freud significantly shifts his position on this throughout his writings, and the oedipal moment gradually ceases to be an automatic process and becomes instead a struggle in which the symbolic position and power of the Father in the oedipal triangulation of mother, father and child, assumes the decisive importance.

Though first discussed in *The Interpretation of Dreams*, the complex makes no direct appearance in the *Three Essays* of 1905, and did not even receive its name until 1910. By 1919, however, it had become the cornerstone of psychoanalysis. Even so until the early 1920s Freud continued to assume a strict parallelism in the impact of the complex on boys and girls: boys desired their mothers, girls their fathers, a heterosexual privileging which allowed Jung, for instance, to invent an Elektra Complex to describe the latter.[29] It was the undermining of this assumption in the 1920s which ironically served to displace Oedipus at the moment of its final theorisation. The discovery between 1922 and 1924 of a pre-oedipal phallic stage in both boys and girls between the oral/anal phases and full genital maturity brought into play the significance of castration in propelling the individual through the oedipal crisis.[30]

The dawning realisation (not fully integrated into his theory of sexuality until the early 1930s) of the common pre-oedipal emotional involvement of both boys and girls with their mothers finally brought home the crucial significance of the *different* journeys through the oedipal crisis of young girls and boys. The vital element then became the threat of castration in breaking or transforming the initial relationship with the mother, a threat represented by the father and operative because of the psychic significance attributed to the anatomical distinctions between the sexes.

Though the importance of castration had first been mentioned in *The Interpretation of Dreams*, it gradually becomes central to Freud because of his realisation of the importance of childhood thoughts and theories. The two papers written in 1908, 'On the Sexual Theories of Children' and 'Family Romances', together with his case history of 'Little Hans' are critical to the development of Freud's third and final theory of sexuality. As Freud put it in a later addition to the *Three Essays*,

> The assumption that all human beings have the same
> [male] form of genital is the first of the many remarkable
> and momentous sexual theories of children.[31]

From others, equally remarkable, stem Freud's concepts of the phallic mother, castration anxiety, female envy for the penis, girls' wish to be boys themselves, as well as explanations for homosexuality.

The theory suggests that what is held to be true in the mind, whether or not the thought is conscious, has a decisive effect on the child's development. A child's sexual researches have revealed to him or her the importance of the penis and the fantasised existence of the penis in both parents. The development of masturbatory activities coincident with the phallic phase of sexual growth has also produced an awareness of genital pleasures and a narcissistic investment in one's own body. The threat of castration imagined or real therefore has a catastrophic effect. And what gives it its particular force is the evidence of castration that gradually dawns on the child through the existence of the 'castrated' female. In the boy it is the deferred effects of the threats of castration (perhaps haphazardly delivered by mothers, nannies and so on) reactivated by the boy's sight of the female genitals and the awareness of its 'inferiority' that propels the child through the crisis. The threat works because the boy has already experienced narcissistic loss, most fundamentally through withdrawal of the mother's breast, but also through learning to defecate.[32]

The girl's recognition of her 'castration' dictates a different, more painful route. Like the boy, she too starts with a love attachment to her mother. But from the first she envies the boy's penis. As Freud notoriously put it, 'her whole development may be said to take place under the colours of envy for the penis.'[33] And she extends her judgment of inferiority from the penis to herself. Not surprisingly, the mother is blamed for her inadequacy, and the girl transfers her love object to her father. But at the same time she is, despite her resentments, necessarily putting herself in the place of her mother; and her wish to have a penis like her father's becomes the wish to have a baby from him. Because the girl is already 'castrated', the oedipal moment is more prolonged and more difficult for the girl. The boy, after all, only has to take his place as the heir to his father and transfer his love for his mother to other women. The girl has to decisively switch her desires from her mother to her father and other men. The differences in this process explain the differences between men and women. In males, therefore,

> the threat of castration brings the Oedipus complex to an end; in females we find that, on the contrary, it is their lack of a penis that forces them into their Oedipus complex.[34]

The threat or fear of castration is thus constitutive of sexual difference. Before the full integration of the complex into Freud's theory, it seemed that the Oedipus Complex simply passed away as a natural development. Accounts within psychoanalysis, such as those of Ernest Jones, which rejected the significance Freud gave to castration, continued to see sexual identity as acquired automatically through the maturation of the drives. Even for ostensibly more radical accounts, such as Reich's, Oedipus appears as a natural stage unless prematurely thwarted. However, for Freud in his mature theory it is castration that alone shatters the Oedipus Complex and hence forces the acquisition of sexed identity. The castration threat is therefore now an embodiment of a cultural imperative which continues to enforce its demands on the mind through the strictures of the superego. Starting with the fantasised, unconscious evaluation of the penis, the child has come to recognise its symbolic importance and organises his or her (and now the pronouns are decisive) identity in relationship to it.

Why, as several generations of feminists and others have asked, should the male organ have such a decisive significance? Why, say, shouldn't male envy for the breast have as cataclysmic an effect? At this point Freud reveals a profound and ultimately crippling hesitation.

The problem resolves itself into a question: is the fear of castration so significant because the penis is naturally the superior organ, or because of its symbolic importance in a male-dominated culture? Freud wavers. His early general explanation is that the genital region achieves hegemony over the sexual organisation because of the high narcissistic investment in it, and hence the powerful effect of a threat of loss. But within the matrix of genital dominance, it is the *male* organ which dominates, and here Freud is ultimately unable to avoid a teleological explanation. The penis, he suggests, taking up a suggestion of his colleague Sandor Ferenczi, 'owes its extraordinarily high narcissistic cathexis to its organic significance for the propagation of the species.'[35] The penis is so significant because it is the organ of generation. In the end, Freud seems to be suggesting, the penis is central because it is the key to the imperative of reproduction which ultimately governs sexuality. Is it possible that after such an elaborately original theory of sexuality Freud in the end succumbs to this most banal of explanations?

The problem with Freud's theory is that it is neither satisfactorily biological nor clearly anything else. The way was opened for endless debate. Ernest Jones dismissed Freud's 1922 paper on 'The Infantile Genital Organisation', with the importance it assigned to the phallic phase, because it gave insufficient emphasis to the complementarity of male and female organs:

Freud does not seem to have taken sufficiently into account the thrusting tendency of the organ and its almost physical search for a corresponding counterpart.[36]

In this criticism is encapsulated one powerful tendency within psychoanalysis, which sought to temper what was seen as the 'phallocentrism' of Freud by suggesting a natural polarity and complementarity between the sexes. Jones, with feminist colleagues such as Karen Horney, sought an explanation, which would not so ostentatiously devalue women, in the *natural* difference between men and women. The ultimate question, Jones felt, was 'whether a woman is born or made', and the answer seemed to him transparent.[37]

The so-called Freud-Jones debate was enormously significant—not least in encouraging Freud to clarify his own view on female sexuality.[38] The arguments of Jones and Horney and Melanie Klein, and others who entered the battle, such as J. Lamph De Groot, Helene Deutsch and Ruth Mark Brunswick, helped shape the analytic views on femininity for a generation, and echoes can be heard in recent feminist psychoanalysis.[39] The feminist break away from Lacan of analysts such as Luce Irigaray in the 1970s replays the schisms of the 1920s and 1930s.[40]

But the enduring problem with these early critiques of Freud's views is that they assume an essential masculinity and femininity and a natural heterosexuality. In psychoanalytic protocols, therefore, no explanation for the girl's turning away from the mother to the father is needed: it is simply an effect of innate heterosexuality.[41] The difficulty of reconciling this with Freud is that he precisely makes the attainment both of heterosexuality and of adult masculinity and femininity (but especially the latter) the problem that psychoanalysis had to explicate. It is, after all, the *psychic* consequences of anatomical distinctions that concerned Freud.

There is a further problem. Freud was clearly concerned with the fragile distinctions between the sexes, which presupposes relationship where the terms masculine and feminine are profoundly problematic and defined only in terms of what they are not. But the very nature of the controversy pushed the debate decisively towards a discussion of the inherent qualities of femaleness, which inevitably led to a search for the essentially feminine, to which a biological argument was always the easiest answer.

In recent debates, by contrast, particularly those stemming from contemporary feminism, it is the structural significance both of Oedipus and of the penis/phallus that are stressed. For Lacanian analysis, the oedipal moment is the point at which the human animal enters the 'Symbolic Order', the order of language, a system of signification which positions the subject within a given structure of meaning organised (in accord with Lacan's adaptation of post-Saussurian linguistics) around the recognition of difference ('meaning is only produced by a systematic arrangement of differences' as Coward and Ellis succinctly phrase it).[42] In this system, the penis, or rather its symbolic representative, the phallus, is the prime signifier, in relation to which meaning is shaped. The phallus is the mark of difference; it symbolises power differences within language and males become the symbolic bearers of power. The phallus represents the 'law of the Father', the controlling exigency within which sexual relations are lived. The effect of the castration complex and the resolution of the oedipal crisis is therefore to structure a recognition of sexual difference as necessary for cultural order. It is not clear from this, however, whether it is patriarchal culture or culture as such that demands the organisation of difference. If the former, then the question of historical agency to produce change looms. If the latter, then sexual difference simply becomes an elaborately new way of describing a nature-given sexual division. Such ambiguities provide the energy for continuing debate—and scepticism.[43] They have their source in Freud's own ambivalence.

His earliest work, the basis of some of his founding speculations, had been with women, especially hysterics, and his first great case history had been of a woman, that of Dora, written soon after *The Interpretation of Dreams* and published in 1905. But much of his writing until the 1920s had been based on male development, with the female seen as basically parallel or complementary. Whatever his protestations, a heterosexual assumption dominated. The exploration of the separate development of female sexuality was therefore absolutely necessary if Freud was to break fully with biological essentialist explanations. His papers on female sexuality between 1920 and 1932 were belated attempts to achieve this. The implications of these relatively late works were profound, for they suggested that femininity and female sexuality were constructed only through struggle, and at a huge psychic cost: a more prolonged, and less easily resolved, passage through the Oedipus crisis, a greater proneness to neuroses, a less successful suppression of bisexuality (because of the girl's prime involvement with her mother) and a less well developed superego. In the process the little girl has become a little woman, but only with pain and at the cost of a fundamental splitting of personality. Jacqueline Rose has argued that:

> Feminism's affinity with psychoanalysis rests above all ... with this recognition that there is a resistance to identity which lies at the very heart of psychic life.[44]

What distinguishes Freud's insights into sexual difference is the perception of the difficulty of femininity which decisively separates it from more conventional accounts of the acquisition of gender. Nancy Chodorow, for instance, in her psychoanalytic account of *The Reproduction of Mothering* assumes that the internalisation of cultural norms of femininity works through the dynamics of parenting.[45] But the most disruptive premise of psychoanalysis is that it does not work. The problem with Freud himself, however, is that he constantly oscillates between this radical insight and his own normalising tendency. Even as he came to grips with the problems of female sexuality in the 1920s, Freud was to write his most notorious sentence:

> ... the feminist demand for equal rights for the sexes does not take us far, for the morphological distinction is bound to find expression in differences of psychical development—'Anatomy is Destiny', to vary a saying of Napoleon's.[46]

What we have in Freud, it would seem, is a theory which can explain the cultural acquisition of sexuality and gender framed in a language and institutional form which obscures its promise. Recent critics have suggested that psychoanalysis represents both the discovery of the mechanisms of desire, and the means of its recodification and control.[47] Sex is the secret which needed to be both discovered and controlled. Freud's analytical work, as opposed to his theoretical constructions, offer some evidence for this recodification even as the moment of discovery. This is strikingly clear if we look at two of his earliest but most famous and influential case histories, those of Dora and Little Hans, works he never repudiated, even as his own development cast new light on the hidden assumptions of psychoanalytic method.

In 'Dora' we can witness, in Freud's honest but incomplete account, both the play of unconscious desires on the part of analysand and analyst, and the conscious role assigned to psychoanalysis by both the client (or at least the person who paid, Dora's father) and the analyst. Dora was eighteen when she went to Freud, suffering from many hysterical symptoms (loss of voice, nervous cough, headaches, depression). She believed (and Freud agreed), that she was being used as a pawn in a game between her father and Herr K, husband of her father's mistress. Dora claimed (and there seems no reason to disbelieve her) that her father sent her to Freud to cure her opposition to his affair with Frau K, as a quid pro quo for which she was expected to take Herr K as her lover.[48]

Freud came to believe that Dora developed hysterical symptoms because she repressed sexual desire, in the first place for her father, then for a substitute for him, in Herr K himself. Freud's treatment therefore consists of repeated attempts to get Dora to admit to her desire, which Dora steadfastly resisted, in the end breaking off the analysis. Lacan, as others, has seen in this insistence, a sign of Freud's counter-transference in the case, his identification with Herr K, and inability to accept that Dora had no desire for him.[49] Freud himself offered a classic example of his ambivalence. He describes how Herr K:

> suddenly clasped the girl to him and pressed a kiss on her
> lips. This was surely just the situation to call up a distinct
> feeling of sexual excitement in a girl of fourteen who had
> never before been approached. But Dora had at that
> moment a violent feeling of disgust, tore herself free from
> the man, and hurried past him to the street door.[50]

To anyone reading this today, Dora's action would seem sensibly precautionary, for Freud it was a sign of her hysteria.

It is apparent that Freud was governed by a set of assumptions which shaped his analysis, the most fundamental of which was the inevitability of heterosexual desire; to him, at this stage, at least of his awareness of the problem of sexuality, it was inconceivable that Dora should not be attracted to Herr K. The second assumption was of his own neutrality in the situation, and his unawareness of his counter-transference. This blinded him to the possibility until too late that far from repressing her desire for Herr K, the source of Dora's problem might be the repression of her desire for Frau K, and behind that her oedipal desire for her mother, who remains an absence in the text. Dora's ultimate dismissal of Freud and abandonment of the analysis was a prototype of many feminists' rejection of Freud. In the complex play of desire, psychoanalysis could hardly claim a neutrality which its own theory undermined.[51]

If 'Dora' represents Freud's failure to produce a normal, healthy woman, his treatment of 'Little Hans' represents an (apparently) wholly successful attempt to create a Little Man. The case of Little Hans is a curious one: it was the first analysis of a child that Freud himself was to make, but it was carried out at second hand. The boy's father, one of Freud's earliest lay supporters, was the crucial intermediary, and Freud himself only intervened personally on limited—but decisive—occasions. The case begins when Hans is three. He appears to be a normal and happy child, and displays what for Freud was clear proof of the normality of infantile perversity and bisexuality. He wants to sleep with his mother, he loves his father, he expresses desire for the servant girl, for his young girl playfriend. He wishes to be a father, believes he can be a mother. He gains pleasure from urination, defecation, and enjoys watching his mother perform her functions. He was, states Freud, a 'positive paragon of all the vices', displaying a 'very striking degree of inconstancy and a disposition to polygamy'.[52]

The project of the next two years is the instillation of a series of assumptions which structure Hans's emotions in the direction of heterosexual masculinity. This is in response to a phobia that Hans develops in relation to horses, accompanied by a fear of venturing out. Freud traces this back to Hans's incestuous desire for his mother, strengthened by his sister's birth, which exiled him from his parents' bedroom and seemed to produce a decreased maternal interest. To this is added his hatred for his father as a rival, the fear of his castrating ability, and a consequential desire for his death. All this is symbolised by Hans's fear of being bitten by a horse; the dread that Hans experiences on seeing a horse stumble is an expression of his death wish against his father. His attempt to escape from the horse is a manifestation of the phobia which was developed as an escape from these fears.

Through the active intervention of the father and Freud, the child resolves the phobia by learning about the significance of his fantasies, and recognising female castration and the differences between the sexes.

From the start Hans displayed two overwhelming and related interests: with genitals ('widdlers') and with childbirth, which aroused both curiosity and anxiety. He seems to accept that girls and boys have different sizes of genitals, but at first this does not bother him.

> [FATHER]: ... You know what Hanna's widdler looks like, don't you?
> [HANS]: It'll grow though, won't it?
> [FATHER]: Yes, of course. But when it is grown it won't look like yours.
> [HANS]: I know that. It'll be the same (*sc.* as it now is] only bigger.[53]

But at Freud's instigation, Hans's sexual enlightenment consists of the breaking of the child's belief that girl children have *different* organs, and the construction of the myth that they have none. Instead, he learns that the function of women is to experience (painfully) childbirth.[54]

Throughout the analysis it is clear that both the father and Freud are insistent on demonstrating to the child what they take to be the natural and correct explanation. Thus Hans is faced by two contradictory explanations of his mother's role in producing children: hers, which stresses her active agency ('If mummy doesn't want one, she won't have one'), and the father's, which attributes the initiatory role not to himself (whose role is continuously obfuscated in the analysis) but to God. And it is the latter explanation that the mother underlines when challenged over the contradiction.[55]

The insistence on the part of Freud that it was Hans's test of normality to accept his masculinity leads him to ignore what becomes apparent in the text itself: both the child's affection for his father, and the father's unconscious jealousy of the child. At a crucial point in the analysis the father explains to Hans what he conceives has been going on: that the boy desires his mother, and is afraid of the father. The parental explanation has the effect both of explicating and of forbidding: the norms of heterosexual desire are clasped onto the growing boy.

Years later Freud by his own account was visited by a strikingly healthy looking young man. To his delight he discovered it was Little Hans—apparently perfectly normal and heterosexual. Freud had every right to be delighted, for he had been instrumental in his normalising adjustment. As Mitchell has vividly described:

> Little Hans finally 'resolved' his castration complex in a paradigmatic way by realising that he would one day be heir to his father's rights, if he gave up his own desires in the infantile present.[56]

This 'epic' in the constitution of sexuality[57] illustrates the potentialities of the psychiatric institution itself in reinforcing cultural assumptions about masculinity and femininity. Running throughout the case study are two central themes of Freud's sexual theory: the unstructured and polymorphous nature of infantile sexuality; and the necessities of the abandonment of this in the accession to heterosexual masculinity and femininity. Freud is saying simultaneously that gender and sexual identities are precarious, provisional and constantly undermined by the play of desires, and that they are necessary and essential, the guarantee of mental and social health. Despite the profound development of his theory of sexual difference Freud never really abandoned this deep ambivalence. It is here, surely, that Freud slips from analysis to prescription, and the well-organised tyranny of the genital organisation becomes the tyranny of psychoanalytic definition.[58]

Homosexuality and perversity

The ambiguous role of psychoanalysis becomes clearer if we explore its response to homosexuality and the 'perverse' efflorescences of sexuality. The perverse was not, on the one hand, a category apart. It was part of all of our infantile heritage, and its effects never escape us: what is neurosis, after all, but a symptomatic manifestation of a repressed perverse wish? But on the other hand, the perversions were obviously the antithesis of the reproductive definition of sexuality that Freud was constantly driven to by his own ambivalence. Not surprisingly, the contradictions in Freud's own attitudes have coloured several generations of psychoanalytic intervention—and consequent hostility from homosexuals themselves.

The reaction to Freud has been shaped by the impact of 'Freudianism'. Given an ambiguous inheritance, contemporary gay politics has, unlike the modern feminist movement, displayed little positive interest in psychoanalysis. Whereas a number of modern feminists have attempted to use concepts derived from a reading of the Freudian tradition to theorise patriarchy, the psychological characteristics of masculinity and femininity, individual psychic differences, or the reproduction of motherhood, with few (usually European) exceptions most theorists of gay politics have either rejected the Freudian tradition totally or have resorted to *ad hoc* appropriations which have often served to conceal rather than clarify contemporary problems.[59]

This is hardly surprising. A form of psychoanalysis has from the 1920s been vital to attempts to deal with homosexuality as a 'social problem'. Since the 1940s, especially with the wholesale medicalisation and psychologisation of the official approach to homosexuality both in Europe and North America, this tendency has been accentuated, underlined by the development of ego psychology, with its insistence on the healthiness of acceptance of normal sexuality and gender identities. There are undoubted sources for this in Freud's own writings. He speaks constantly of homosexuality as a 'perversion', an 'abnormality', a 'disorder', as 'pathological', as a 'flight from women', and so on. This ambivalence, very closely related to similar ambiguities in his attitude to female sexuality, need not invalidate his major insights, but it has unfortunately lent credence to the work of his more conservative *epigones*, especially in America.

Perhaps the most striking feature of recent psychoanalytically inclined studies of homosexuality has been their explicit abandonment of key elements of Freud's own theory to sustain their case. Thus Bieber and Socarides, both of whom have published substantial studies of homosexuality in men, have rejected the central notion of bisexuality, with Socarides, for example, arguing that the concept of bisexuality has 'outlived its scientific usefulness'.[60] So instead of seeing an original bisexuality of which both heterosexuality and homosexuality are, in complex ways, derivatives, this approach sees heterosexuality as the given natural state, from which homosexuality emerges as a result of the blockage of the heterosexual impulses.

The inevitable consequence of this perspective is an emphasis on the importance of the norm.

> One of the major resistances continues to be the patient's misconception that his disorder may be in some strange way of hereditary or biological origin or, in modern parlance, a matter of sexual 'preference' or 'orientation', that is, a normal form of sexuality. These views must be dealt with from the very beginning.[61]

It follows that the main test of psychoanalysis is therapeutic success, and Socarides duly parades his catalogue of such 'successes', having no doubt dealt with the problem in the process.

Freud himself had no such illusions. He put the term 'cure' carefully into quotation marks in the *Three Essays* and was even more emphatic elsewhere (as for example in his study of a female homosexual). Though he did believe an adjustment was possible, depending on the degree of resistance encountered, it is clear that Freud was sceptical:

> In general, to undertake to convert a fully developed homosexual into a heterosexual does not offer much more prospect of success than the reverse, except that for good practical reasons the latter is never attempted.[62]

Therapeutic zeal within psychoanalysis has obviously increased since Freud wrote. What for Freud was an abnormality of object choice, that in the first place needed explanation, has since taken on the characteristics of an illness which demands curing. Guy Hocquenghem has noted that Freud's speculation in the Schreber analysis that repressed homosexuality was a cause of paranoia has been simply reversed into the notion that paranoia is a cause of homosexuality.[63] The way was prepared early on, however, when others working either within or from a position only recently severed from psychoanalysis were more conservative. For Stekel and Adler the perversions *were* a sign of neuroses, not their negative. Adler, in a monograph in 1930, saw homosexuality basically as a failure of social learning reinforcing a fear and hostility towards the opposite sex. Even the generally orthodox Ernest Jones criticised Freud for his tolerant attitude to his lesbian patient and commented that 'Much is gained if the path to heterosexual gratification is opened.'[64]

Several important consequences have flowed from the shift of emphasis within psychoanalysis. Firstly, it is clear that the psychoanalytic institution, especially in America and parts of Europe, has played a vital part in that repressive categorisation of homosexuality as an illness or condition, which is increasingly seen as the core of the oppression of homosexuality. Secondly, this form of Freudian theorising has had conservative social implications, and has been mobilised against potentially more radical approaches, from the work of Kinsey onwards. Thirdly, its impact has not exhausted itself, even amongst sexual radicals themselves, where little use has been made of the potentially disruptive insights of Freud on sexuality, at the cost of a viable theory of desire.

The extension of the theory of sexuality that Freud sought inevitably forced him to confront the issue of homosexuality. His position was, in outline at least, straightforward.

> From the psychoanalytic standpoint, even the most eccentric and repellent perversions are explicable as manifestations of component instincts of sexuality which have freed themselves from the primacy of the genitals. . . . The most important of these perversions, homosexuality, scarcely deserves the name. It can be traced back to the constitutional bisexuality of all human beings . . .[65]

So what is the distinctive quality of homosexuality? In the *Three Essays* Freud noted that:

> The most striking distinction between the erotic life of antiquity and our own no doubt lies in the fact that the ancients laid the stress upon the instinct itself, whereas we emphasise its object ... we despise the instinctual activity in itself, and find excuse for it only on the merits of the object.[66]

This cultural shift points to the organising function of object choice in modern society. Starting with a notion of the original undifferentiated nature of the libido, Freud argues that homosexuality is a peculiarity of object choice, not of a constitutional, perverse instinct. The implication then is that homosexuality is not absolutely separable from heterosexuality for 'one must remember that normal sexuality too depends upon a reduction in the choice of object'.[67] Both are compromises from the range of possibilities, and it follows that:

> from the point of view of psycho-analysis the exclusive sexual interest felt by men for women is also a problem that needs elucidating and is not a self-evident fact based upon an attraction that is ultimately of a chemical nature.[68]

Homosexuality, then, was not a thing apart. Not only were many of its forms (especially object choice and genital organisation) continuous with those of heterosexuality, but homosexual feelings were manifested in apparently normal people, either latently or unconsciously. Everyone, he wrote in his essay on Leonardo, was capable of a homosexual object choice,[69] while sublimated homosexual feeling was an important factor in binding groups together, from the sanctity of priestly orders to the masculine ethos of military organisations.[70]

Freud's main interest was not in homosexuality as a deviation from an unquestioned social norm, but in the psychic mechanisms of homosexual object choice; and, as a corollary to this, he used homosexuality to illustrate general psychic processes. Several consequences flowed from this approach. Firstly, he consciously distances himself from the notion that homosexuality was a product or sign of 'degeneracy', the favoured late-nineteenth-century term to describe the 'abnormal'. This was, he suggested, no more than a 'judgement of value, a condemnation instead of an explanation'. Such concepts were inadequate because perverts often showed no other signs of mental or social inefficiency apart from their sexual preferences.[71] Also, quite obviously, the hypothesis of an original polymorphous perversity in both race and individual infant necessitated the abandonment of any concept of degeneracy.

Secondly, he rejected the distinction, favoured by Havelock Ellis amongst others, between acquired and congenital homosexuality as a 'fruitless and inappropriate one'.[72] He avoided any concept of the innateness of homosexuality on the grounds of the existence of non-absolute forms and its widespread nature; and he made no play with the distinction between 'inversion' (innate) and 'perversion' (a product of corruption) which was to be significant in later social policy debates.[73] Homosexuality could not be explained (as apologists from Ulrichs to Hirschfeld held) in terms of male souls in female bodies or vice versa,[74] nor understood simply as a result of infantile seduction (though this *could* result in a certain fixation of the libido). The general explanation had to be found in the universal bisexuality of human beings.

Thirdly, Freud rejects any simple association of sexual inversion with gender inversion:

> The literature of homosexuality usually fails to distinguish clearly enough between the question of the choice of object on the one hand and of the sexual characteristics and sexual attitudes of the subject on the other. ... A man in whose character feminine attributes obviously predominate ... may nevertheless be heterosexual. The same is true of women.[75]

Like Ellis, he felt that this was less true in women than in men, for he noted a distinct flirtation with masculine characteristics. Freud, like Ellis, was commenting on what appeared to be a sociological fact, and like the English sex psychologist sought an explanation within his own theory.[76] The 'mystery' of homosexuality for Freud could not be solved by any of the rival theories, whether congenital or environmental, and could only be sought in the general theory of the psychic apparatus. Homosexuality had to be understood as a particular combination of three phenomena: physical sexual characteristics, mental sexual character, and kind of object choice, and the form of the combination was shaped by particular psychic experiences. So the greater gender inversion of female homosexuals as opposed to males was explicable for Freud only in terms of the different relationship of men and women to the processes of psychic development.

Even at this point Freud was reluctant to offer a monocausal explanation: there could be no single cause because so many factors in individual development varied:

> What we have thrown together, for reasons of
> convenience, under the name of homosexuality may derive
> from a diversity of processes of psychosocial inhibition.[77]

Homosexuality can only be understood, Freud argued, in terms of the psychic conflicts of identity and identification generated in the advent to culture. As we know Freud had a clear notion of what that meant, and above all it did mean differences between the sexes. Inevitably, therefore, Freud opened the way to a series of emphases which saw homosexuality in men and women as a failure of achieved normality. But the problem lies not so much with the account of the mechanisms that shape sexual desire, but with his assumptions about the route they should direct the child along. Freud's accounts of the genesis of homosexuality read today as unfortunately opprobrious and moralistic. But if psychoanalysis is to have any contemporary significance the real lesson that needs to be learnt is that both heterosexuality and homosexuality are peculiar compromises, partial organisations of the flux of sexual desires which are shaped, in complex ways, by the cultural organisation of sexual difference, and the centrality assigned to heterosexuality.

Freud was a liberal of his time in his attitude towards homosexuality. He favoured law reform, and his attitude to homosexual individuals was humane. Even his response towards his young lesbian patient was cautiously sympathetic. He affirmed that 'the girl was not in any way ill', and he accepted her passionate statement that 'she could not conceive of any other way of being in love.'[78] But inevitably, there are certain normalising assumptions in his attitudes. These can be summed up with a quotation from his famous letter to the mother of a young homosexual:

> Homosexuality is assuredly no advantage; but it is nothing to be ashamed of, no vice, no degradation; it cannot be classified as an illness; we consider it to be a variation of the sexual function produced by a certain arrest of the sexual development.[79]

Here we have simultaneously the demythologising effect of Freud's theory of psycho-sexual development, *and* a certain normative stance, for the 'arrest' presupposes a proper and 'normal' 'development'. There is already, contained in the language here, a series of major cultural assumptions. The normal pattern is towards a heterosexual object choice and a genital organisation of sexual aim; and the two are locked together. As Laplanche and Pontalis have put it, when all reservations are made:

> The fact remains that Freud and all psychoanalysts do talk of 'normal' sexuality. Even if we admit that the polymorphously perverse disposition typifies all infantile sexuality, that the majority of perversions are to be found in the psychosocial development of every individual, and that the outcome of this development—the genital organisation—'is not a self-evident fact' and has to be set up and governed not by nature but by the process of personal evolution—even if we admit all this, it is still true that the notion of development itself implies a norm.[80]

So the question inevitably occurs: does this simply mean that Freud's theories return us, by an elaborately different route, to the same categories of perversion as in orthodox sexology?

The difficulty with Freud (especially for someone who wants to use his critical insights) was that in the end he did believe that a heterosexual genital organisation of sexuality was a cultural necessity, so that although he could readily concede that all of us have 'seeds' of perversion, a healthy development demanded their subordination to the norm.

Freud certainly knew that norms could be changed. But he

also believed that civilisation in all its tragic glory demanded repression of desires: the free play of polymorphous perversity could never be compatible with cultural order. Attitudes towards homosexuality could, indeed would, change, but it would always have to be judged by the norm set by heterosexual genitality. That was the organisation of sexuality that culture demanded and there seemed to be no alternative to that.

Here was the point where the theory of the unconscious clashed with the politics of desire, and where the conservative cast of psychoanalysis obscured its radical impulse.

CHAPTER 7

Dangerous desires

> Our concern is not with a corrected or improved
> interpretation of Freudian concepts but with
> their philosophical and sociological implications.

> HERBERT MARCUSE, *Eros and Civilisation*

> Psychoanalysis is like the Russian Revolution.
> We don't quite know when it started going bad.

> GILLES DELEUZE AND FELIX GUATTARI, *Anti-Oedipus*

> Desire is no longer viewed as a desire *for* something
> ... desire no longer has a precise substance or a meaning.

> JACQUES DONZELOT, review of *Anti-Oedipus*

Civilisation and repression

'Desire' dances on the precipice between determinism and disruption. After Freud, it cannot be reduced to primeval biological urges, beyond human control, nor can it be seen as a product of conscious willing and planning. It is somewhere ambiguously, elusively, in between, omnipotent but intangible, powerful but goal-less. Because of this it can lay claim to universality, to being out of time and beyond identity, infiltrating the diverse spaces of our social lives, casting out delicate strands which embrace or entrap, isolate or unify. *But* it also has a history. The flux of desire is hooked, trapped and defined by historical processes which far from being beyond understanding, need to be understood. The difficulty that has plagued the Freudian tradition is of pinpointing those processes, identifying that history, without falling prey to the mythopaeic universalism of a Jung, for whom cultures seem little more than emanations of archetypal forms, or the sociological relativism of post-Freudian dissidents like Erich Fromm or

157

Karen Horney for whom Oedipus, repression and libido theory are little more than cultural emanations.[1]

Freud sought to close part at least of that gap by his famous (or infamous) 'Just-so' story in which history and biology come perilously close to being identified with one another. Building upon post-Darwinian biology and evolutionary anthropological explanations, he produced what he himself recognised as a 'fantastic' hypothesis about a society which 'has never been an object of observation'.[2] He postulated the prehistoric existence of small hordes of people living together under the leadership of an all-powerful male, who had sole property in women, and who drove out or castrated all the sons who challenged him. Eventually, fuelled by sexual jealousy, the sons banded together to overpower the father, and devoured him raw. But, as with 'primitives of the present day', or indeed all of us in our emotional make-up, the sons were ambivalent in their attitudes to their father. They hated and feared him, but they also loved and honoured him, and wished to take his place. This ambivalence was the origin of the guilt which actually increased the father's powers over them. But they also sought for themselves their father's inheritance. Out of the chaos, a 'social contract' was eventually agreed, to form a new social organisation in which the role of the father was restored and honoured through the totemic meal and totemic symbol, and to which the sons submitted, in the knowledge that they were heirs of his place and power. This was a drama at the dawn of history but its effects were transmitted through each individual. Individual characteristics are precipitates of prehistoric experiences. We all, Freud suggested, carry within us a phylogenetic memory trace of this 'real event' as our 'archaic heritage', so that the individual micro-dramas of infantile progress through the Oedipus Complex are little more than recapitulations of this founding moment. In our biology we bear marks of this history, and our history is a working through of this heritage. It is, at the same time, a drama of renunciation, sacrifice, and non-satisfaction, based on the realisation that 'civilisation' and the satisfaction of all drives are antagonistic. Subordination to the law of this murdered primal father is a guarantee of civilised life.

The theory may have its absurdities but it also had its advantages as a 'scientific myth', and Freud held tenaciously to it. At the very least it saved Freud from the embarrassment of having to prove that each individual saw the genital equipment of the opposite sex, or was threatened by (or recognised) castration, or hated the father. The power of the castration threat could be read simply as a memory trace of that original, and real, castration threat. Even more significantly, the theory liberated Freud both from the sociological relativism of some of his critics, and from the universalism of Jung, though at the expense of a different sort of universalism. Moreover, it opened the way to a later, structuralist, interpretation of this attempted juncture between individual and social experience. For Juliet Mitchell, following the anthropologist Claude Lévi-Strauss, there are structural necessities of human culture—the law of exogamy, the prohibition of incest, the 'exchange of women'— which must be repeated in each culture for culture to survive. There is no need now for any hypothesis of a racial memory. The laws of culture are embedded in kinship structures, which in turn are analogous with linguistic relations as described by structural linguistics.[3] In this system women are exchanged by men as signs. The problem with this structuralist account is that like Freud's it assumes much of what it is trying to explain. Lévi-Strauss's account of the founding significance of the exchange of women already presupposes that it is men who, as naturally promiscuous, are in a position to exchange their women. This repeats the difficulty that Freud's phylogenetic account leaves unanswered. The Oedipus Complex in Freud is intended to be constitutive of sexual identities, but the primal event already presupposes distinct sexual identities, at the start of history, with the Father already in his symbolic position. What Freud's account at best can do is to explain the reproduction of that symbolic position, not why it came about. Certain differentiated psychic structures are already in place at the founding moment of cultural taboos, and it is difficult not to see these taboos as products for Freud of basic psychic needs.[4] In other words, Freud is forced to derive cultural forms from individual structures which he implies are biologically given.

Despite all his elaborate theoretical efforts Freud's founding myth relies solidly, in the end, on a heterosexual psychic structuration. Desire, far from being unconstrained, is tightly contained right from the start.

The uneasy marriage of Marx and Freud

The main attempt to provide a more fully social and historical account of the organisation of desire has come from the chief rival of psychoanalysis as the dominating intellectual discourse of the twentieth century, Marxism. But a synthesis of the two approaches has proved far from easy to achieve. Classical Marxism had as its major concern the movement of economic forces; its dominating interest could never be gender and sexual differences. Freud on the other hand was conservative over many issues, and looked unfavourably on attempts to link psychoanalysis with radical political positions, especially Marxism.[5]

Nevertheless, many socialists have seen in Freudianism since the early part of the century a powerful contribution to radical analysis. As Jacoby has observed, even if Freud in the end justified civilisation he said enough in the interim about its antagonistic and repressive essence to put it in question. Alfred Adler made an early attempt to relate Marx and Freud even before his break with the latter. In 1909 he delivered a paper 'On the Psychology of Marxism' to Freud's Vienna Psychoanalytic Society, which did not, it seems, arouse overwhelming enthusiasm. From 1919 Paul Federn was writing as a socialist Freudian, and he was to be a major influence on Wilhelm Reich. By the 1930s there were a number of 'Freudo-Marxists' in Central Europe and they even produced offshoots in the rather more unfavourable climate of Britain.[6]

The background to this new intellectual formation was essentially political. Freudo-Marxism grew in the first place out of theoretical attempts to understand the failure of the revolution in the west in the early 1920s. Psychoanalysis and in particular the theory of repression was viewed as a powerful analytical tool in understanding the perpetuation of passive and/or authoritarian values. Herbert Marcuse's work was a direct outgrowth of the Frankfurt School, which from its establishment in the early 1920s was instrumental in exploring the possibilities of a Marxism more sensitive to ideology and values (and has continued to do so to the present in the form of 'critical theory' and the work of Habermas).[7] The seçond factor was the actual rise of authoritarian and fascist politics in the 1920s and in social conditions of economic depression in the 1930s which propelled someone like Wilhelm Reich away from orthodox Freudianism towards a new psychology which could explain sexual misery. Reich's political radicalism in the Vienna of the 1920s and his move towards communism offer a paradigm of a particularly passionate, and in the end thwarted, intellectual project. Marcuse's movement towards Freudo-Marxism was slower. During the 1930s he left much of the exploration of the instinctual sources of oppression to colleagues like Erich Fromm and Horkheimer. It was not until the 1940s that he began seriously to explore Freud. But as with Reich, the motivating force was the need to explain reaction—though this time as much the continuation of Stalinism as the efficacy of the unconscious appeal of Fascism.[8] In a sense Reich and Marcuse represent opposite movements: the first moving from Freud towards revolutionary socialism, the second moving from Frankfurt School Marxism towards a rendez-vous with Freud. But they have both in different ways been enormously influential in the development of radical sexual theory. They also represent the limits of Freudo-Marxism, the ultimate impossibility of the attempted synthesis in the terms offered.

The focus of Reich's work was the theory of the orgasm. For Reich, people fell ill because of a failure to achieve satisfactory release. Many neurotics, of course, had apparently satisfactory sex lives, but not every orgasm lived up to its true potential. It had to be heterosexual, accompanied by appropriate fantasy, of the correct duration—and to lead to a complete release of dammed-up libido. The libido for Reich was a biological force, and the key to individual and social health was its full release and orgastic potency: 'Not a single neurotic individual possesses orgastic potency.'[9] Such a theory involved several major breaks with Freudian orthodoxy. Firstly, it abandoned Freud's view of the complex structuration of the drive in favour of a biologistic theory, which saw the libido as a concrete force—later called Cosmic Orgone Energy—which was both measurable and visible. By the 1940s Reich was able to detect the colour ('bluish') as visible in the bluish coloration of sexually excited frogs, and to measure orgonic energy with the aid of the Orgone Energy Field Meter. This libidinal force, moreover, was inherently genital and heterosexual in its nature, so that there was a natural, not as in Freud, a conflict-ridden progress through the oral, anal and genital phases. Whereas for Freud the oedipal moment enforced a tragedy of separation and denial, and the genital organisation was a restriction of the drive, for Reich the resolution of the Oedipus Complex into genital heterosexuality was a natural development: only inhibition to this development by repressive forces could prevent its natural, healthy efflorescence and resolution. At the heart of Reich's theory was a natural man and a natural woman whose sexual urges were basically heterosexual and genital; and essentially complementary:

> Beneath these neurotic mechanisms, behind all these dangerous, grotesque, unnatural phantasies and impulses I found a bit of simple, matter-of-fact, decent nature.[10]

Secondly, what caused neurosis according to Reich was a disturbance of this natural genitality. Freud believed that it was the repression of desires attached to polymorphous sexuality that caused neuroses in the conflict between sexuality and necessity. For Reich it was the survival or encouragement of these partial sexual activities, that is the failure to achieve genitality, that was central. Neurosis was caused by a direct disturbance of healthy sexuality.

Thirdly, following from this, it was logical for Reich to see the main aim of therapy as the restoration of orgastic potency. But this ran counter to Freud's specific injunctions that the aim of psychoanalysis was not to be a mentor for sexual release: 'A recommendation to the patient to "live a full life" sexually could not possibly play a part in analytic therapy',[11] Freud wrote, precisely because sexuality was only one of the forces in mental conflict. To emphasise the sexual at the expense of other forces might merely lead to the appearance of opposite symptoms—but would not cure the neurosis.

Finally, for Freud the unconscious was constituted in the development of the child from a combination of inherited memories and repressed ideas. It was a product of mental repression. But for Reich, the unconscious was constituted from the repression of healthy biological instincts by a sex negative culture. For Freudian orthodoxy repression was a complex mental process, for Reich it was a social and political phenomenon, of social-economic and not of biological origin.[12] The factors which inhibited genitality had economic and social sources in poverty, inequality, authoritarianism. The implication was that if the carapace of repressive social institutions were destroyed, man's natural and spontaneous sociality (and sexuality) would lay the basis of a better society.

If the orgasm theory was the prime element in Reich's revolutionary sexual politics, the second was his political theory, derived from an eclectic appropriation of Marxism. He argued in his essay, *Dialectical Materialism and Psychoanalysis* (1929) that there was a dialectical affinity between psychoanalysis and Marxism: just as Marxism represented man becoming conscious of the laws of economics and the exploitation of a majority by a minority, so psychoanalysis was the expression of man becoming conscious of the social repression of sex.[13] Both Freudianism and Marxism were deficient, however, the one because of its acceptance of bourgeois morality, the other because it ignored the ideological basis of capitalist rule, the internalisation of bourgeois morality, which was anchored in the character structure of the masses. And the fundamental mediating term between individual and repressive society was the family: a product of definite economic forces, it created through child rearing the type of character structure which supported the political and economic order of society. Character-analysis was thus the crucial analytical tool for Reich in analysing repression.

It demonstrated above all that the family was a factory for the production of submissive personalities. From this flowed Reich's analysis of the *Mass Psychology of Fascism*.[14] Nazism, he argued, was grounded in the character structure of the German masses, and especially in those of the German petite bourgeoisie. The economic and social forces produced a family pattern which encouraged the authority of the father, discouraged sexuality, and created an ambivalent authoritarian fixation. If the bourgeois family produced submissiveness through sexual repression, it followed that communism necessitated sexual liberation. In his book the *Sexual Revolution* he traced the failure of the social revolution in Russia directly to its unwillingness to go further in the direction of radical sex reform; its negative stance made Stalinism inevitable.[15]

In these two books there is much that is perceptive and historically of value—and they have been influential. The *Mass Psychology* was a prototype of a number of works that sought an explanation of fascism in psychic structuring through the family, and its influence continues in sexual politics (as in the work of Gilles Deleuze and Felix Guattari). His analysis of the failure of the Russian Revolution has similarly influenced contemporary critiques (Kate Millett's *Sexual Politics* is a good example). Perhaps even more influential has been the emphasis on the family as a factory for the reproduction of submissive personalities; its influence is traceable both in cultural theory and in the more personalist and libertarian critiques of the 1960s (Laing and Cooper especially).[16] But the real focus of this theory, the theory of the orgasm, has had more dubious political effects. Reich himself came to place increasing emphasis on this aspect of his theory as he sloughed off his more radical politics. In the 1940s he saw in organic energy a universal life force, which if collected in his Orgone Energy Accumulator could be utilised to cure numerous psychic ills from hysteria to cancer. Libidinal energy became a cure-all. But as Horowitz has observed: 'Reich's orgasm theory, the fount of his radicalism, was also the expression of his repressive super genitality.'[17] The effects of this are still visible both in personal therapy and in the theory of certain forms of radical sexual politics. In the USA of the 1970s it was still possible for a well-publicised work on homosexuality (by Kronemeyer) to justify a normative attitude towards homosexuality by reference to the therapeutic adages of Reich. And what was claimed to be a major intervention into American Marxism, by Bertell Ollman, relied entirely on a Reichian model of repression to advocate sexual transformation (as long as it was genital and heterosexual). Even the emphasis in Masters and Johnson's work on marital orgasmic harmony can be seen as a covert (even unconscious) adaptation to Reich.[18] Reich, perpetually the exile during his lifetime, has found a warm bed in a certain type of contemporary sexual radicalism.

Though following Reich in many of his contemporary concerns, Marcuse in his major intervention into Freudo-Marxism, *Eros and Civilization*, carefully distinguished himself from his predecessor. He followed the line of his own colleagues within the Frankfurt School in rejecting the naturalism and primitivism of Reich. In a postscript to *Eros and Civilization* Marcuse criticised in particular Reich's inability to distinguish between different types of repression, which prevented him from seeing the 'historical dynamics of the sex instinct and of their fusion with the destructive impulses'.[19] As a result, Reich was led to a simplistic advocacy of sexual freedom as an end in itself. Interestingly, Marcuse's critique of the culturalist Erich Fromm ends up with the same point. He praised Fromm's early work, especially his opposition to patriarchal (or 'patricentric-acquisitive') society, which he saw as parallel to his own rejection of the 'performance principle'. But he argued that Fromm, like the other neo-Freudians, had succumbed to the idea that true happiness could be achieved in this society. In a repressive society, individual happiness and productive development were in contradiction to society; if they become defined as values to be realised within contemporary society, they become themselves repressive. They ignored the pain and alienation at the heart of civilisation.[20]

Against both Reich and Fromm, Marcuse proposed a radical redefinition of Freud, which began by accepting the most extreme of his theories, especially his latent biologism, the conflict of Eros and Thanatos, the primal horde and the necessity of sexual repression, but using them to reach a more utopian conclusion than either Reich or Fromm (or Freud). Where Reich put a conflict between orgastic potency and repression, Marcuse saw a conflict between a false or distorted sexuality and a true sexuality. The theory was no less essentialist than Reich's but the moral position that resulted pointed to a different type of sexual liberation, a flourishing of polymorphous pleasures.

Marcuse accepts in *Eros and Civilization* that some form of restriction on the free flow of sexuality is a prerequisite of civilisation (basic repression). On it depends the internalisation of restrictions on the desires which is the basis of the attainment of individual autonomy and subjectivity. But over and above that, different forms of society have imposed a surplus repression, a result of the economic necessities and social ordering (resulting from class exploitation) of these societies. In modern society the larger part of repression is in the service of domination—and unlike Freud's critique of civilisation, it is surplus, not basic, repression that is the primary cause of discontent.[21] This opens the way for an exploration of the *historical* roots of sexual misery and oppression; and the possibility of the transcendence of limitations on human happiness.

This is the point of Marcuse's critique of the 'performance principle'. Capitalist society inevitably induced sexual repression since its continued existence depended on the postponement of gratification in the work process, precisely because most work under capitalism is unpleasurable and routine. Marcuse argued that the performance principle took the form of the repression of a particular type of sexuality—the secondary or partial sex drives—which led to the complete desexualisation of pre-genital sexual zones. This enforced total genitality, resulting in a radical reduction of man's potentiality for pleasure, and a simultaneous harnessing of the body to the exigencies of exploitative labour.

Resexualisation is therefore a major goal of human history. From this perspective it was clear that Reich's emphasis on genitality offered no real alternative to repressed sexuality. Marcuse argued that the repression of sexuality in all its multitudinous forms was one of the factors leading to the significance of the death instinct. Only if Eros was given a freer reign could the effect of Thanatos be minimised. 'Civilisation arises from pleasure', he stated in a 1955 lecture, 'we must hold fast to this thesis, in all its provocativeness.'[22] And one of the major provocative elements was his argument that the 'perversions' express a rebellion against the hegemony of procreative, genital sexuality, were a 'great refusal' of enforced normality harnessed to the performance principle. This is perhaps the most important aspect of Marcuse's analysis, for unlike Freud it radically questions the necessity of the heterosexual and genital norms.

For Marcuse the 'perversions' upheld sexuality as an end in

itself against the demands of surplus repression. They were upholders of the pleasure principle against the performance principle, for the perversions pointed to a polymorphous sexuality which was not limited by space and time or object choice or organ, and hence threatened the partially desexualised individuals necessary to contemporary civilisation. Marcuse is not suggesting that 'anything goes', because he clearly believes that some form of instinctual renunciation will always be necessary.[23] But with that qualification Marcuse endorses the 'perversions' as offering the possibility of a new community of humans, based on spontaneity and the release of hitherto repressed human possibilities. Such phenomena as narcissism and homosexuality, tabooed in bourgeois societies (and as 'perversions' in Freud) contained a revolutionary potential. The perverse sexualities (even paedophilia) were a revolt against the procreative norm, pointing to a fuller meaning of Eros, where the drive towards life represented the realisation of the full possibilities of the body.[24]

This is a powerful image of a transformed sexuality, and one that has had a major resonance in post-1960s sexual politics. It is a clearly utopian vision, though one which in *Eros and Civilization* Marcuse believed to be on the road to achievement. Tendencies in automation, the elimination of unnecessary expenditure of human labour through reduction of working hours and the fading away of the family as a factor in repression, seemed in the 1950s to offer the possibility of the reconciliation of labour and Eros, of sex and civilisation. By the 1960s the optimism had dimmed. *One-Dimensional Man* is a famously more pessimistic tract: technological rationality seemed destined to bind the individual even more closely to the status quo. The work opens with the ominous sentence: 'A comfortable, smooth, reasonable, democratic unfreedom prevails in advanced industrial civilisation, a token of technical progress.'[25] One of the forms of this 'unfreedom' was the controlled liberalisation of sexuality through which the conflict between the pleasure principle and the reality principle had been repressively negotiated so that 'pleasure' generated submission. This partial or 'repressive desublimation', far from being an advance, is a guarantor of the survival of oppression and exploitation. It is now a form of sexual freedom, not sexual denial, that binds people to their oppressions. As Reimut Reiche put it crudely but representatively, 'Sexuality is given a little more rein and thus brought into the service of safeguarding the system.'[26]

But the vision of *Eros and Civilization* does not disappear from Marcuse's work. It now operates as a moral counterpart to what is, the book of revelation as opposed to the critical analysis. It becomes an 'educational utopia' and not simply a free-floating vision. Marcuse came to see it as embodied in the ideals of the new radicalism of the late 1960s, the revolt of the marginals (women, gays, blacks) in the absolute refusal of capitalism. His political chiliasm here was no less romantically conceived than the vision of the earlier writings, and possibly as misplaced. Yet what stands out now is not the political ingenuousness but the status of his writings as a moral critique of the excesses of the 'sexual revolution'.[27]

Nevertheless, if Marcuse provides an ultimately more satisfying and relevant moral vision than Reich, his conceptual framework is no less inadequate. Freudo-Marxism suffers from a number of problems which in the end takes it no further than the Freudianism it claims to supplant. It depends in the first place on a theory of sexuality which, because of its rigid biologism, is ahistorical to a degree which Freud's actually is not. Reich and Marcuse both have different views of what the sexual drive is, and both agree it is modifiable by repression, but they also agree on the existence of a common instinctual structure across all cultures. They are thus unable in the end to transcend the traditional dualism between man and society. Sexuality is not shaped within history, but outside and beyond it, whatever its contingent forms. Some recent 'critical theorists' have seen in this biological framework the real materialism of Freudo-Marxism,[28] and there can be no doubt that while biological theories have tended to ignore the social, culturalist interpretations of psychoanalysis have ignored the body. But in Reich and Marcuse 'biology' takes on a different status: not as the indispensable basis of psycho-sexual development, but as coterminous or identical with it.

Following on from this, it has led secondly and inevitably to an identification of social and sexual liberation. The release of sexual energy is seen as beneficent and liberating in a way which is strongly reminiscent of the pre-Freudian romantics. This has been an important emphasis against a socialist tradition which has tended to ignore issues of sexuality and sexual difference, but it has also led to a moral position which has been as normative and restrictive in its implications as the bourgeois forms it aims to challenge.

Reich's emphasis on genital normality is one example. In the case of some recent adherents of critical theory, monogamy and familial values reassert themselves more or less surreptitiously. Though Reimut Reiche is ostentatiously Marcusean in his analysis, his attitude to homosexuality (at least in his earliest writings) is close to Reich's, while Jacoby, following Lasch, sees the traditional family as a battered haven in a corrupted, consumerised world, against which a healthy nature alone might assert itself.[29]

There is a further danger: that in posing the opposition as one between an undifferentiated sexual force and society, the differentiation along lines of gender are totally lost. Unlike the later Freud, none of the Freudo-Marxists are particularly concerned with the shaping of female sexuality (in fact, the Frankfurt School as a whole has shown little interest in gender division). The result, inevitably, is to fall into the assumption that masculinity and femininity are simply active and passive forms of the same sexual drive. The concentration on a simple antinomy of sexuality and culture avoids the complex but crucial question of the psychic and social shaping of masculinity and femininity (and it is indicative that whereas Reich sees the Oedipus Complex as more or less a natural process, Marcuse almost ignores it).

The final problem is implied in this: the reduction of the contradictions of sexuality to one polar opposition: sex and repression, with 'liberation' as the point of transformation. Sexuality itself is seen as a critical opponent of power, resistant to its workings, the refusal of repression and the embryo of its transcendence. What is missing is any notion of the plurality of forms of control in a complex history. The constructive, creative modes of the operation of power, which Foucault has particularly emphasised, are strikingly absent. As a result, Freudo-Marxism concentrates to an overwhelming extent on the dream of 'liberation' rather than on the diverse forms of struggle which all the time shift the definitions and relations of sexuality. This drastically undermines the possibility of realistically analysing the status quo (leading in both Reich and Marcuse to false projections of what was happening conjuncturally, though as it happens in different directions). The overemphasis on 'liberation' either has the effect of postponing sexual change to the never never of the moment of transcendence; or of breaking the link between social and sexual change, for it becomes all too easy to slip from an awareness of the necessary links between the two to a concentration on *personal* liberation (a danger illustrated in Reich's later work).

The crucial contribution of Freudo-Marxism has been to reassert the centrality of sexual transformation to a wider social transformation. Its moral energy and vigour has allowed the regeneration of a largely abandoned nineteenth-century tradition. But the forms of that revival have been no less ahistorical than Freud's. In seeking a totalising theory in which the social and the sexual are seen as differentiated manifestations of a single process of repression, the specifics of sex regulation are irreparably lost. Within this discourse Freud and Marx make uneasy bedfellows: to the detriment of both.

Politics and desire

The living history of desire disappears when grasped too firmly either to a transhistorical biology or to a class-reductionist view of social regulation. It was the perceived inadequacy of this approach that directed many sexual radicals in the 1970s towards an engagement with the work of Jacques Lacan and the Lacanian school of psychoanalysis. Lacan offered a 'recovery' of Freud from the biological encrustation of both immediate post-Freudians and the Freudo-Marxists; and a critique of the dominance of the psychoanalytic institution, particularly in the form of institutionalised ego psychology as it had developed in the United States.[30] The most telling aspect of Lacan's work related to his account of the complexity of subjectivity and the fragility of sexed identities. Society does not influence an autonomous individual; on the contrary the individual is constituted in the world of language and symbols, which come to dwell in, and constitute, the individual. So Lacan's theory of the construction of the subject within the symbolic order belies the boundary between self and society. 'Man' becomes social with the induction into language. Such an approach offered a way of theorising the relationship between the individual and society which the biologism of Reich and Marcuse could not. 'Natural man' disappears in the Lacanian discourse. Subjectivity is formed as individuals become aware of their alienation from themselves, in the pre-oedipal imaginary realm which always remains with them; and then as through the oedipal process, individuals become aware of the structures of human sexuality which they acquire through the acquisition of language. What this means in regard to sexuality is that there is no insistent sexual desire which pre-exists the entry into the structures of language and culture. 'Desire' is constituted in the very process of that induction, predicated upon absence or lack.

Lacanian psychoanalysis has had an influence way beyond the limits of clinical discourse: in anthropology, within Marxism and widely in other post-structuralist writing (for instance the work of Gilles Deleuze and Michel Foucault).[31] But more relevantly here it has been widely appropriated within feminism and contemporary sexual politics. The work of Kristeva, Cixous, Irigaray, in French feminist writings, whatever the ultimate fate of their allegiance to Lacan, and the work of Juliet Mitchell, Rosalind Coward and Jane Gallop, amongst others, in Anglo-American discourse, testifies to the vitality of the Lacanian contribution.[32] Juliet Mitchell's *Psychoanalysis and Feminism* has been particularly important in offering an account of the patriarchal construction of femininity under the reign of the 'law of the Father'. The problem inevitably has been that of attaching this account to the living fabric of historical processes. Mitchell has attempted to move away from the phallocentricity which besets Lacan's work, but at the expense of adding to the power structures of capitalism, as explained in fairly orthodox terms, another set of relationships, those of patriarchy, which are not transparently congruent with them. The problem remains of how to theorise the relationship between desire and the social, between the ideological categories which address and construct a particular subject, and the processes, real historical processes, by which individual meanings and identities are shaped.

Some writers going beyond Mitchell, and heavily influenced by semiological theory, have argued that the idea of the unconscious and subjectivity as produced in language simultaneously proposes their pluralism, diversity, heterogeneity and contradictoriness. Coward's subtle evocation of 'female desire' pursues the 'lure of pleasure across a multitude of different cultural phenomena, from food to family snapshots, from royalty to nature programmes'.[33] Here desire is both ingratiating and polyvocal, a potentiality for change, for breaking out of the cage of expectations, and for co-option, for sustaining things as they are. Desire is pluralistic, but the political consequences that flow from that are complex and cannot simply be read off from the analysis. It is as easy to drift into a new emphasis on the cultivation of self as to sustain collective activity for change. The fate of a Kristeva in France, who drifted from Maoism and the psychoanalytic avant garde to an agnostic liberalism and semi-mystical religiosity, testifies to the insubstantiality of some versions of the new politics of desire.[34]

There is a fine dividing line between recognising the powers of desire and surrendering to their intoxicating energy. One significant step has been the questioning, against Lacan, of the category of 'the Symbolic', the world of language itself. For a Marxist like Althusser, the entry of the individual into the order of language was an entry into the human. But for many it was precisely this human (and patriarchal) order that was an imposition.[35] For these, leaving the world of flux that preceded 'oedipalisation' and acculturation is the real human tragedy, for in that flux desire was polymorphous and hence 'revolutionary'. Out of this stance grew what has been called 'a political naturalism' not unlike, in fact, Marcuse's which urged a return to 'man's' freedom, spontaneity, and unmediated desire, represented by the pre-symbolic. Drawing on a range of writers and movements from Hegel and Nietzsche, to Dadaism and Sartre—but above all Nietzsche—the new political mode rebelled against a linked set of targets: left puritanism as much as right-wing authoritarianism, the 'fascism of the mind' as much as of the streets. Lacan may have been present at the conception of this politics of desire, but his fate was to be that of the rejected Father.

This philosophy of desire distances itself from that of the Frankfurt-American Schools by its acceptance of Lacanian linguistic theories of how 'the individual' becomes social. But now the society itself is condemned, along with Lacan's phallocentrism, the family, the 'oedipalisation of society'—and psychoanalysis itself, which is crucially seen as the agent for the imposition of Oedipus and the control of desire. The main exponents of this position in the philosophical field have been Gilles Deleuze and Felix Guattari in their book *Anti-Oedipus*, first published in French in 1972, and in subsequent writing, and Jean-François Lyotard; and in the field of historical investigation pre-eminently Michel Foucault and Jacques Donzelot.[36]

Like Lacan, whose writing is deliberately complex and unconventional, rejecting the stylistic simplicity of Freud in pursuit of the real complexities and turmoil of the unconscious, Deleuze and Guattari attempt to challenge ordinary language as well as conventional theory, with the result that in *Anti-Oedipus* we are presented with a world whose complexity and flux defy language. For them any acceptance of Oedipus implies artificial restriction on a field, the unconscious, where everything is in fact infinitely open. There is in this flux no given self, only the cacophony of 'desiring machines', desiring production. This flux is like the early stages of sexual development as described by Freud, with a child as a blob of partial drives seeking satisfaction through part objects. For Lacan, this is a stage of alienation, predicated already on absence. But for Deleuze and Guattari the fragmentary impartial drives are the core of human reality. Desire is not a striving for the lost unity of the womb, but the core of a reality which is a state of constant flux.[37] In this world fragmentation is universal, and is not the peculiar fate of what society conventionally defines as a schizophrenic. But this flux is too much for capitalist society to endure, for it simultaneously encourages and abhors this chaos, and cannot live with the infinite variety of potential interconnections and relationships. It needs to impose constraints regulating which desires are to be allowed, and these are of course those centrally relating to reproduction in the family.

So oedipalisation is a key moment in this constant effort to recode and control:

> The Oedipal triangle is the personal and private territoriality that corresponds to all of capitalism's efforts at social reterritorialisation. Oedipus was always the displaced limit for every social formation, since it is the displaced representative of desire.[38]

Psychoanalysis, by accepting the familial framework, is trapped within capitalist concepts of sexuality, concepts which distort the production of desire. By concentrating on an oedipal triangulation of parents and child, it accepts the social, political and religious forms of domination in modern society, and is complicit with how capitalism has constructed social order. So the Oedipus Complex, instead of being, as in Lacan, a necessary state of the development of a human individual, is seen by Deleuze and Guattari as the only effective means of controlling the libido in capitalist societies. And Freudianism plays a key role under capitalism: it is both the discoverer of the mechanisms of desire and the organiser of its control. For Deleuze and Guattari the individual consciousness is not determined by a closed or autonomous family system, but by a historical situation. The corollary of this is that desire becomes an element in the social field, an active participant in social life, not simply an element in the individual psyche. This is the point of their difference from Reich. They applaud his analysis of fascism, for taking the desires of the masses into account:

> The masses were not innocent dupes; at a certain point, under a certain set of conditions, they *wanted* fascism, and it is this perversion of the desires of the masses that needs to be accounted for.[39]

But Reich himself could never provide a satisfactory explanation of this, because he insisted on splitting the psychic and the social: he never found the common denominator. For Deleuze and Guattari, desiring production is one and the same thing as social production, 'for desire produces reality'.

The Deleuzian approach has been described as partaking of a 'classic irrationalism'[40] and there is clearly an element of truth in this, for against the ordered pattern of the symbolic, the glorification of desire is deeply disturbing of our conventional ways of conceiving of reality. In part this stems from a surprising affinity with the sort of naturalism that Freud's work sought to displace. Despite its genealogical relationship to the Lacanian tradition, its main axis of speculation is the body and its apparently unbounded possibilities and pleasures, not the processes of language; while its relationship to the real world of exploitation and material hardship remains unspecified. It never becomes clear why desire is productive in the sense deployed by Deleuze and Guattari. There is a real danger therefore that 'desire' merely becomes an evocative appeal to a Dionysian spirit to counter the smooth technological rationalities of contemporary society. In this 'desire' there is neither rational order, nor gender (a category significantly absent from the approach), nor 'sexuality' in any conventional sense, nor identity; only the flux of possibilities. There is no longer a recognition of the pain of sacrifice that is integral to Freud (and Lacan)—only a glorification of polymorphous perversity. The coherent ego, in any meaningful sense, disappears, and with it reason—and choice. Even more subversively, this latent naturalism produces a strong displacement of all ethical and moral systems. For if desire is multifarious and multi-vocal, and the criteria by which it has conventionally been organised and controlled are social, and prohibitive, then the theory itself contains no internal criteria by which to judge the moral and the immoral, the permitted and the impermissible. Against the moralism of a Reich or a Marcuse we now have an amoral celebration of pleasure. Whose pleasure, at what expense, are questions scarcely whispered.

Jameson has made the point that post-structuralism has in fact an opposite effect from the Frankfurt School's work. The latter (and Marcuse's critique of one-dimensionality embodies this) feared American capitalism. The former, however, have turned towards America as an exemplum of the explosion of desire—in commodification:

> Both accounts share a secret referent, whose identity they rarely blurt out as such, both aim implicitly to come to terms with the same troubling and peremptory reality. This we can now identify as *American* capitalism.[41]

It is a strange fate for an ostensibly transgressive theory, to be half in love with the easy pleasures of the American way of life. The question that immediately arises is whether constraint is indeed, after all, a necessary adjunct of 'civilisation', whether humanistic values may get abandoned in the amoralism of desiring politics.

There are still, however, disturbingly challenging elements in this 'politics of desire', for it undermines any idea that accepted social definitions of sexuality reflect a deeper reality or truth. It suggests that social categories of sex are imposed upon a sexual flux, a ceaseless turmoil of sexual possibility organised by social forces: the various erotic possibilities of the body are organised through a multiplicity of social practices that work to produce categorisations and definitions that regulate, constrain and limit. This insight has not been peculiar to French theoretical work. A prime development has indeed come from a different theoretical area, that of post-Kinsey sexual research in the United States and Britain.[42] But what is now added is a recognition of psychic reality in tandem with a broadening of the concept of power, exemplified especially in the later work of Michel Foucault.[43]

Foucault's chief concern in writing the 'history of sexuality' has been with the very processes of subjectification by which we today can claim to know ourselves by knowing our sex. It is this which has enabled Foucault to argue very powerfully, in lines parallel to Deleuze, that the psychoanalytic institution itself has become a site of power, a form of power/knowledge which simultaneously organises and controls, where the techniques of psychoanalysis are at one with the confessional techniques of a Christian tradition which seeks the (sinful) truth of an individual through his (or her) minutest manifestation of desire. Subjectivity for Foucault is thus a function of the operation of particular discursive practices, not the constituting elements in them. In the later volumes of his *History* he takes this to a logical conclusion by shifting his focus away from the discourses and practices which have shaped the modern domain of sexuality to the genealogy of the 'man of desire' in pre-Christian Greece and Rome. The key problem now becomes that of understanding how the question of desire becomes the central object of moral concern in the Christian era, and how this contributes to the construction of self.[44] In that process, inevitably, the question of unconscious processes and of drives is displaced in favour of the intricate discursive practices which organise the subject of desire. By a curious paradox, a theoretical approach which had one source at least in the revolution within psychoanalysis has ended by tracing the emergence of the preconditions of that very discourse. But in doing so it forces us to think again about the context in which meaning is generated.

The meanings of desire

If there is a lesson we can draw from this debate, it is that sexual meanings are not neutral, objective phenomena, but are the bearers of important relations of power. 'Sexuality' plays upon, ideologically constructs and unifies, as Foucault has suggested, 'bodies, organs, somatic localisations, functions, anatomo-physiological systems, sensations and pleasures ...' which have no intrinsic unity or 'laws' of their own.[45] The body is a site for the deployment of power relations, a limit, for the possibilities of sexualisation, and in the end only an ambiguous source for sexual expression.

This implies a new centrality for the order of meaning, of social definition—and of language. Meaning does not arise from its reflection of something more real gliding silently below the surface of words; meaning is constructed through languages, through the relation of terms to each other. 'Men' and 'women', 'normal' and 'abnormal', 'heterosexual' and 'homosexual', all key terms in the sexological vocabulary, each derives its meaning from the existence of the other. Sexuality is relational; it exists through its relation to other concepts (the non-sexual). It is a linguistic unity.

Language, of course, does not determine reality, or create the erotic simply by its existence. Meaning never floats free: it is anchored in particular sets of statements, institutions and social practices which shape human activity through the social relations of power. These forms nevertheless naturalise and universalise, so that alternatives seem impossible. To take an obvious example, language as such is not male, and it does not simply exclude women by its fiat. But particular organisations of meaning do shut out women:

> There is a discourse available to men which allows them
> to represent themselves as people, humanity, mankind.
> This discourse, by its very existence, excludes and
> marginalises women by making women the sex.[46]

The construction of categories defining what is appropriate sexual behaviour ('normal'/'abnormal'), or what constitutes the essential gender being ('male'/'female'); or where we are placed along the continuum of sexual possibilities ('heterosexual', 'homosexual', 'paedophile', 'transvestite' or whatever); this endeavour is no neutral, scientific discovery of what was already there. Social institutions which embody these definitions (religion, the law, medicine, the educational system, psychiatry, social welfare, even architecture) are constitutive of the sexual lives of individuals. Struggles around sexuality are, therefore, struggles over meanings—over what is appropriate or not appropriate—meanings which call on the resources of the body and the flux of desire, but are not dictated by them.

This approach fundamentally challenges any idea of a simple dichotomy between 'sex' and 'society'. Sex and sexuality are social phenomena shaped in a particular history. But also called into question is any idea of a unitary 'society' which can construct 'sexuality'. An important body of recent work has attempted to show that the idea of 'the social' is itself a historical construction, amounting to a unification into an apparently coherent entity of what ultimately is no more than a diverse set of relationships, institutions and practices, each with its own history. What we conventionally designate as 'society' is therefore a contradictory unity with no single dynamic shaping its form. Instead there are:

> aggregates of institutions, forms of organisation, practices
> and agents which do not answer to any single causal
> principle or logic of consistency, which can differ in form
> and which are not all essential one to another.[47]

This does not mean that the experience of 'society' is chimaeric. The 'social' exists as a network of relations, which are ever growing in complexity. There are constant efforts at unification, around major articulating principles. But these are always simultaneously partial and challenged.

If this is so, then we need to pay attention to the intricate, often microcosmic practices, which construct the dense labyrinth of social relations which shape sexual subjectivities into what Gayle Rubin has called the 'sex-gender' system.[48] In *Sex, Politics and Society* I described five areas which can serve as guidelines for investigation. Firstly, there are the kinship and family systems, which specify different types of relationships between different cultures, and within a particular culture, and which provide the fulcrum in which sex and gender identities are shaped. Secondly, there are the economic and social changes which form class relations, ethnic diversity and sexual patterns, change the relationship between men and women, and set the limits of material possibility. Thirdly, we must recognise the changing forms of social regulation, informal and formal, from the operations of churches and state to the forms of popular morality. Fourthly, the political context provides the means by which popular passions can be mobilised, legal changes proposed and enacted, relationships constructed between the domain of sexuality and other areas of the social. Finally, there are the cultures of resistance, too easily forgotten in the analysis of sexuality, but the rock on which many forms of sexual regulation have crashed.[49]

There are many sources which shape sexual patterns. The corollary is that many forms of sexuality result, differentiated along lines of class, generations, geography, religion, nationality, ethnic and racial grouping. There are sexualities, not a single sexuality. In the western world today all definitions of the erotic are hegemonised by the prime importance imputed to 'the sexual' (as a source of identity, pleasure and power), and in particular to male heterosexuality. Sexology has played a major part in legitimising these definitions. But this dominance is in reality but a precarious welding together of a huge sexual diversity. A product of a living past, this underlying pluralism provides the opportunity for change in the future. Here at last we can refind the dangers of desire, many-sided, polymorphous, malleable but disruptive—and historical.

We may, after this long detour, be no nearer a resolution of the teasing problem of the actual relation between desire and social forms. But at least the problem has been reformulated. We are no longer addressing a question which can be answered by a calculation of the exact relationship between a given 'sex' (biology) and a self-explanatory 'society' (cultural). We have found or rediscovered a third term, which can be reduced to neither, that of unconscious desire. As the tortuous debates within the psychoanalytic discourse have illustrated, it has been difficult to hold the delicate balance between the three terms. Tip the weight too much one way and we fall back into biologism. Tip it too far the other, and we return to culturalism. And if we ignore both right term and left term we fall into the trap that finally ensnared the founding father himself, of seeing social forms as themselves the emanation of a psychic constitution whose origins can never be described or accounted for, only assumed.

I do not intend, in a final flourish, to magically resolve what has seemed unresolvable. I tend, indeed, to believe that part of the problem has been the belief that the problem is resolvable in the ways it has hitherto been approached. The basic difficulty seems to have lain in the search for a single method that would explain both desire and social forms. It may be that we should be more modest, and find appropriate methods to explore each specialised domain.

What I hope to have established is that no theory of sexuality can be complete which ignores the lessons of the discovery of the dynamic unconscious. Two lessons particularly stand out. Firstly, psychoanalysis has established the problematic nature of identity. This was clearly there in Freud; the message had a curious trajectory through the work of other writers; it has been reaffirmed in the recent celebration of the flux of sexuality by feminist writings and by Deleuze and Guattari in their different ways. Whatever the vagaries of their thought, ranging from the pessimism of Freud to the anarcho-amoralism of recent writers, here is a gain which theorists of sexuality must increasingly take into account. Secondly, the debate around psychoanalysis has also demonstrated the potency of social norms and institutional formations. The possibility exists within the discourse of accepting them (as Freud did to some extent) or rejecting them (as many sexual radicals have sought to do). What cannot be done is to ignore them.

This points to the importance of seeing sexual identities as social products. They draw on the biological possibilities of the body, which are made meaningful through psychic activity. But they are 'fixed', in so far as they can ever be fixed, not by Nature but within defined social relations, and are subject to critical political mediations. Sexual definitions are historically formed, are sites of contradiction and of contestation, and can therefore be socially changed. The organisation of sex does not operate through a single strategy of control. On the contrary, power relations addressing sexuality operate through a multiplicity of practices and of apparatuses (medicine, psychology, education, the law), each of which has its specific structures of regulation. If power in relationship to sexuality operates through such varying and often contradictory modes then the political problem becomes one of recognising the best forms of intervention necessary to change the relations of power.

It is clear that there is no transforming essence of sexuality that has to be released in a definite 'liberation'. There are instead various relations of sexuality and conflicting definitions of sexuality which are sustained by and embedded in a variety of social practices. Once we recognise this, then the road is open for development of alternative practices and definitions of sexual behaviour, definitions which would owe more to choice than to tradition or inherited moralities. This throws the debate on to quite a different level, for it opens up the question of who is to produce the new definitions; how they are to be articulated; by what means can they be attained; and how they relate to the multifaceted nature of desire.

The very statement of the problem in these terms challenges the dominance which sexology has had in defining the appropriate form and realities of sexuality. This perhaps is the most profound and unsettling legacy of the recent revolution in theoretical approaches to sexuality. The sexologists sought in Nature a true sex; the dissenting voices produced by the political movements of the last twenty years have sought a multiplicity of truths—and in doing so they have succeeded in redrawing the boundaries of sexuality along new, highly political, lines.

PART FOUR

The boundaries of sexuality

Communities are to be distinguished, not by
their falsity/genuineness, but by the style in
which they are imagined.

BENEDICT ANDERSON, *Imagined Communities*

CHAPTER 8

'Movements of affirmation': identity politics

> Sexual identity is the public representation
> of sensual aims and objectives as integrated
> into the personality.
>
> ROSALIND COWARD, *Patriarchal Precedents*

> Identity must be continually assumed and
> immediately called into question.
>
> JANE GALLOP, *Feminism and Psychoanalysis.
> The Daughter's Seduction*

> ... the movements labelled 'sexual liberation'
> ought to be understood as movements of affirma-
> tion starting with sexuality. Which means two
> things: they are movements that start with
> sexuality, with the apparatus of sexuality in
> the midst of which we are caught, and which
> make it function to the limit; but, at the same
> time, they are in motion relative to it,
> disengaging themselves and surmounting it.
>
> MICHEL FOUCAULT, in an interview in *Telos*, 1977

Identity and community

Recent sexual politics have been a politics of identity. For very many people in the modern world knowing who we are involves knowing our sexuality, recognising, in Christopher Isherwood's phrase, to which 'tribe' we are affiliated, where we really belong. As Michael Denneny has put it:

> I find my identity as a gay man as basic as any other
> identity I can lay claim to. Being gay is a more elemental
> aspect of who I am than my profession, my class, or my
> race.[1]

185

The recognition of true location shapes the way we see, and live, our lives, releasing feelings and energies that we scarcely knew existed. For Pat Califia:

> Knowing I was a lesbian transformed the way I saw,
> heard, perceived the whole world. I became aware of a
> network of sensations and reactions that I had ignored my
> entire life.[2]

From this renewed sense of identity, of belonging, has flowed a reorientation both of personal commitment and of political identification. For Charlotte Bunch, 'Feminism is at the root of my personal identity and my politics.'[3] Many involved in radical sexual politics over the past decade and a half have uttered similar sentiments, and made identical alignments.

Yet we know, simultaneously, and often from the same people who so passionately affirm their sexual identity, that such an identity is provisional, ever precarious, dependent upon, and constantly challenged by, an unstable relation of unconscious forces, changing social and personal meanings, and historical contingencies:

> There was no such thing as a Castro clone, a lesbian
> feminist or a Kinsey 6, a century ago, and 100 years from
> now, these types will be as extinct as *Urnings*.[4]

There is a troubling paradox here. We are increasingly aware that sexuality is about flux and change, that what we call 'sexual' is as much a product of language and culture as of nature. But we earnestly strive to fix it, stabilise it, say who we are by telling of our sex—and the lead in this conscious articulation of sense of self has been taken by those radically disqualified for it by the sexual tradition. Since the late nineteenth century most western societies have witnessed a prolonged effort to realise a lesbian and homosexual identity, or identities. As the homosexual ways of life have become more open and variegated, more consciously political, so in their wake other claims to valid sexual identity have been heard. 'The mobilization of homosexuals', Gayle Rubin observed, 'has provided a repertoire of ideology and organisational technology to other erotic populations.'[5]

Transvestites, transsexuals, paedophiles, sado-masochists, fetishists, bisexuals, prostitutes and others—each group marked by specific sexual tastes, or aptitudes, subdivided and demarcated often into specific styles, morals and communities, each with specific histories of self-expression—have all appeared on the world's stage to claim their space and 'rights'.[6] In the larger metropolitan communities of the west, from San Francisco to Sydney, London to Toronto, Amsterdam to New York, Paris to Los Angeles, sexual identities have been struggled for within emergent sexual communities, which often have material weight and political clout, and house a vast range of facilities to satisfy the most minutely specialised sexual needs and possibilities.[7] Most of these sexual identities have been constructed on the basis of the categories of the sexologists. But as lived they have become more. As John D'Emilio has argued in relation to homosexuality:

> The group life of gay men and women came to encompass not only erotic interaction but also political, religious, and cultural activity. Homosexuality and lesbianism have become less of a sexual category and more of a human identity.[8]

But this undoubtedly correct historical appraisal only draws us more tightly back to the central problem: why are we so preoccupied with sexual identity? At stake, I suggest, are fundamental issues about sexual relations and choices. Which is why the debate is not an arcane one confined to 'sexual minorities'. It casts light on the very nature of masculinity and femininity today.

There is an ambivalence in the very concept of 'identity'. It professes to inform us of what we have in common, what makes us all alike and recognisable, what is true about ourselves. When it is allied to the prescriptive work of religion, psychiatry, medicine or the law it also works to tell us what makes us truly 'normal'. It is in this sense that the imposition of identity can be seen as a crude tactic of power, designed to obscure the real human diversity with the strict categorisations of uniformity. Michel Foucault's edition of the tragic memoirs of the mid-nineteenth-century hermaphrodite, Herculine Barbin, is a gentle hymn to the 'happy limbo of a non-identity' and a warning of the dire consequences of insisting upon a true identity hidden behind the ambiguities of outward appearance.[9]

The seeking out of a 'true identity' is here a threat and a challenge, because it is the negation of choice. It claims to be finding what we *really* are, or should be. Its reality is of restriction and force.

But at the same time, 'identity is differentiation',[10] it is about affinities based on selection, self-actualisation and choice. It is therefore something we have to search for, something that has to be attained in order to stabilise the self, ward off anomie and despair. For Erikson who gave a name to the problem ('identity crisis') after the Second World War, personal identity roughly equals individuality.[11] It is a reality that has to be struggled for against the awesome weight of the social, and is found in the interstices of society, in the crevices forgotten by weightier social forces. Dennis Wrong has suggested that terms such as 'identity' and 'identity crisis' have become 'semantic beacons of our time, verbal emblems expressing our discontent with modern life and modern society'.[12] They point towards the need for 'authenticity' against the life denying impulsions of contemporary society. For Cohen and Taylor, 'identity work has to be done against or in spite of the institutional arrangements of society', challenging the weight of 'paramount reality'.[13] 'Identity' is something that is really there, but has to be enforced; is the ultimate truth about ourselves but has to be found. Its ambiguity reinforces our modern anxiety.

Yet for the sexually marginal it seems to be an essential ideal. In 1925 the artist F.O. Matthiesson wrote to his new lover Russell Cheney:

> Of course this life of ours is entirely new—neither of us know of a parallel case. We stand in the middle of an uncharted, uninhabited country. That there have been other unions like ours is obvious, but we are unable to draw on their experience. We must create everything for ourselves. And creation is never easy.[14]

Here an 'identity' scarcely exists. There is certainly little community of knowledge. But a sense of self does exist and a sense of need and desire; the urgent note of striving and self-activity is unmistakable. The quest for identity has characterised the history of homosexuality during this century. The finding of it has invariably been described in terms of homing in on an ultimate self buried beneath the detritus of misinformation and prejudice. It is like finding a map to explore a new country. Such a discovery has been the precondition for a sense of personal unity. Categorisations and self-categorisations, that is the process of identity formation, may control, restrict and inhibit but simultaneously they provide 'comfort, security and assuredness'.[15] And the precondition in turn for this has been a sense of wider ties, of what we can best call sexual community. It is in social relations that individual feelings become meaningful, and 'identity' possible.

The most obvious reason for this emphasis on identity is that for countless numbers of people it is their sexuality that is in question. Modern society is fractured by many divisions, along lines of class, race, religion, ideology, status and age. These intersect with, and complicate, but do not cause, two other major divisions, of gender and sexual preference. It is only at certain times, in certain cultures, that these divisions became the central foci of political controversy. Though feminism has swept the west (and parts of the Third World) since the late 1960s, by and large more specific questions of sexual choice have not become major mobilising issues. In countries like Britain and France issues of class and ideology weigh heavier than sexuality. But in the United States, where class loyalties are less fixed, politics more coalition-minded, 'minority' politics, especially the struggles of blacks, better established, and social loyalties more fluid sexuality *has* become a potent political issue, and sexual communities have become bases for political mobilisation, affirming diverse sexual identities.

This preoccupation with identity cannot be explained as an effect of a peculiar personal obsession with sex. It has to be seen, more accurately, as a powerful resistance to the organising principle of traditional sexual attitudes, encoded in the dominant and pervasive heterosexual assumption of the sexual tradition. It has been the sexual radicals who have most insistently politicised the question of sexual identity. But the agenda has been largely shaped by the importance assigned by our culture to the 'correct' sexuality, and especially to the correct sexuality of men. Ethel Spector Person has noted 'the curious phenomenon by which sexuality consolidates and confirms gender in men, while it is a variable feature in women'.[16] For modern men, masculinity is in part at least expressed through their sexuality. The impotent man feels that his masculine identity as well as his sexuality are threatened. Sexuality and sexual performance are among the most vital ingredients of male heterosexual identity. This message was always implicit in the writings of the sexologists who took the aggressive male drive as the very model of what sexuality was. Yet though dominant in the sexual texts, so that women are always presented as the other and sexual minorities the to-be-explained deviants, male heterosexuality has been little explored as a historical and social phenomenon. The odd result is that we know that in our culture male sex and gender identities are, and are expected to be, welded together—but not very clearly how that came about, or even in detail how it is lived today.

Though the tortuous history may not be transparent, its effects are. Sexual self-confidence is seen as one of the yardsticks of masculinity—to such an extent that performance anxiety is a leading cause of secondary impotence. At the same time the overemphasis on sexual success by men is clearly an indicator of a 'relative gender fragility'.[17] Masculinity or the male identity is achieved by the constant process of warding off threats to it. It is precariously achieved by the rejection of femininity and of homosexuality. Male violence against women, and the taboo against male homosexuality may both be understood as effects of this fragile sense of identity, rooted both in the psychic traumas of childhood (in which boys must break their identification with women in order to become 'men') and in the historical norms which have defined male identity as counterposed to the moral chaos of homosexuality.

The early male homosexual culture was like a negative of this. It was frequently characterised by a gender inversion, a self-conscious 'effeminacy' where homosexual people either saw themselves as having 'women's souls in men's bodies' or as being 'effeminate men'. They were not 'real men' because they had too much of the woman in them. But simultaneously, there was a recognition of the contingent nature of this association. The characteristic style and humour of the early homosexual subcultures, 'camp', showed, as Richard Dyer has indicated, 'a great sensitivity to gender roles *as* roles and a refusal to take the trappings of femininity too seriously'.[18]

Such a subcultural style played with gender definitions as they existed, accepting the limits of the apparently natural dichotomies, but in doing so sought to subvert them, treat them as inevitable but ridiculous.

In recent years we have seen a sharp break with this historic identification of male homosexuality and effeminacy. Increasingly sexual variants have been defined and have defined themselves less as gender deviants and more as variants in terms of object choice. *Sexual* identity, at least in the lesbian or gay subcultures of the west, has broken free from *gender* identity. You can now be gay and a 'real man', lesbian and a true (or even better) woman. But the rise of the macho-style amongst gay men in the 1970s can also be read as another episode in the ongoing 'semiotic guerrilla warfare' waged by sexual outsiders against the dominant order. As Dyer has suggested:

> By taking the signs of masculinity and eroticising them in a blatantly homosexual context, much mischief is done to the security with which 'men' are defined in society, and by which their power is secured. If that bearded, muscular beer drinker turns out to be a pansy, how ever are they going to know the 'real' men any more?[19]

There is some evidence that the macho-style in male gays arouses *more* hostility than effeminacy in men. It gnaws at the roots of a male heterosexual identity.

But politicised sexual identities are not automatic responses to negative definitions. They need complex social and political conditions for their emergence—to produce a sense of community experience which makes for collective endeavour. Five conditions seem to be necessary for this: the existence of large numbers in the same situation; geographical concentration; identifiable targets of opposition; sudden events or changes in social position; and an intellectual leadership with readily understood goals.[20] Each of these has been present in the emergence of the most spectacularly successful of politicised sexual identities, the lesbian and gay identities. Most European countries witnessed the embryonic stirrings of subcultures organised around male homosexual activity in early modern times, if not earlier, but the nineteenth century saw qualitatively new developments. The medical model of homosexuality as it emerged in Europe and America in the late nineteenth century was in large part a response to groupings of 'sexual perverts' already being discovered in major cities. An American book of 1871 referred to congregations of 'men in women's attire, yielding themselves to undesirable lewdness', and by 1911 the Chicago Vice Commission had uncovered 'whole groups and colonies of these men'. The lesbian presence was less obvious, but certainly emergent in various forms. In many American cities 'passing' women mingled easily with homosexual men. By the turn of the century substantial networks of like feeling people existed to provide a solid basis for confident self-identification. By 1915 one observer of the American homosexual scene was even able to observe 'a community distinctly organised'. Between the 1850s and the 1930s a complex sexual community had developed in many American as well as European cities, which crossed class, racial, gender and age boundaries, and which offered a focus for identity development.[21]

Since the Second World War the expansion of these subcultures has been spectacular, with one of the unlikely heroes of this growth being the gay bar. For homosexuals, it has been suggested, 'bars and discos play the role performed for other groups by family and church'. Unique among the expressions of a homosexual way of life the bars encouraged an identity that was both public and collective, and they become, 'seed beds for a collective consciousness that might one day flower politically'.[22] The growth of an open male gay subculture in cities such as San Francisco and New York in the 1950s and 1960s paved the way for the emergence of a mass gay movement at the end of the 1960s. By comparison, the frequently privatised nature of lesbian bonds, the slower development of a bar scene and the conscious political distancing of themselves by lesbian leaders in the 1950s and 1960s from the organised lesbian subculture were crucial factors in the separate, slower, but distinctive development of a lesbian identity.

Without large numbers and geographical concentration a 'sexual minority' is, as Schur puts it, a 'community of latent interests' which is not able to realise its potential political weight.[23] By corollary, erotic groupings which can never expect to achieve obvious social weight or whose tastes apply only to a minority of a minority—sado-masochists, paedophiles, transvestites, prostitutes come to mind—have to rely in large part on association with related sexual groupings. Only in a city like San Francisco has it been possible for a sizeable subculture of sado-masochists to emerge. It is inconceivable that there could be geographical concentration of the highly stigmatised networks of paedophiles. By and large, these groups have relatively small natural constituencies to appeal to and their political emergence is dependent upon alliances with more powerful movements.

Numbers and geographical concentration are vital conditions for the growth of politicised sexual identities, but these only become crucial when there is a felt sense of oppression to combat. Despite the long-standing taboo against homosexuality, social conditions have varied enormously, and many homosexual people have been content to 'pass for straight' throughout the century. Moreover, the conditions necessary to mobilise people around sexual issues are difficult to attain. All sexual groupings are bisected by class, racial, national, age, intellectual and taste differences. Sexual desire is a fragile bond for political identification, and especially one that in the nature of things is oppositional and challenging to the status quo. It is not surprising, therefore, that sexual political groupings frequently tend to be fractious and sectarian in their practices.[24] What is surprising is their success in a difficult social climate. And yet, the past decades have witnessed recurrent and often successful mobilisations around sexual issues. The major reason for this has been the perception of oppression. Witch-hunts against sexual deviants in the 1950s and 1960s, purges in the armed forces and public services, police clamp-downs on sexual misdemeanours, raids on bars and stigmatising trials, have all failed to obliterate the sexual minorities. On the contrary, as was historically likely, they served to solidify the sense of identity of those attacked.

Wider changes in society have encouraged this. A more open climate for the discussion of sexuality, a burgeoning literature of sexual information, more relaxed attitudes of some of the churches, greater liberalism in the airing of sexual issues in the media—all these have helped the articulation of a sexual identity. Even more vitally, they have aided the creation of a new community of knowledge amongst the marginalised sexual minorities. Ironically, the work of sexual medicine and sexology has contributed to this. Even the obsessive wartime searching out of homosexual proclivities amongst the military helped:

> For homosexual soldiers, induction into the military forced
> a sudden confrontation with their sexuality that
> highlighted the stigma attached to it and kept it a matter
> of special concern.[25]

Here the medicalising intervention *made* sexuality important to individual identity. More widely the work of the liberal sexologists had an enormous impact, from the relativism of Kinsey to the investigation and reassessments of psychoanalysts such as Judd Marmor, clinical psychologists like Evelyn Hooker, and sociologists of deviance like Howard S. Becker, Edwin Schur and Erving Goffman. New ethnographies of the urban homosexual subcultures—such as Martin Hoffman's *The Gay World* (1968)—were not only dispelling myths but also providing cool appraisals and knowledge. And the long tradition of discussing homosexuality simply in terms of aetiology, which of course emphasized its deviant nature, was giving place to discussion of homosexual roles and categorisations, that is to understanding the social processes of identity formation.[26] These did not displace the works of the Biebers and the Socarides, but for the first time they began to challenge their hegemony. They helped change the climate in which homosexuality could be discussed. But they also had practical effects: alerting people to the diversity of human sexuality, informing individuals of where they could meet others, even occasionally intervening themselves in political or practical issues.[27]

All these factors provided fertile ground for a transformation in attitudes towards sexuality. It was, however, the emergence in the 1960s of a new, politically conscious layer of activists, often schooled in direct grass-roots activity, whether in the black, anti-war or feminist movements, but simultaneously rooted in the burgeoning urban gay communities, which made the rise of a radical sexual politics possible. There was a long tradition of politically aware homosexual activity, in large pressure group activities as in Hirschfeld's Germany, in semi-secret activity as in Carpenter and Ellis's Britain, in initially left-wing groupings as with the US Mattachine Society in the early 1950s, or in respectable parliamentary lobbying politics as in Britain in the 1960s.[28] These had enjoyed varying degrees of success. The more spectacular achievement of the new generation of activists was predicated upon a crucial juncture between the politics of sexuality and the mass weight of the burgeoning gay subcultures. Political energy combined with a new community strength were the crucial components shaping the new sexual identities of the 1970s.

Three elements have come together in the modern gay consciousness: a struggle for identity, a development of sexual communities, and the growth of political movements. Today, each appears necessary to the other. The sense of community is the guarantor of a stable sense of self; while the new social movements have in an important way become expressions of community strength, emanations of a material social presence. But these developments have changed the experience of homosexuality, posing new issues, personal and political. Today it is not clear what homosexuality is: an orientation or a preference, a social role or a way of life, a potentiality in all of us or a minority experience. The debates on these issues offer important insights into the changing meanings of sexuality.

The idea of a 'sexual minority'

Many openly homosexual men today see themselves as belonging to a 'sexual minority', a term that has been taken up and used more recently by other sexual groupings, such as paedophiles and sado-masochists. As an idea it has a powerful resonance. 'Minorities' can lay claim to 'rights'. There is a hallowed tradition in liberal democracies of recognising (even if they never satisfy) the claims of minorities, who are usually oppressed and discriminated against. More—there is a vested interest in recognising such rights for in some degree we are all members of minorities. 'The majority' is a mythical construct, stitched together out of fragments of lives on the basis of the lowest common denominator (which does not mean it lacks power). It seems appropriate, therefore, that 'sexual minorities' should enter the discourse of rights and seek the same social, and even constitutional, safeguards as other minorities.

One difficulty is that not all homosexually inclined people want to identify their minority status—or even see themselves as homosexual. Sexologists since at least Kinsey have pointed out that there is no necessary connection between sexual behaviour and sexual identity. According to Kinsey's best-known statistic some 37 per cent of men had homosexual experiences to orgasm; but perhaps less than 4 per cent were exclusively homosexual—and even then did not necessarily express a homosexual identity, a concept of which, in any case, Kinsey disapproved.[29] More recent surveys of homosexually inclined men have revealed a frequent 'flight from identity' with substantial numbers of people—up to a third in some earlier samples—wishing they could swallow a magic pill and not be homosexual. Some prefer to stress their 'homosocial' links as members of the same gender rather than their sexual identity as 'gay people'. To relate as a man to other men or as a woman to other women is more important than the sexual nature of the contact. Others affirm their identity as black people over and above their sexual preference. On this argument more separates a black gay from a white than colour of skin. There is a world of cultural and political dissonance.[30]

Sexual identification is a strange thing. There are people who identify as gay and participate in the gay community who do not experience or wish for, homosexual activity. And there are homosexually active people who do not identify as gay. Obviously as Barry Dank has argued, 'the development of a homosexual identity is dependent on the meanings that the actor attaches to the concepts of homosexual and homosexuality.'[31] These processes in turn depend on the person's environment and wider community. Many people 'drift' into identity, battered by contingency rather than guided by will. Some choices are forced on individuals, whether through stigmatisation and public obloquy or through political necessity. But the point that needs underlining is that *identity* is largely a choice if it is not dictated by internal imperatives.

Nor does the acceptance of a particular identity necessarily imply the adoption of a particular lifestyle. The idea that there are 'homosexualities' rather than a single 'homosexuality' is now a familiar one. As Bell and Weinberg have suggested, 'homosexual adults are a remarkably diverse group'.[32] Differences in sexual tastes and behaviour, in opportunity and desire, in political affiliations and economic status, in racial attitudes and origins, in religion and national traditions—these are the hallmarks of the modern gay communities, not uniformity and common feelings.

Is it appropriate, therefore, to see all these people as belonging to the same 'sexual minority'?

The history of the concept illustrates its ambiguity. It was implicit in the earliest pro-homosexual arguments in the early part of this century, in the idea that 'homosexuals' constituted a 'third sex'. The writings of Edward Carpenter in Britain and Hirschfeld in Germany were focused on this notion, and were essentially appeals for 'Justice' for this minority 'sex'. The idea of homosexuals as a fixed minority of the population is a subtext of most discussions of homosexuality thereafter. But it was the post-war homophile movement in the United States that recognised its political significance. The Mattachine Society, formally founded to advance homosexual rights in 1951, reflected its origins in the leftist experience of its founder members by developing an analysis of homosexuals as an oppressed cultural minority, though one yet unconscious of itself. The task of the society was therefore to raise consciousness and to emphasise the importance of identifying as homosexual as a way of self-liberation. The initiating proposal for the society, in November 1950, drafted by Harry Hay, declared as its purpose: 'the heroic objective of liberating one of our largest minorities from ... social persecution.'[33] Central in this was the idea that homosexuals had a common cause with other minorities fighting against oppression. As Donald Webster Cory put it in his influential *The Homosexual in America*, the homosexual was 'similar in a variety of respects to that of national, religious and other ethnic groups'.[34] This suggested a *radical* agenda of progressive struggle, and as such it was bitterly opposed by the more conservative elements in the Mattachine Society, who by 1953 were dominant. The idea of homosexuals constituting a distinct minority cut across *their* integrationist ethic; and the drive of the society moved from the mobilisation of a homosexual constituency to an appeal for help and assistance from those in a position of power. It was not a strikingly successful appeal.

In the embryonic stirrings of the post-war gay movement, then, the idea of a 'minority' status was a radical one because it stressed self-activity, self-consciousness and political alliances. The concept was intended as a mobilising call, stressing what homosexuals had in common rather than what divided them.

But when the hoped-for mass gay movement did at last emerge in the late 1960s the idea of a gay minority had a different fate. The chief radical intent of the early gay liberation movement was to disrupt fixed expectations that homosexuality was a peculiar condition or minority experience. Building in large part on the celebration of a polymorphously perverse sexuality in the work of Marcuse and the radical Freudians, homosexuality was perceived as a potentiality in all of us. Early theorists of gay liberation looked forward to the 'end of the homosexual', the breaking down of socially constructed divisions between sexual subjects.[35] A radical separation was proposed between homosexuality, which was about sexual preference, and 'gayness', which was about a subversively political way of life. Now in a neat ruse of history it was the less radical elements in gay liberation who took up the idea of a gay minority. A polymorphously perverse 'gayness' looked forward to a breakdown of roles, identities, and fixed expectations. But the new spokespeople, acting openly for the 'gay minority', argued for 'rights', for the legitimate claims to space of what was now an almost 'ethnic' identity, and became the new integrationists. The consolidation of a minority status has obvious advantages. It fits easily into the common discourse of liberal pluralist societies. It offers legitimacy to the claims of the oppressed minority and can act as a spur for legal and other reforms. It is also, as the ex-Communist founders of Mattachine saw, a mobilising idea: it might be a myth, but it is a powerful and believable one.

It has, of course, become more than an idea. In the creation of urban communities throughout the cities of the west gays have *become* an effective minority force, with a complex culture, varied politics and material resources. Gay people have invested a great deal in coming out as homosexual, have often risked careers, friendships and family ties. They have also gained much by their openness, political activity and culture-constructing work: they have consolidated their personal and social identities. In such circumstances challenges to the fixity and permanence of the gay identity and the idea of a gay minority seem a fundamental undermining of all that has been achieved.

There are, however, disadvantages. A number of writers have pointed to the paradox that gay activists began by challenging the naturalness and inevitability of received roles and identities, but have themselves become key definers of a homosexual role, and hence their own source of regulation:

> 'Homosexuals' were once regulated and defined by
> 'experts'; now these experts need no longer do it, for the
> homosexual has assumed that role for himself or herself.[36]

The result could be a new sort of sexual conservatism, where little can be risked because too much is at stake. Moreover, in the process, the work of challenging the hegemonic definitions of sexual normality is abandoned: sexual minorities by definition can never become majorities. The acceptance of homosexuality as a minority experience deliberately emphasises the ghettoisation of homosexual experience and by implication fails to interrogate the inevitability of heterosexuality. The emphasis on minority status may be a necessary phase of gay mobilisation, but it is doubtful whether it can be the last word.

The theoretical and political debates within the gay communities have reflected this tension. On the one hand, the supporters of the idea that gays constitute a fixed minority have indulged in a remarkable feat in resurrecting from the semi-dead the notion of a fixed sexual orientation, often aided by the intoxicating charms of sociobiology. Whitham, a major defender of the idea of a fixed orientation, has vigorously challenged the view that there is a constructed 'homosexual role'. He sees homosexuality as a 'non-dominant, universal manifestation of human sexuality'. Through comparing three different societies (United States, Guatemala and Brazil) Whitham discovers that on at least six indicators (such as dressing up and playing with dolls as a child) homosexuals differed from heterosexuals in all three cultures.[37] To back up this there is certainly evidence of frequent homosexual feelings in children in their early years and for the fairly definite establishment of exclusive homosexuality by adolescence. The importance of a deep-rooted sense of sexual preference for many individuals cannot easily be denied.[38]

On the other hand, there is also a good deal of evidence for the idea that 'homosexuality is a complex, diffuse experience that anyone may have'. Both the Freudian tradition and the work of Kinsey and his followers tend to support this. For the more radical Freudians specialised object choice is something that is tenuously achieved or imposed, not something in-born. For the socio-sexual studies inspired by Kinsey, exclusive homosexuality is only one extreme of a continuum of sexuality whose organisation is social not essential. Kinsey's own seven-point scale, ranging from the minority of exclusively heterosexual people at one extreme through to the extreme of exclusive homosexuality at the other, powerfully made this point, even as he attempted to subdivide the continuum into neatly demarcated blocks (which some of his successors have attempted to reify into scientific categories).[39]

The essentialist view lends itself most effectively to the defence of minority status, to the consolidation of recent gains and to the enhancement—even celebration—of gay community. The more extreme constructionist view tends to reject the value of a fixed identity and to glory in the subversive effects of alternative lifestyle and of a plurality of sexual practice, in breaching the norms of sexual orthodoxy.[40] The irony is that in practice both positions are dependent on the growth of the subculture and the enhancement of a sense of self in recent years. Without the *historically* conditioned rise of the new gay communities and the 'modern homosexual' the debate about the merits of a homosexual orientation or preference would be irrelevant. And without the new sense of community and identity it would scarcely be possible to indulge in the joys of 'polysexualities'.

The 'sexual outlaws' of old have constructed a way of life, or more accurately ways of life, which have reversed the expectations of sexology. They have disrupted the categorisations of the received texts and have become thinking, acting, living subjects in the historical process. The implication of this is that the modern gay identities, whether they are the outgrowth of essential internal characteristics (which I do not believe to be the case) or of complex socio-historical transformations (which I think is more likely), are today as much *political* as personal or social identities. They make a statement about the existing divisions between permissible and tabooed behaviour and propose their alteration. These new political subjectivities above all represent an affirmation of homosexuality, for by their very existence they assert the validity of a particular sexuality. This surely is the only possible meaning of the early gay liberation idea of 'coming out' as homosexual, of declaring one's homosexuality as a way of validating it in a hostile society. Arguments that this merely confirms pre-existing categories miss the point.[41] The meanings of these negative definitions are transformed by the new, positive definitions infusing them. The result is that homosexuality has a meaning over and above the experience of a minority. By its existence the new gay consciousness challenges the oppressive representations of homosexuality and underlines the possibilities for all of different ways of living sexuality. This is the challenge posed by the modern gay identity. It subverts the absolutism of the sexual tradition.

The challenge of lesbianism

Amongst feminists the debate about identity has taken a different direction. For gay men the question has fundamentally been about sex, about validating a denied sexuality. In recent discussions on lesbianism, on the other hand, there have been heated exchanges about the necessary connection of a lesbian identity to sexual practices. Conventional wisdom, and even more stringently, sexological expertise, have defined lesbianism as a sexual category. But increasingly it has been proposed by feminists primarily as a political definition, in which sexuality plays a problematical role. Lillian Faderman argues that 'Women who identify themselves as lesbians generally do not view lesbianism as a sexual phenomenon first and foremost.'

It is instead a relationship in which two women's strongest emotions and affection are directed towards one another.[42] It becomes a synonym for sisterhood, solidarity and affection, and as such a basic aspect of feminism.

The difficulty is that for many self-declared lesbians who are not feminist, lesbianism *is* about identity and sex. Joan Nestle has even wondered whether:

> We lesbians from the 1950s made a mistake in the early
> 1970s ... we allowed our lives to be trivialised and
> reinterpreted by feminists who did not share our culture.
> The slogan 'Lesbianism is the practice and feminism is the
> theory' was a good rallying cry, but it cheated our
> history.[43]

Feminism and lesbianism have never been coterminous. Many of the pioneering lesbian activists were only dubious feminists, while feminism has historically tended to shy away from any association with overt lesbianism defined in sexual terms. Most feminists in the first wave of feminism in the late nineteenth century stressed their sexual respectability, and the early days of the 'second wave' in the 1960s were marked by hostility towards the traditional lesbian bar scene. The 1980 declaration of the US National Organisation for Women on Lesbian and Gay Rights carefully distinguishes lesbianism from any association with dubious sexual practices.[44] The result has been a rupture amongst self-identifying lesbians between those who see themselves first and foremost as feminists, who see their politics as reflected in their lesbianism; and those who identify as lesbians whose political expression may or may not be feminism. In the process crucial questions have been raised about the nature of female sexuality, and the appropriate feminist attitude towards sex.

Traditionally female homosexuality has been seen almost exclusively in terms derived from the experience or study of male. Male homosexuality has invariably been more closely observed and researched than lesbianism—partly because of its greater public salience, partly because it challenged the dominant definitions of male sexuality, partly because female sexuality has usually been studied only in so far as it was responsive to male sexuality, and lesbianism was hardly understandable in those terms. More recently, ethnographies of female homosexuality have tended to adopt research techniques honed in investigation of male behaviour, concentrating, for example, on 'coming out', contact patterns, sexual expression and duration of relationships. The impact of this was to conceptualise lesbianism, like male homosexuality, as a specific minority experience little different in its implications from male patterns. This inevitably had the effect of establishing male homosexuality as the norm, while ignoring the implications of lesbianism for feminism.[45]

There is a good deal of evidence now accumulating for the differences between the lesbianism and homosexual male experiences. Recent studies of female relationships have stressed the strength and consistency of ties between all women in which sexual bonds may or may not have played an important part. A specific lesbian sexual identity emerged later than the male; subcultural development was slower; and relationships patterns are different. Lesbians and gay men are not two genders within one sexual category. They have different histories, which are differentiated because of the complex organisation of male and female identities, precisely along lines of gender. But this still leaves open the question of whether lesbianism should be seen as a distinct sexual identity of some women, or a political identity for all women. This is the heart of the problem.

The most influential exponent of a political lesbian position has been Adrienne Rich. In her powerful essay 'Compulsory Heterosexuality and the Lesbian Existence' she argues that a distinction has to be made between the 'lesbian continuum' and 'lesbian existence'.[46] The latter is equivalent to a lesbian identity, but its character is not defined by sexual practice. It is the sense of self of women bonded primarily to women who are sexually and emotionally independent of men. In turn this is the expression of the 'lesbian continuum', the range through women's lives of woman-identified experience. Such experiences go beyond the possibility of genital sex, to embrace many forms of primary intensity, including the sharing of inner life, the bonding against male tyranny, practical and political support, marriage resistance, female support networks and communities.

Such possibilities of bonding between women are denied by 'compulsory heterosexuality', which is the key mechanism of control of women, ensuring in its tyranny of definition the perpetuation of male domination. Lesbianism is the vital point of resistance to this heterosexual dominance; its central antagonistic force. Lesbianism is thus about the realisation of the male-free potential of women, and in drawing on this essence, male definitions are cast aside. Rich sharply dissociates lesbianism from male homosexuality because of the latter's presumed relationship, *inter alia*, to pederasty, anonymous sex and ageism (denunciations culled, it must be said, from the pathologising literature Rich elsewhere rejects). Lesbianism, on the other hand, she argues, is a profoundly *female* experience, like motherhood, and she looks forward to a powerful new female eroticism:

> as we deepen and broaden the range of what we define as lesbian existences, as we delineate a lesbian continuum, we begin to discover the erotic in female terms: as that which is unconfined to any single part of the body, or solely to the body itself, as an energy not only diffuse ... but an 'empowering joy'.[47]

Few protagonists in recent debates have attempted to deny the varied potentialities of female sexuality. The experience of the women's movement seems to have been that many women have been enabled and emboldened to express their homosexual desires who were not previously self-identifying lesbians, while many women have been prepared to identify with lesbianism for feminist-political reasons. But against the passion and conviction of Rich's position several fundamental criticisms have been made.

In the first place it is based on a romantic-naturalisation of female bonds. It is not always clear whether Rich sees the 'lesbian continuum' as a powerful solidarity that is there but constantly suppressed, or as a potentiality that could be realised in a mythical future, but in either case it stretches towards an essentialism about femininity which can distort the complexities of the construction of women, and obscure the necessary politics.

On the most immediate level, Rich herself succeeds in dichotomising women. As Cora Kaplan has noted, in Rich's scenario:

> female heterosexuality is socially constructed and female homosexuality is natural ... Political lesbianism becomes more than a strategic position for feminism, it is a return to nature.[48]

Nature now is benign, female and affectionate, sensual and creative, revolutionary and transcendent—and lesbian. But all the problems we have already observed in naturalistic explanations of sex still come to the fore: its untheorised and untheorisable claims to truth, its transhistorical pretensions, and its strong moralism: this is how you must behave because Nature tells us so.

The result is a narrowing in political focus, and this is the second major objection. The view that attributes all women's oppression to 'compulsory heterosexuality' suggests that somehow women are always socially controlled by men, who stand outside history, towering over it like Zeus with his hands around the globe. Women are inevitably presented, in consequence, as perpetual sufferers and victims.[49] The struggles of women, the resistances they have offered and changes they have fashioned, are silenced in the portrayal of the timeless rule of heterosexual domination. But we know that forms of heterosexuality *have* changed; that male power has been challenged and sometimes undermined; that women have changed the conditions of their lives. Oppression is not monolithic, nor is it exercised purely through sexual control; and the diverse and contradictory forms of domination do allow space for challenge and change.

'Political' as opposed to 'sexual' lesbianism sees men rather than male-dominated institutions as the enemy. It conflates 'compulsory' heterosexuality with any form of heterosexual practice and reifies male characteristics so that male sexuality in itself becomes a 'perversion'.[50] Above all, it focuses on sexual *practices* rather than the form of sexual relations as the chief target of attack. At its most extreme it can lead to the belief that every act of heterosexual penetration serves the function of punishing and controlling women and that 'Heterosexual women are collaborators with the enemy.'[51] There does not seem much room for sisterhood in this.

Finally, the political lesbian position tends to deny the specifics of lesbian sexuality. As Pat Califia sees it: 'Lesbianism is being desexualised as fast as movement dykes can apply the whitewash. We ... are pretending that the words "feminist" and "woman" are synonymous for "lesbian".'[52] Lesbian activists such as Califia are suggesting that there is a history of a specific lesbian eroticism which has been historically derived, and which has produced its own forms of struggle and institutionalisation. According to such feminist positions, the elevation of female sexuality in general into a semi-mystical bonding, where bodily contact and genital pleasure are secondary or even non-existent, denies the possibilities of female eroticism, including the real potentiality of lesbianism for affirming female identity and autonomy.[53]

The immediate background to this controversy over sexuality is clearly the 1960s and its mythical attributes. As many feminists have pointed out, sexual liberation is not the same as female liberation, and the relaxation of female sexual norms in that period has been seen as reactionary in its 'imposition' of a male-defined sexual liberation on women. But what has also been challenged are the chief emphases of the early phases of contemporary feminism on what Beatrix Campbell has called the 'quality of the act'. The main impact of sexological writing on women since Kinsey has been to emphasise the orgasmic potentiality of female sexuality. Kinsey stressed the clitoral focus of female sexuality, Masters and Johnson demonstrated its huge potentiality for multiple orgasms, and Mary Jane Sherfey, following as a feminist in their footsteps, postulated a male necessity to repress this protean potentiality in the interests of reproduction and male domination.[54]

But there were dangers in this modernised vision of female sexuality. It portrayed female sexuality as rather akin to male, both in the weighting given to orgasm, and in the affinity of physiological response in men and women. Men and women, Masters and Johnson have repeated recently, 'are incredibly similar not different, in facility to respond to effective sexual stimuli.'[55] Theories such as this seem to undermine the grounds for a specifically *feminist* politics around *female* sexuality. Moreover, there was, as Shere Hite suggests, a new pressure on women to have orgasm—and to enjoy 'sex'—just like men. Many feminists saw this as a dangerous recuperation of female eroticism by men.[56]

But the debates about the nature of lesbianism have a wider resonance. They are part of the dilemma about female sexuality that has run like a tangled thread through feminist debates since the early nineteenth century: must sexuality be held at bay, as source of danger; or must it be embraced, as site of feminist pleasure? Most nineteenth-century feminists, from Mary Wollstonecraft onwards, sought to advance women's claim to justice by emphasising the rational control of sexuality, which respectable women already exercised and which must be extended to men. This suggested caution toward birth control and abortion, sympathy but often distant solicitude for 'fallen women', and frequent support for social purity campaigns and legislation. Part of this was undoubtedly a result of political caution. Part of it was a rational response to the real dangers that did confront women (sexual diseases, poor contraception, the economic necessity of marriage, the force of moral opinion). The sexual radicals, on the other hand, were usually libertarian in their ethos, challenging towards the respectable status quo, firm supporters of contraception, and even occasionally of lesbians. They remained a minority, but an important one.[57]

The libertarians emphasised pleasure at the expense of the danger. The more sexually conservative feminists emphasised the dangers at the risk of losing any emphasis on pleasure. The polarisation has continued to the present, taking a new form in current debates. Political lesbians emphasise the dangers of contemporary male sexuality. From this stems the violence of their denunciations of pornography, promiscuity, even male homosexuality. Some modern radical feminists have cultivated what has been called a 'politics of rage', in which feeling, 'anger', is pivotal. This type of politics offers, Lisa Orlando has suggested, 'a comprehensive vision of a world in which the smallest contact with male-dominated culture is—and must be—a source of suffering'.[58]

The 'pro-sex' feminists, on the contrary, have tended to see sexuality as a positive force, which can be used to increase female autonomy, even at the cost of challenging the 'good girl'/'bad girl' distinction. As Califia said about her coming out as a lesbian sado-masochist:

> I like S/M because it is not lady-like. It is a kind of sex
> that really violates all the things I was taught about being
> a nice little girl and keeping my dress clean.[59]

There does not seem much common ground between the romantic mysticism of a Rich and the erotically charged iconoclasm of a Califia, yet each lays claim to being a lesbian spokesperson and a defender of female sexuality.

Clearly a great deal is at stake in this controversy, not just an account of the past but a programme for the present and the future, and it has been marked by sharp clashes. The heated exchanges between pro-sex and sexually conservative feminists that surrounded the Barnard Conference on Sexuality organised by the former in 1982 represented perhaps the low point of the debate. Ironically, given the anathemas launched at the organisers of the conference, one of them, Carole S. Vance, had proposed an approach which need not exclude anyone. She argued for a 'dual focus' which would acknowledge that sexuality is simultaneously a domain of restriction, repression and danger as well as one of exploration, pleasure and agency.[60] Underlying this is the belief that female sexuality, lesbian or heterosexual, is historically constructed, which means it is open to investigation and judgment—and change. The emphasis on feminism as choice prioritises the quality of the relationship over the nature of the sexual act. It is not so much what you do, but how you do it that counts. By implication, it is not heterosexual activity as such that constitutes a problem but the forms in which it is currently embodied. Equally, lesbianism in itself is neither good nor bad. It is the quality of relationship it reveals that matters most.[61]

If we accept this then we can approach once again the question of the lesbian identity. It clearly is not appropriate to equate it with feminism as such. It does not, and cannot, express the essence of femininity, for such an essence does not exist. It is an identity of choice, one related historically to a set of sexual practices, and institutionalised in cultural forms both inside and outside the modern women's movement. Not all lesbians are feminist; all feminists cannot be expected to be lesbians. For Ferguson:

> *Lesbian* is a woman who has sexual and erotic-emotional ties primarily with women or who sees herself as centrally involved with a community of self-identified lesbians whose sexual and erotic emotional ties are primarily with women; and who is herself a self-identified lesbian.[62]

A lesbian identity is obviously not an easy phenomenon to describe, though it is clearly related to sexual practice. It is an identity that is changing, but it is changing because of the self-activity of those who define themselves as lesbians. Like the gay male identity, the lesbian identity has a political as well as a social and personal implication. That means that there need to be no necessary relationship between sexual practice and sexual identity. On the other hand, the existence of a specific identity testifies to the historic denial of a particular form of female desire—and the struggle necessary to affirm it. As with the homosexual male, the lesbian identity is historically contingent—but seemingly inevitable; potentially limiting—but politically essential.

Making relationships

Identity is not a destiny but a choice. But in a culture where homosexual desires, female or male, are still execrated and denied, the adoption of lesbian or gay identities inevitably constitutes a *political* choice. These identities are not expressions of secret essences. They are self-creations, but they are creations on ground not freely chosen but laid out by history. So homosexual identities illustrate the play of constraint and opportunity, necessity and freedom, power and pleasure. Sexual identities seem necessary in the contemporary world as starting points for a politics around sexuality. The form they take, however, is not predetermined. In the end, therefore, they are not so much about who we really are, what our sex dictates. They are about what we want to be and could be. The lesbian and gay identities are ultimately concerned, as Bell and Weinberg suggest, with 'a way of being in the world', or about 'trying to work out and evolve a lifestyle', as Foucault be-lieves.[63] But this means they are also about the morality of acts, the quality of relations, the possibilities of pleasure: about the making of sexualities.

An examination of the evolution of oppositional sexual identities reveals the degree to which they are social inventions. In turn this confirms the degree to which the edifice of sexuality that envelops us is a historical construction, and what has been historically constructed can be politically reconstructed. This is the real challenge that the feminist and radical sexual move-ments pose to the sexual status quo. They reveal its contingent and changeable nature, and point to alternatives.

But there are many alternatives. It clearly cannot be the case that all manifestations of non-orthodox sexuality are equally valid; that no real distinctions can be made. To argue that 'anything goes' is to fall back into an easy libertarianism which ignores questions of power and the quality of relationships. We need to tread carefully between the scylla of a new puri-tanism and the charybdis of a cold amoralism. This is not an easy task, and there is a danger that any attempt at a golden mean will be prescriptive, and hence proscriptive.

A way through can only be found if we begin with the recognition of human diversity. There exists a plurality of sex-ual desires, of potential ways of life, and of relationships. A radical sexual politics affirms a freedom to be able to choose between them. Sex is not a fatality, it's a possibility for creative life.[64] That belief, starting with sex, but going beyond it, is the indispensable foundation of a contemporary politics of sexual-ity. But for a variety of historical reasons, the cement of those foundations comes from a recognition of identity. Identity may, in the end, be no more than a game, a ploy to enjoy particular types of relationships and pleasures. But without it, it seems, the possibilities of sexual choice are not increased but diminished. The recognition of 'sexual identities', in all their ambivalence, seems to be the precondition for the realisation of sexual diversity.

CHAPTER 9

The meaning of diversity

It is when man is at his most purely moral
that he may be most dangerous to the
interests, and most callously indifferent
to the needs of others. Social systems
know no fury like the man of moral
absolutism aroused.

ALVIN GOULDNER, *For Sociology*

There is certainly a branch of the sex
field that is progressive. Many women,
even feminists, even dykes, work in that
field. Instead of assuming that sex is
guilty until proven innocent these people
assume that sex is fundamentally okay until
proven bad.

GAYLE RUBIN, *Talking Sex*

Erotic diversity

The most intractable problems in contemporary sexual debates
stem from the obvious but politically contentious facts of erotic
diversity. The early sexologists sought to contain the problem
within their proliferating but neatly drawn taxonomies, label-
lings and definitions, where subtle (and to the untutored eye
often imperceptible) distinctions demarcated perversions from
perversity, inverts from perverts, abnormalities from anomalies
and degeneration from deviation. The categories of the perverse swelled to embrace the marginal and marginalised, de-
spised and despicable sexualities that flourished exotically in
the interstices of a normative sexual order (flourished in part
because of that order) while much effort was steadfastly and
self-consciously devoted to the searching out, in the deepest
recesses of the human body, blood, chromosomes, genes
or psyche, of the aetiologies of these erotic disorders. As
each new breakthrough in knowledge occurred—hormones,

211

chromosomes, genetics, the power of the dynamic unconscious—they were harnessed to the work of bolstering the edifice of sexuality, in all its majestic certainty, and to the provision of a scientific justification for moralistic and medical
intervention into people's lives.

But there was always a dangerous gap between the relatively
narrow range of theoretical explanations of sexual behaviour
and the actuality of an immensely broad range of sexual variations. The sexological descriptions and aetiologies yanked
together into broad categories many disparate sexual practices,
to create sexual dichotomies which while seeming to help us
understand human sexuality actually trapped individuals in
mystifying compartments, where morality and theory, fear and
hopes were inextricably and dangerously enmeshed. The gap
became a void, filled by contending moral and political values.

Kinsey, as ever, was a key figure in transforming this debate.
He noted that traditionally there had been a gap between two
antagonistic interpretations of sex, the hedonistic, which justifies sex for its immediate, pleasurable return, and the reproductive, where sex is only to be enjoyed in marriage. But Kinsey suggested—coming close, as he rather reluctantly admitted,
to Freud's notion of a polymorphous perversity—that there
was a third possible interpretation which had hardly figured in
either general or scientific discussion: 'of sex as a normal bio-
logic function, acceptable in whatever form it is manifested.'[1]
From our point of view, the *biological* justification is clearly
inadequate. But its essential message has become crucial to
contemporary controversies. Few mainstream sexologists today
—with the exception of conspicuously conservative analysts
and psychologists, or openly right-wing moralists—would be
easy with the use of a term like 'perversion' to describe
homosexuality or even the wide range of other sexual practices. For the most authoritative modern study of the subject,
that of Robert Stoller, 'perversion' is the 'erotic form of
hatred', defined not so much by the acts ('*the* perversions') but
by the content, hostility, while the word 'pervert' is cast out of
the sexological lexicon virtually completely.[2] Even for the de-
terminists of sociobiology, it is no longer the silent whispers
of genetic malfunction that are listened for but the genetic
functionalism of the 'sexual variations'. In part this is a result

of theoretical changes, of which Freud and Kinsey are key exponents. In part, it is a result of political pressure. The decision of the American Psychiatric Association to delete homosexuality from its published list of sexual disorders in 1973 was scarcely a cool, scientific decision. It was a response to a political campaign fuelled by the belief that its original inclusion as a disorder was a reflection of an oppressive politico-medical definition of homosexuality as a problem.[3]

Not surprisingly, the retention of the term 'perversion' is more clearly now a political stroke and it is as a term of political abuse that it is most commonly used, whether in the insidious tones of the 'New Morality', 'we hate the perversion but love the pervert', or in the assertions of some moral feminists that 'male sexuality' is a perversion.

The speaking perverts, first given a carefully shaded public platform in the volumes of early sexologists, have become highly vocal on their own behalf. They no longer need to ventriloquise through the Latinate and literary prose of a Krafft-Ebing or a Havelock Ellis, or engage in the intricate transference and counter-transference of analyst and analysand. They speak for themselves in street politics and lobbying, through pamphlets, journals and books, via the semiotics of highly sexualised settings, with their elaborate codes of keys, colours and clothes, in the popular media, and in the more mundane details of domestic life. There is a new pluralism of sexual styles—styles which have not by any means broken the dominance of the heterosexual norm, but which have thrown its normalising claims into some relief. There no longer appears to be a great continent of normality, surrounded by small islands of disorder. Instead we can perceive huge clusters of islands, great and small, which seem in constant motion each to the other, and every one with its peculiar flora and fauna. This is the material basis for our contemporary relativism.

The questions that insistently arise from this ecological chaos go something like this: can each desire be equally valid; should each minute subdivision of desire be the basis of a sexual and possibly social identity; is each political identity of equal weight in the corridors of sexual politics, let alone wider politics? Sex, where is your morality? the moral authoritarian can cry. Sex, where are your subtle distinctions? the weary liberal might whisper.

The inherent difficulty of responding to these interrogations is compounded by the absence of consensus on them within the radical sexual movements themselves. There is little solidarity amongst the sexually oppressed. Lesbians dissociate themselves from the 'public sex' of gay men. Gay leaders dissociate themselves from paedophiles. Paedophiles can see little relevance in feminism. And the ranks of feminism are split asunder by divisions on topics such as pornography, sado-masochism and sex itself.

Does pornography constitute an act of violence against women or is it simply a reflection of wider problems? Is inter-generational sex a radical disruption of age expectations or a traditional assault by older people on younger? Is transsexuality a question of control over one's body, or another twist in the medical control of it? Is promiscuity a challenge to sexual repression or a surrender to its consumerised form? Is sado-masochism no more than a ritualised and theatrical enactment of power relations or is it a sinister embrace of socially constructed fantasies? Are butch-fem relations the erotic working through of chosen roles or the replication of oppressive relations? These are not always heated debates in the wider society. They excite enormous controversy in the ranks of the sexually oppressed.[4]

None of the existing discourses of sexual regulation provide easy passages through these dilemmas. The liberal approach implicitly accepts diversity but flounders in many of the dilemmas it poses. The appeal to the right of free speech might be a useful tool in opposing censorship of erotica, but in practice few liberals would take that right to an absolutist extreme. Historically, there has been liberal acquiescence in the censorship of fascist and communist material, racist literature, horror comics and kiddie-porn. There does not seem any fundamental principles for refusing censorship of the obscene. The same difficulty applies to the question of the 'right to privacy'. It was not until the 1960s that even the American Civil Liberties Union was prepared to take up the issue of discrimination against homosexuals on these grounds.[5] Many still baulk at the prospect of having to defend *public* forms of homosexual interaction, or paedophilia or sado-masochism. The meaning of free speech and of rights varies, though we speak of them as if they have absolute value.

The historic nature of the categories that liberal arguments depend on, especially the private/public distinction, have been most clearly underlined in the debates surrounding the 'Wolfenden' approach in Britain. The two classic propositions on which this approach relies are derived from John Stuart Mill: that no conduct should be interfered with unless it involves harm to others; and that it is not the law's business to enforce morals. The assumption is that intervention should only be contemplated if the harm caused by it will be less than the damage caused by the continuation of a given condition.[6]

But clearly this is a matter for decision-making and calculation. In some cases, as in the British sex-reforms of the 1960s, the operation of what Stuart Hall has called a 'double taxonomy' of freedom *and* control[7] becomes apparent as a result of political shifts, where a move towards a greater freedom in the private sphere was balanced by a tightening of control in some aspects of the public sphere. In the Wolfenden approach, the law's role is to hold the ring, to provide the public conditions which would allow the privately contracting citizens ('consenting adults') to decide on their actions ('in private'). But categories, such as 'exploitation', 'corruption', and 'harm', which must be controlled, and the 'vulnerable' or the 'young', who must be protected, are obviously flexible and changing ones.

The difficulties with the libertarian response are as acute. Here sex is too often regarded as in itself in opposition to power. As Califia wrote of her book, *Sapphistry*, a controversial look at lesbian sexuality, 'This book carries a subversive message. It presents an alternative to conformity.'[8] The assumption seems to be that the enactment of an outlawed practice is itself oppositional. What counts is the morality of the act. Charles Shively writes as a gay activist of the merits of 'pure sex' and endorses a:

> morality of participants in which being 'good' is giving a
> good blow job or rim job, being 'good' is being hot and
> hard, being 'good' is letting it all come out: sweat, shit,

> piss, spit, cum; being 'good' is being able to take it all,
> take it all the way.[9]

At stake here, clearly, is a politics of romanticism where desire exists to disrupt order, and where disruption and transgression are the keys to pleasure. Much of the iconography and style of the sado-masochist movement is of this type. The lesbian s/m book, *Coming to Power*, begins deliberately: 'This is an outrageous book.'[10] The outrage comes from its self-conscious snapping of our usual assumptions about the connections between sex and love, sex and relationships, sex and pleasure; sex and emotions. Developments within capitalism, Tim McCaskell has suggested, have 'untangled' the emotions and the erotic: 'Where traditionally one need existed, capitalism has produced two. Erotic life and emotional life have come apart. They are now distinct human needs where before they meant the same thing.'[11]

There is genuine insight here which underlines the new opportunities for pleasure and self-realisation provided by consumer capitalism. But as the Frankfurt Marxists were arguing from the 1930s, the other side of this has been the incorporation of old desires into, and the manufacture of new needs by, consumerism. The selective co-option of the sex radical movements by capitalist society has been widely observed by activists. The aspirations of the gay liberation movement for an alternative sexual-political culture has been answered by the organisation of a huge gay market, with profits to be had in everything from poppers to perfumes, leather accoutrements to orgy houses. The radical transgression implied by the presence of the embryonic s/m subcultures of North America has been paralleled and partly overshadowed by the rise of a sort of leather s/m chic where style obliterates content.[12] The new libertarianism can easily fall into a celebration of the now individual self-realisation today. Its opportunities for providing guidelines for *social* change are therefore obviously limited.

The ambiguities of the liberal and libertarian positions inevitably prepare the way for the rise of new certainties. Moral absolutism, as Gouldner suggests, 'serves to cut the Gordian knot of indecision'.[13] It magically wipes out ignorance and the resultant anxieties, and makes possible the onward march. The decision of the (American) National Organisation of Women Convention in October 1980 to sharply distinguish lesbianism from any association with 'other issues (i.e. pederasty, pornography, sado-masochism and public sex) which have been mistakenly correlated with Lesbian/Gay rights by some gay organisations and by opponents of Lesbian/Gay rights who seek to confuse the issue'[14] was more than a tactical retreat in the face of a colder climate. It marked the acceptance by a significant body of feminists of a new absolutism which attempts to prescribe appropriate behaviour as the test of legitimate incorporation into the army of the good. The problem with correct ideas is that they can all too readily become correctional ideals. Moral absolutism, Gouldner concludes, 'invariably manifests an edge of punitiveness, a readiness to make others suffer. There is, in short, an edge of sadism in moral absolutism.'[15] The moral feminism that emerged in the late 1970s has many differences from the old absolutism. On pornography, the most emotive of issues, its ostensible concern has not been, as it was on the moral right, with the effect of explicit sex on the viewer, but its impact on women, and with the power relations inherent in pornography. But on pragmatic politics they have often marched hand in hand with the old morality in favouring censorship, sometimes in tones not radically dissimilar to traditional ones. 'Feminists must demand that society find the abuse of women both immoral *and* illegal.'[16] Social purity reformers of the nineteenth century would not have put it very differently. The effect is to support moves to strengthen social authority against sexual dissidents.

The moral absolutists, old and new, have another similarity. In an exact mirror image of the libertarian position, they too concentrate on a morality of acts, where sin or salvation resides in the activity itself. The litany of activities and variations —pornography, promiscuity, paedophilia, sado-masochism—is a checklist of original sin, which does not, in the end, seem very different from the old thesaurus of ecclesiastical anathemas or medical definitions. Political alliances are never neutral. In a context where sex has become a political front line, where moral issues become the displaced arena for arguing about what sort of society we want to live in, then these alignments and divisions are of crucial importance. Their effect in shaping the climate in which the erotic minorities have to live can be decisive. On certain issues many feminists have objectively allied with the Right. Ellen Willis has commented that 'as the sexuality debate goes, so goes feminism.'[17] Equally, it seems, as feminism goes, so goes sexuality.

The radical pluralist approach is more tentative than the absolutist or libertarian traditions, though it draws inspiration from the sex positive elements of the latter. And it is more decisively aware of the network of power-relations in which sex is embedded than the liberal approach, though being properly aware of the mobilising force of the discourse of rights and of sexual choice. Its aim is to provide guidelines for decisions rather than new absolute values, but two inter-related elements are crucial: the emphasis on choice and relations rather than acts, and the emphasis on meaning and context rather than external rules of correctness.

Foucault makes a useful distinction between 'freedom of sexual *acts*' and 'freedom of sexual *choice*'. He is against the first, because it might involve endorsement of violent sex-related activities such as rape which should never be acceptable whether between man and woman or man and man. But he is for the second, whether it be 'the liberty to manifest that choice or not to manifest it'.[18] The implication of this is that the nature of the social relationships in which choice becomes meaningful is of crucial importance. There has long been a weak version of this in the idea that certain types of sexuality (usually homosexuality) become justified only when they are embedded in a 'loving relationship'. It is in this form that a limited acceptance of non-reproductive sexualities has been incorporated within liberal Christianity. The underlying assumption is that gay sex has to be justified by the relationship it is expressed in.[19] But a stronger version of this position reverses the terms: now we would start with an assumption of the merits of an activity unless the relationship in which it is embedded can be shown to be harmful or oppressive: in Rubin's terms, instead of assuming that sex is guilty until proven innocent we would assume 'that sex is fundamentally okay until proven bad'. This implies in turn the acceptance of what Foucault calls a 'relational right', a claim to break out of the narrow confines of traditional patterns of relationships to invent and explore new forms of communication and involvement.[20]

It is at this point that the second set of elements are important, meaning and context. If we endorse the radical approach that no erotic act has any intrinsic meaning this suggests that, though they may not be the conclusive factors, subjective feelings, intentions and meanings are vital elements in deciding on the merits of an activity. The decisive factor is an awareness of context, of the situation in which choices are made.

Using these criteria—choice, relationship, context and meaning—I want now to look more closely at some of the most controversial issues that have riven the world of radical sexual politics in recent years. But rather than simply treating them as unproblematical sexological categories, I want to explore each of them in relationship to the wider issue they most clearly illuminate: the public/private division in relation to gay promiscuity; the question of male power in relation to pornography; intergenerational sex and the issue of consent; and sado-masochism as a problem of choice. In this way I hope to be able to confront key difficulties in existing approaches. My aim is not to 'resolve' intractable problems, rather to indicate the issues that must be confronted in facing sexual diversity.

'Public sex' and the right to privacy

For a long time we have cherished sex as the most private of secrets. We talked about it incessantly but shrouded its details with a discreet veil. For several hundred years now, especially in the Anglo-American heartlands of puritanism, the entrepreneurs of social morality have strenuously engaged in struggles against public manifestations of sexual vice in order to reinforce this private domain. Behind the fights against alcoholism, obscenity, prostitution and homosexuality lay a profound belief that while individual moral reformation was the key to salvation, religious and secular, a cleaning up of public spaces, a remoralisation of public life, was a decisive element in encouraging personal change. The moral panics, purity crusades, police interventions and state regulation that punctuate the history of sexuality are the results of such evangelical fervour.

Their effects are manifest in the shifting and ambiguous divisions between public and private life that we inhabit today.

Homosexuality has always posed a threat to these distinctions. It does not fit easily into the usual neat divisions between home and family and work. The characteristic forms of picking up, social interaction and erotic relating of most male homosexuals and many lesbians radically cut across conventional forms of courtship and sexual partnership. So it is not surprising that the social regulation of homosexuality often took the form of attempts to outlaw its expression altogether, both in public and private. Unlike prostitution, with which it was often legally linked, it was not the form of its organisation but homosexuality as such that was regularly perceived as a threat.[21]

It seems that public displays of gayness still arouse fear and anxiety. The consolidation of lesbian and gay lifestyles within gay communities in recent years has meant that it is more difficult now to attack homosexuality itself. But homosexual practices are much easier to challenge. Significantly, in the trail of the anti-gay backlash that developed in the United States from the late 1970s, alongside the even more predictable accusations of child corruption, it was the 'public sex' of homosexuals that was most vociferously excoriated by the Moral Right.[22]

Behind 'public sex' lies the threat of rampant promiscuity. Promiscuity implies a frequent change of partners, but it also suggests cruising haunts, meeting places and most insistently during the 1970s the proliferating growth of bath houses, backroom bars, fuck houses, establishments offering varied facilities and degrees of comfort and luxury, but all of them having one purpose: sex, sex for its own sake, sex in isolation, or in couples or in multiples, sex for pleasure, detached from all conventional ties and responsibilities.

Gay men in particular have regularly been attacked for their promiscuity. It has been seen as a fundamental marker dividing lesbians from gay men, while suggesting lines of continuity between homosexual and heterosexual men. Male homosexuality, as the sociobiologists have recently affirmed, is the quintessence of male sexuality. The reality has always been more complex. The various surveys of homosexual behaviour have all suggested that, while gay men might have more partners than heterosexual men, they generally tended to have less frequent sex. Many gay radicals have argued as a result that historically gay men far from being hyperactive have been sexually deprived so that the 1970s celebration of promiscuity was by way of a historic compensation.[23] On the other hand there is no reason to believe that gay men are any less able or willing to form relationships than heterosexual. Spada found that 90 per cent of his respondents preferred sex with affection—but did not regard it as necessary that that affection should be long term.[24] The split between emotional loyalty and casual, but affectionate, sexual ties may be different from conventional modes of behaviour, but it is not in itself a sign of social pathology, more a sign of an alternative way of life.

The deeply rooted injunctions against homosexual sex have had the effect, nevertheless, especially amongst gay men, of focusing attention upon the act of sex itself. The expansion of *publix* sex in the 1970s was an expression of an intensified *personal* need, representing, it has been argued, a search for a kind of affirmation of a denied sexuality. Altman saw in the gay bath houses two phenomena: an increased sexual expectation in the light of changes since the 1960s, and the more problematic result of a 'commercialisation of desire'. This suggested a dual impact. On the one hand the new patterns tended to undermine conventional morality, for they were predicated neither on the subordination of women to men (as say in heterosexual brothels) nor on the direct exchange of sex for money (as in prostitution). Instead they relied on a 'silent community' of desires, creating a sort of brotherhood of sexual outlaws: 'a sort of Whitmanesque democracy, a desire to know and trust other men in a type of brotherhood far removed from the male bondage of rank, hierarchy, and competition that characterises much of the outside world.'[25]

On the other hand, the bath houses represented an intricate incorporation of gays into consumer capitalism, with all its ambiguities. At best, there were opportunities as never before: 'Imagine, instant sex without any hassle, all for a few dollars.' At worst, there was the risk of a commodification of relationships: 'It's like going into a candy store and saying "I'll have this one, and this one and this, and this ..."' consumer sex. Sex

on the installment plan.'[26] Sex was freer than ever, but everywhere it was commoditised and commercialised as never before.

By the turn of the decade every fair-sized American city had
its bath house or houses, as did cities across the continent of
Europe (with the exception of Britain) and Australasia. Yet
already, before the mid-1980s, they were beginning to look like
historical accidents, products of a sudden spectacular, but brief,
breakthrough in the life opportunities of homosexuals rather
than of an evolution of new sexual forms. The widespread
emergence of AIDS after 1981 posed a major challenge to the
easy acceptance of promiscuity. Even if there was nothing in
the lifestyle of male gays themselves that produced AIDS, it
seemed likely that its spread was facilitated by close sexual
contact. The easy solidarity of the baths and similar places
ironically began to appear as a source of weakness for the
wider gay community. But the challenge posed by the emergence of these commercialised emporia of sex remained. We can
observe in operation a series of what can best be described as
'consensual communities' whose members know the rules and
act according to them. A kind of consent to enter the community operates, least formal but perhaps most rigid in the
most public places, say a public square, carefully formalised in
terms of entry criteria or membership in the most private, such
as a bath house. Within these contexts a consent to 'co-pres-
ence', in Laud Humphreys' phrase, operates. Such places break
with the conventional distinctions between private and public,
making nonsense of our usual demarcations. As Humphreys
points out, 'It is the safeguarded, walled-in, socially invisible
variety of sex we have to fear, not that which takes place in
public.'[27] It is in the home that most sexual abuse of small
children takes place and it is relatives or neighbours who
are most likely to rape women. Most ostensibly public forms
of sex actually involve a redefinition of privacy—a definition
based not on received distinctions built around the home/work
dichotomy but on a tacit but firm agreement about the conditions for entry and the rules of appropriate behaviour. In this
context campaigns for the 'right to privacy', as in Toronto in
1981 and 1982 following a series of police raids on gay bath
houses,[28] go beyond the traditional implications of that phrase

—the rights of individuals in private. Instead they placed on the agenda the question of collective decisions about privacy. Such arguments, of course, do not close the issue, they merely shift its focus. Just as public interest in sexual behaviour cannot in practice stop at the door of the private house (otherwise there would be no social regulation of incest and sexual abuse) so there can be no absolute privacy in 'consensual communities'. Commercial exploitation, racist exclusions, the subordination of women or of the young and old are no less important issues when practised amongst the sexually marginal as when displayed by the majority.[29] Nor could acceptance of the conditions of entry involve an abdication of personal responsibility, especially in matters relating to transmittable disease—a topic which became of great importance in the wake of the panic over AIDS. In San Francisco in 1984 the city authorities tried to institute new controls on public bath houses, backed by sections of the gay community. The call for a wider concept of the 'right to privacy' does not exclude other criteria of decision making. But neither is it necessary to wait until all other problems are resolved before confronting the issue.

The point to note is that the demand for the 'right to privacy' can transcend its liberal antecedents and become a radical demand for change in the relationship between private and public life. This is the real threat posed by so-called 'public sex'—and why it will remain an important issue in debates about sexual choice.

Intergenerational sex and consent

If public sex constitutes one area of moral anxiety, another, greater, one, exists around intergenerational sex. Since at least the eighteenth century children's sexuality has been conventionally defined as a taboo area, as childhood began to be more sharply demarcated as an age of innocence and purity to be guarded at all costs from adult corruption. Masturbation in particular became a major topic of moral anxiety, offering the curious spectacle of youthful sex being both denied and described, incited and suppressed. 'Corruption of youth' is an ancient charge, but it has developed a new resonance over the past couple of centuries. The real curiosity is that while the actuality is of largely adult male exploitation of young girls, often in and around the home, male homosexuals have frequently been seen as the chief corrupters, to the extent that in some rhetoric 'homosexual' and 'child molesters' are coequal terms. As late as the 1960s progressive texts on homosexuality were still preoccupied with demonstrating that homosexuals were not, by and large, interested in young people, and even in contemporary moral panics about assaults on children it still seems to be homosexual men who are investigated first. As Daniel Tsang has argued, 'the age taboo is much more a proscription against gay behaviour than against heterosexual behaviour.'[30] Not surprisingly, given this typical association, homosexuality and intergenerational sex have been intimately linked in the current crisis over sexuality.

Alfred Kinsey was already noting the political pay-off in child-sex panics in the late 1940s. In Britain in the early 1960s Mrs Mary Whitehouse launched her campaigns to clean up TV, the prototype of later evangelical campaigns, on the grounds that children were at risk, and this achieved a strong resonance. Anita Bryant's anti-gay campaign in Florida from 1976 was not accidentally called 'Save Our Children, Inc.'. Since these pioneering efforts a series of moral panics have swept countries such as the USA, Canada, Britain and France, leading to police harassment of organisations, attacks on publications, arrests of prominent activists, show trials and imprisonments.[31] Each panic shows the typical profile, with the escalation through various stages of media and moral manipulation until the crisis is magically resolved by some symbolic action. The great 'kiddie-porn' panic in 1977 in the USA and Britain led to the enactment of legislation in some 35 American states and in Britain. The guardians of morality may have given up hope of changing adult behaviour, but they have made a sustained effort to protect our young, whether from promiscuous gays, lesbian parents or perverse pornographers.[32]

From the point of view of moral absolutism intergenerational sex poses no problem of interpretation. It is wrong because it breaches the innocence necessary for mature development. The English philosopher, Roger Scruton, suggested that we are disgusted by it 'because we subscribe, in our hearts, to the value of innocence'. Prolonged innocence is the prerequisite to total surrender in adult love. Erotic love, he argues, arises from modesty, restraint and chastity. This means 'we must not only foster those necessary virtues, but also silence those who teach the language which demeans them.'[33] So 'intolerance' is not only understandable but virtually necessary—there are no liberal concessions here.

Liberals and radicals on the other hand have found it more difficult to confront the subject. It does not easily fit into the rhetoric of rights—whose rights, and how are they to be expressed: the child's, the adult's? Nor can it be dealt with straightforwardly by the idea of consent. Kinsey argued that in a sense this was a non issue: there was no reason, except our exaggerated fear of sexuality, why a child should be disturbed at seeing the genitalia of others, or at being played with, and it was more likely to be adult reactions that upset the child than the sexual activity itself.[34] This has been echoed by the advocates of intergenerational sex themselves. David Thorstad of the North American Man-Boy Love Association (NAMBLA) argued that 'if it feels good, and the boy wants it and enjoys it, then I fail to see why anyone besides the two persons involved should care.' Tom O'Carroll, whose *Paedophilia: The Radical Case* is the most sustained advocacy of the subject, suggested that:

> The usual mistake is to believe that sexual activity, especially for children, is so alarming and dangerous that participants need to have an absolute, total awareness of every conceivable ramification of taking part before they can be said to consent ... there is no need whatever for a child to know 'the consequences' of engaging in harmless sex play, simply because it is exactly that: harmless.[35]

There are two powerful arguments against this. The first, put forward by many feminists, is that young people, especially young girls, do need protection from adult men in an exploitative and patriarchal society, whatever the utopian possibilities that might exist in a different society. The age of consent laws currently in operation may have degrees of absurdity about them (they vary from state to state, country to country, they differentially apply to girls and boys, and they are only selectively operated) but at least they provide a bottom line in the acceptance of appropriate behaviour. This suggests that the real debate should be about the appropriate minimum age for sex rather than doing away with the concept of consent altogether.[36] Secondly, there is the difficult and intricate problem of subjective meaning. The adult is fully aware of the sexual connotations of his actions because he (and it is usually he) lives in a world of heavily sexualised symbols and language. The young person does not. In a recent study of twenty-five boys engaged in homosexual paedophile relations the author, Theo Sandfort, found that 'Potentially provocative acts which children make are not necessarily consciously intended to be sexual and are only interpreted by the older persons as having a sexual element.'[37] This indicates an inherent and inevitable structural imbalance in awareness of the situation. Against this, it might be argued that it is only the exalted cultural emphasis we place on sex that makes this an issue. That is undoubtedly true, but it does not remove the fact of that ascribed importance. We cannot unilaterally escape the grid of meaning that envelops us.

This is tactily accepted by paedophile activists themselves who have found it necessary to adopt one or other (and sometimes both) of two types of legitimation. The first, the 'Greek love', legitimation basically argues for the pedagogic value of adult-child relations, between males. It suggests—relying on a mythologised version of ancient Greek practices—that in the passage from childhood dependence to adult responsibilities the guidance, sexual and moral, of a caring man is invaluable. This position is obviously paternalistic and is also often anti-homosexual; for it is not the gay nature of the relationship that is stressed, but the age divide and the usefulness of the experience for later heterosexual adjustment. The second legitimation relies on the facts of childhood sexuality. O'Carroll carefully assesses the evidence for the existence of childhood sex to argue for the oppressiveness of its denial.[38] But of course an 'is' does not necessarily make an 'ought', nor does the acceptance of childhood sex play inevitably mean the toleration of adult-child relations.

It is difficult to confront the issue rationally because of the series of myths that shroud the topic. But all the available evidence suggests that the stereotypes of intergenerational sex obscure a complex reality.[39] The adult is usually seen as 'a dirty old man', typically 'a stranger' to the assaulted child, as 'sick' or an 'inhuman monster'. Little of this seems to be true, at least of those we might describe as the political paedophile. He is scarcely an 'old man' (the membership of the English Paedophile Information Exchange, PIE, varied in age from 20 to over 60, with most clustered between 35 and 40); he is more likely to be a professional person than the average member of the population (only 14 per cent of PIE members were blue collar workers); he is more often than not a friend or relation of the child; and to outward appearances is not a 'special type of person' but an apparently healthy and ordinary member of the community. His chief distinguishing characteristic is an intense, but often highly affectionate and even excessively sentimental, regard for young people.[40]

The sexual involvement itself is typically seen as being an assault on extremely young, usually pre-pubertal, people. The members of PIE, which generally is preoccupied with relations with pre-pubertal children, seem chiefly interested in boys between 12 and 14, though heterosexual paedophiles tended to be interested in girls between 8 and 10. This is less startling than the stereotype of babies barely out of the cradle being assaulted but poses nevertheless difficult questions about where protection and care ends and exploitation begins. Most members of NAMBLA, on the other hand, which has attracted obloquy in the USA as great as PIE has attracted in Britain, have a quite different profile. They appear to be chiefly interested in boys between 14 and 19. As Tom Reeves, a prominent spokesman for man/boy love, has put it:

> My own sexuality is as little concerned with children, however, as it is with women. It is self-consciously homosexual, but it is directed at boys at that time in their lives when they cease to be children yet refuse to be men.[41]

Self-identified 'boy-lovers' like Reeves scarcely fit into any conceivable picture of a 'child molester'. They carefully distinguish their own practices from sex between men and girls which 'seems to be a reprehensible form of power tripping as it has been reported by women'; and stress the beneficial aspects for adult and young partners of the sexual relationship.

When the official age of consent in France is 15 for boys and girls in heterosexual and homosexual relations (compared to 16 for girls in Britain, and 21 for male homosexuals), and when in the 1890s Krafft-Ebing fixed on 14 for the dividing line between sexually mature and immature individuals,[42] the fear that NAMBLA is attempting a corruption of young people seems excessive.

The young people themselves are typically seen as innocent victims. Certainly, many children are cruelly assaulted by adults, but in relations involving self-identified paedophiles or 'boy lovers' there seems to be no evidence of either cruelty or violence. Sandfort found that in his sample the boys overwhelmingly experienced their sexual activities as positive. The most common evaluative terms used were 'nice', 'happy', 'free', 'safe', 'satisfied', and even 'proud' and 'strong'; and only minimally were negative terms such as 'angry', 'sad', 'lonely' used. Even when these negative terms were used, it was largely because of the secrecy often necessary and the knowledge of hostile norms and reactions, not because of the sexual contact itself.[43] There is strong evidence that the trauma of public exposure and of parental and police involvement is often greater than the trauma of the sex itself. Moreover, many adult–child relations are initiated by the young person himself. A young member of NAMBLA was asked 'You can be desperate for sex at 13?' He replied, 'Oh yes'.[44] Force seems to be very rare in such relations, and there is little evidence amongst self-declared paedophiles or 'boy lovers' of conscious exploitation of young people.

All this suggests that intergenerational sex is not a unitary category. Brian Taylor has distinguished eight possible categories which pinpoints the existence of 'paedophilias' rather than a single 'paedolphilia'. There are the conventional distinctions between 'paedophiles' (generally those interested in prepubertal sex partners), 'pederasts' (those interested in boys) and 'ephobophiles' (those interested in adolescents). But distinctions can also be made on gender of the older person or the younger person and along lines of homosexuality and heterosexuality. This variety suggests we need to be equally discrete in our responses.[45] There are three continuums of behaviour and attitude which interweave haphazardly. Firstly, there is a continuum of beliefs and attitudes, from the actual violent assaulter at one end to the political paedophile at the other. These can not readily be put in the same class for approval or disapproval. Most people brought before the courts for child abuse are heterosexual men who usually view their girl victims as substitutes for real women. Most activists who court publicity (and risk imprisonment themselves, as happened to Tom O'Carroll of PIE in 1981) have adopted a political identity, which sometimes does not coincide with their actual sexual desires (both NAMBLA and PIE had members interested in older teenagers) but is built around an exaggerated respect for children.[46] It is not obvious that all people involved in intergenerational sex should be treated in the same way by the law or public opinion if intentions or desires are very distinct.

A second continuum is of sexual practices. Some researchers have found coitus rare. It seems that the great majority of heterosexual paedophilia consists of 'sex play', such as looking, showing and fondling, and much homosexual involvement seems to be similar. Tom O'Carroll has suggested that these sexual distinctions should be codified, so that intercourse would be prohibited before a certain minimum age of twelve.[47] But bisecting these nuances, problematical in themselves, are two other crucial distinctions, between boy partners and girl, and between heterosexual and homosexual relations. There is a strong case for arguing that it is not the sex act in itself which needs to be evaluated, but its context. It is difficult to avoid the justice of the feminist argument that in *our* culture it is going to be very difficult for a relationship between a heterosexual man and a young girl to be anything but exploitative and threatening, whatever the sexual activity. It is the power asymmetry that has effect. There is still a power imbalance between an adult man and a young boy but it does not carry the socio-sexual implications that a heterosexual relation inevitably does. Should these different types of relation carry the same condemnation?

The third continuum covers the age of the young people involved. There is obviously a qualitative difference between a 3-year-old partner and a 14-year-old and it is difficult to see how any sexual order could ever ignore this (even the PIE proposals, which first sparked off the panic about paedophile cradle snatching in Britain, actually proposed a set of protections for very young children). 'Sex before eight, or it's too late', the reputed slogan of the American René Guyon Society, founded in 1962 to promote intergenerational sex, is not likely to inspire widespread support, because it imposes sex as an imperative just as now our moral guardians would impose innocence. There is a strong case for finding non-legal means of protecting young children, as Tom O'Carroll has suggested, because it is clear that the law has a damaging and stigmatising impact.[48] But protection of the very young from unwanted attentions will always be necessary. The difficult question is when does protection become stifling paternalism and 'adult oppression'. Puberty is one obvious landmark, but the difficulty of simply adopting this as a dividing point is that physiological change does not necessarily coincide with social or subjective changes. It is here that it is inescapably necessary to shift focus, to explore the meanings of the sex play for the young people involved.

Kate Millett has powerfully underlined the difficulties of intergenerational sex when adult/child relations are irreducibly exploitative, and pointed to the problems of a paedophile movement which is arguing for the rights of adults. What is our freedom fight about? she asks. 'Is it about the liberation of children or just having sex with them?'[49] If a progressive sexual politics is fundamentally concerned with sexual self-determination then it becomes impossible to ignore the evolving self-awareness of the child. That means discouraging the unwelcome imposition of adult meanings and needs on the child, not simply because they are sexual but because they are external and adult. On the other hand, it does mean providing young people with full access to the means of sexual knowledge and protection as it becomes appropriate. There is no magic age for this 'appropriateness'. Each young person will have their own rhythms, needs and time scale. But the starting point can only be the belief that sex in itself is not an evil or dirty experience. It is not sex that is dangerous but the social relations which shape it. In this context the idea of consent takes on a new meaning. There is a tension in consent theory between the political conservatism of most of its adherents, and the radical voluntarism implicit in it.[50] For the idea of consent ultimately challenges all authority in the name of free self-determination. Certain categories of people have always been deemed incapable of full consent or of refusing 'consent'—women in marriage, certain children, especially girls, under a certain age, classes of women in rape cases. By extending the idea of consent beyond the narrow limits currently employed in minimum age or age of consent legislation, by making it a positive concept rather than simply a negatively protective or gender-dichotomised one, it may become possible to realize that radical potential again. That would transform the debate about intergenerational sex, shifting the focus away from sex in itself to the forms of power in which it is enmeshed, and the limits these inscribe for the free play of consent.

Pornography and power

'Power' is an amorphous concept. If it is not something that we hold, or a force that is immanent in any particular institution, or the exclusive property of one social class or caste, then its tentacles seem everywhere—and potentially its reality can be found nowhere. The usefulness of 'pornography' as an object of feminist anger and evangelical mobilisation is that it offers a clear visual target: here, it appears, is the most graphic representation of female sexual exploitation, floating like detritus out of a huge industry of sexual fetishisation and commoditisation, and providing a searchlight into the heart of male power over women.

It is scarcely surprising, then, that pornography should be a major issue in sexual politics. Long a concern of the moral right, it has become a crucial preoccupation of contemporary feminism. In the United States by the early 1980s the feminist campaigns against pornography were perhaps the best organised and financed in the movement's history and, though they did not have the same salience, there were similarly energetic groupings in countries like Britain and Australia. But at the same time the campaign against pornography seemed to divide the women's movement, for it posed fundamental questions about the nature of female subordination, and hence of the forms of power in contemporary society. Pornography, as

Deirdre English has said, 'pushes people's buttons. They polarise and go to their corners very fast.'[51]

One of the reasons for this is that 'pornography' is an exceptionally ambiguous yet emotive term, which takes on different meanings in different discourses. For the traditional moralist pornography is a thing in itself—'explicit sexual images' which incite sexuality in the vulnerable and immature. For the liberal pornography is a movable feast, a product of shifting interpretations of taste and acceptability. For the radical feminist opponent of porn it is a visual demonstration of male power. Yet, as Rosalind Coward has argued, pornography can have no intrinsic meaning, for it is a product of shifting definitions and historically variable codes. It is not an act or a thing but a 'regime of representations'.[52] These representations do not, however, float free, for they are anchored in concrete forms. Pornography is simultaneously a legal definition, a historically shaped, and changing product, and a sociological phenomenon, organised into a particular industry in various social locations. It exists as a historical phenomenon because of the regulation and control of what can and cannot be said in relation to sexuality, and thrives on the belief that sex is naughty and dirty, that what is being purveyed is being distributed *because* it is illicit. The institution of pornography results from the designation of certain classes of representation as in some way 'objectionable'.[53] But what is defined as 'objectionable' changes over time, so that the themes of pornography vary, like the technology of representation on which it relies, and the opportunities for production and consumption are variable. There is no doubt that there has been a vast increase in the pornography industry in recent decades. By the early 1980s it was estimated that in the USA pornography constituted a $5 billion industry, organised in some 20,000 'adult bookshops' and 800 full-time sex cinemas, but it is by no means clear what the real impact of this was. It may even be, as some have argued, that a large part of the pornography and 'sex aids' industry was dedicated simply to improving marital sex. Such clear distinctions exist within the pornography industry—for example between heterosexual and gay pornography, between sadistic pornography and kiddie porn—that it is difficult to generalise about markets or impact. Even amongst feminists there is no clear agreement on the merits of pornography. Some feminists have found in a minority of pornography, 'a challenge to the puritanical bias of our culture', 'a set of models antithetical to those offered by the Catholic Church, romantic fiction, and my mother'.[54] Pornography is a complex historical phenomenon and has contradictory effects.

This is not, however, as it appears to the radical feminist opponent of pornography. 'When we're talking about pornography', Andrea Dworkin has said, 'we are fighting for our lives ... dealing with a life and death situation', for pornography both represents violence against women and *is* violence against women. Pornography is 'Material that explicitly represents and describes degrading and abusive sexual behaviour so as to endorse and/or recommend the behaviour as described.' *Simultaneously* it is the reality behind the representation: 'I feel my responsibility in this area is to insist on what I know. And what I know is that pornography is reality.' At the heart of the feminist anti-porn project, fuelling it and giving it passion, is 'female anger'—for pornography is, Brownmiller proposed, 'the undiluted essence of anti-female propaganda'. Pornography is the theory, said Robin Morgan, and rape is the practice. It is part of the male backlash against women, an expression of male fear at the potential power of women. So pornography itself is not so much about sex as about power and violence. 'Erotica is about sexuality', Gloria Steinam wrote, but 'pornography is about power and sex as weapon.'[55] Pornography is important, these feminists believe, because it is the distillation of male power over women, the cutting edge which ensures female subordination. It is this which justifies the fervour and moral passion which infuses the anti-porn campaign. At stake is women's survival.

The danger of this position is that it might exaggerate the power of pornography, and elide crucial distinctions which exist within the pornography industry. Violence against women—economic, social, public and domestic, intellectual and sexual—is endemic in our culture and some of this is portrayed in pornographic representations. But not all pornography—perhaps not even the major part—portrays or encourages violence, while the most violent representations themselves may carry their own forms of irony. One of the most notorious images that has recurrently been attacked is of a *Hustler* front cover which shows a woman being pushed through a meat grinder. The image is appallingly distasteful but it is not clear that *Hustler* is either doing this to a victim (it is, after all, a posed picture) or advocating that it should be done. Deirdre English calls it a 'self parody ... gross but ... satirical, a self critical joke ...'[56] Jokes are never neutral, and attempts at a reasoned view of pornography should not lead to the condoning of highly offensive images or humour. But a critique of the form and context in which such representations appear should not, either, lead us to believe that a specific image can in itself, detached from context, harm either the viewer or women as a whole.

The question of 'harm' has been a central one in debates on pornography. In effect, moral absolutists have sought to demonstrate that pornography is harmful to the viewer, through a general degeneration of moral susceptibilities, a divorcement of sex from context, and an actual stimulant to sexual violence. Liberals on the other hand have attempted to deflate these claims, or at least demonstrate that they are simply 'not proven'. Both the USA's President's Commission on Pornography of 1970 and the British Williams Committee Report on Obscenity and Film Censorship of 1978 made great play with weighing the evidence and came out of their deliberations agnostic or downright sceptical of any causal relationship between pornography and sexual harm. This is increasingly a domain of experts who can tease out the implications of contingent relations, statistical analyses and laboratory tests. Anti-porn feminists on the whole have bypassed the debate in favour of a categoric emphasis that pornography must be harmful. But in so doing they shift the terms of the argument to the effects not on the male viewer but on the climate of opinion, in which women live.[57]

It would be foolish to dispute the power of representation. Images help organise the way we can conceive of the external world and can shape our intimate desire. But there is no reason to believe that the effects will be unilinear or uniform. Susan Barrowclough has pointed out that the feminist anti-porn discourse makes three assumptions: that the male viewer's fantasy is the same as the pornographic fantasy; that the pornographic image directly influences behaviour; and that there is an undifferentiated mass of male viewers, all of whom act in the same way and identify with the same point of view.[58] Each of these assumptions is counterable. The huge variety of porn attests to the variety of tastes and desires. Not all men enjoy pornography. And there is very little evidence for any direct correlation between fantasy and behaviour. The shifts in the content of pornography or the changes in its organisation and incidence may indicate important changes in the social relations of sexuality, including attitudes towards women. But it is difficult to see how pornography as a contradictory practice could be instrumental in producing these changes.

In the end, for old and new moral absolutists, for left and right, it is difficult to avoid the conclusion that the real objection to pornography is moral, however this is coded. That is fair enough if all that is at stake is a personal position, but it seems a poor ground for making proposals which may have universal effects either through the censoring of pornography, or through a fierce attack on those who consume it, whoever they are and whatever their motives. 'We must', wrote Ellen Willis,

> also take into account that many women *enjoy* pornography, and that doing so is *not only* an accommodation to sexism, but also a form of resistance to a culture that would allow women no sexual pleasure at all.

Pornography, Lisa Orlando has suggested,

> may represent women as passive victims, but it also shows us taking and demanding pleasure, aggressive and powerful in a way rarely seen in our culture.[59]

Gay men and lesbians, too, have seen in pornography positive aspects which the critics would reject. They argue that gay porn offers images of desire which a hostile society would deny and are therefore real encouragements for a positive sense of self.[60] Just as pornography has to be seen as a contradictory phenomenon, riven by ambiguities, so the response to pornography, the appetite for it, has to be seen as an ambivalent one.

The anti-pornography crusades act on the assumption that

it is an undifferentiated male sexuality that constitutes the social problem from which women need to be protected. In the crisis of feminist politics that has been caused by the intractability of female oppression and the rise of the New Right, and in the midst of continuing violence against women, the anti-porn campaigns provide a rallying point. But, the feminist writer B. Ruby Rich has suggested, pornography is really a 'soft issue': fear of escalating violence has led to a displacement of anxieties, and produced a will not to see the real dangers. Pornography makes sex explicit; sexism on the whole is not explicit in our culture.[61] It becomes an easy move to reduce sexism to sex, with the result that: 'In using explicit sex to demonstrate explicit sexism the anti-porn movement locates itself within the discursive framework of pornography itself.'[62] It takes for granted the sense of illicitness and a fear-dominated attitude to sex which gives rise to pornography in the first place.

A singular concentration on pornography gives it a political centrality it does not deserve, and in the process the real strategic problems of radical sexual politics are downplayed or ignored. By concentrating on the power of the image in pornography alone the manifold ways in which sexual oppression is produced and reproduced in our culture—in law, medicine, religion, the family, psychiatry—are lost sight of. Ironically, it also means that the pervasive interpretation of sexist imagery throughout the culture, in advertising and the media, even in 'romantic fiction', is largely ignored in favour of a dramatic assault on pornography.[63] The sexual oppression and exploitation of women cannot be reduced to pornography, and it is unlikely that a mass assault on the pornography industry will do much to change the position of women.

The sexual fringe and sexual choice

Our discussions have focused on the effects of power on or in shaping sexuality. The debate on sado-masochism which was stimulated by the emergence of explicit subcultures and activist groupings of gay and lesbian S/Mers in the 1970s[64] takes this a radical step further: to the eroticisation of power itself.

Sado-masochism (S/M) places itself at the extreme fringe of

acceptable sexuality. 'S/M is scary', Pat Califia, one of the leading spokespeople for lesbian sado-masochism admits. But it is more: it is a 'deliberate, premeditated, erotic blasphemy', 'a form of sexual extremism and sexual dissent'.[65] The style of the statement emphasises two key characteristics of S/M politics: its subjectivity, with its emphasis on the meaning of the situation as seen by the participants, and its emphasis on choice, on the right to involve yourself in extreme situations to realise pleasure. Subjectivity and choice imply each other, for the argument proposes that S/M is only really valid in consensual situations between equals—knowing your partner's wishes and desires, and responding to them—while choice is crucial to the eroticisation of the situation, because for the S/M enthusiast sado-masochism is not about suffering or pain but about the ritualistic eroticisation of the wish for suffering and pain, about pleasure as the realisation of forbidden fantasies, and about power differences as a signifier of desire:

> We select the most frightening disgusting, or unacceptable activities and transmute them into pleasure. We make use of all the forbidden symbols and all the disowned emotions ... The basic dynamic of S/M is the power dichotomy, not pain. Handcuffs, dog collars, whips, kneeling, being bound, tit clamps, hot wax, enemas, and giving sexual service are all metaphors for the power imbalance.[66]

Sado-masochism becomes a theatre of sex, where the consenting partners freely engage in extreme activities, from bondage to fist fucking, mixing 'shit, and cum and spit and piss with earthiness', all on the borderlines of endurance, to attain an intensified sense of release and pleasure.[67] The political advocates of S/M take many of the beliefs of the early sexologists —that courtship, power, pain and pleasure are intimately connected, as Havelock Ellis for one suggested—and attempt to transform them by taking them from the penumbra of individual pathology and placing them in the glare of publicity as daring acts of transgressive sex.

S/M activists make three distinct claims for their practices: that they provide unique insights into the nature of sexual power, that they are therapeutic and cathartic, and that they show the nature of sex as ritual and play. Let's look at each in turn.

S/M, Califia suggests, is 'power without privilege'. The dominant roles in sado-masochistic sex are not so much inscribed as won, achieved by performance and trust: 'The dominant role in S/M sex is not based on economic control or physical constraint. The only power a top has is temporarily given to her by the bottom.' But this intense preoccupation with power differences, the ritual enactment of their erotic possibilities does, S/Mers suggest, provide crucial insights into the nature of power, for it shows the way in which *repressed* sexuality lies behind the formal front of oppressive forces. S/M, Califia suggests: 'is more a parody of the hidden sexual nature of fascism than it is a worship or acquiescence to it.'[68]

By tearing the veil from the face of authority, S/M reveals the hypocrisy at the heart of our sexual culture—the bulge under the uniform—and therefore contributes to its exposure and to the dissolution of its effects.

But can the enactment of fantasies that arise from a repressive culture ever be free of the taint of that culture? Two Australian feminists, broadly sympathetic to the lesbian S/M grouping Samois, have written:

> The main problem for us is when the fantasies and the
> play involve scenes with highly reactionary political
> meanings—e.g., nazi uniforms or slave scenes. We wonder
> if there is a limit to how far the individual context of
> sexual sex can transform their social meanings.[69]

Perhaps even more powerful critiques of political S/M have come from black lesbians who feel the whole issue an irrelevance when confronted by the real oppression of Third World women, an oppression which has led to the intricate involvement of sexism and racism and its attendant imagery of white master, black slave, which S/M sometimes plays with.[70]

There are effective arguments, the force of which are tacitly acknowledged by S/M activists through their deployment of a second major legitimation—that S/M is intimately therapeutic and cathartic in its effects, that it releases people from the power of violent and potentially asocial fantasies. 'A good scene doesn't end with orgasm', Califia argues, 'it ends with catharsis.'[71] It breaks the spell of a forbidden wish, and allows for release of repression: 'Fantasies and urges that are not released in some way are more likely to become obsessions.'[72] The living through of fantasies, on the other hand, can produce a new feeling of health and well-being, even states of ecstasy and spiritual transcendence. But, critics have argued, is it really necessary to go to the limits of physical possibility simply because we think we want it? Do we really have to live out each fantasy to be free of it?

This is where the third form of legitimation comes in. S/M, it is proposed, throws new light on to the nature of sexuality itself. Sado-masochism, Ardill and Neumark have suggested,

> stands as an explicit example of the political construction
> of sex—making it clear that the sexual delight caused by a
> tongue in the ear is as socially constructed as the thrill of
> being 'tickled' by a leather whip or the joy of fingering
> your lover's black knickers ...[73]

It demonstrates that pleasure is not confined to one part of the body, one orifice, or one set of sexual activities, but that we can eroticise diverse practices in highly ritualised situations. The rituals in fact are a key to the heightening of pleasure, and the practices, however diverse and exotic, forbidden and extreme, become 'metaphors for abandoning oneself to sexual pleasure'.[74]

Sado-masochism itself is a tiny minority activity, and is likely to remain so. The latent imperialism of its claims—that S/Mers have a special insight into the truth of sexuality, that extreme forms of sexuality are peculiarly cathartic or revelationary, or that we must go to the limits to experience heightened pleasures—is never likely to win over the reluctant and the hesitant. Nor are the arguments entirely convincing or consistent. There is an inherent contradiction between the almost Reichian tones of the argument that sexual repression is a key to social authoritarianism and the explicit social constructionism of the case for the eroticisation of new parts or regions of the body. The case for S/M oscillates constantly between an essentialisation of sex, power and pleasure, and a relativism which suggests that in certain circumstances 'anything goes'. But there is nevertheless a very important challenge in the politics of sado-masochism: it is the most radical attempt in the field of sexual politics to promote the fundamental purpose of sex as being simply pleasure. Sado-masochism is the quintessence of non-reproductive sex; it 'violates the taboo that preserves the mysticism of romantic sex';[75] pleasure becomes its own justification and reward. It is this, rather than the mystical or therapeutic value of S/M, that is the real scandal of sado-masochism.

Sado-masochistic practices dramatise the graphic relationship between context, and choice, subjectivity and consent in the pursuit of pleasure. The starting point of political S/M is the belief that two (or more) people can freely consent to engage in practices which break with conventional restrictions and inhibitions. A contract is voluntarily agreed the sole purpose of which is pleasure. But the condition is equality between contracting partners. It is this condition which, Samois, the Californian-based lesbian S/M grouping, believed made its activities compatible with feminism, while Mark Thompson has spoken of 'the responsibility, trust and clarity required for ritualised sex'.[76] Only amongst members of the same sexual caste is this possible. The debate that this claim has sparked off—most vehemently amongst feminists and other sex radicals but extending into the popular media—has had implications wider than the subject of S/M itself. In the wake of its claims other feminists have re-emphasised their claim to a freedom of sexual self-determination and choice, and have tried to break the 'sexual silences in feminism' whatever the taboos they violate. 'Feminism is a vision of active freedom, of fulfilled desires, or it is nothing', Ellen Willis has stated.[77] That means embracing the range of desires that feminists are beginning to articulate. The S/M debate, by breaking a taboo on what could be said or done, has made it possible to think through again the implications of sexual needs and sexual choice amongst consenting partners.

One implication of this stands out, and that is the way in which traditional definitions of sex have been downgraded in the debates on S/M. It is no longer *the* act and its perversions that is the object of concern but the context and relational forms which allow erotic practices to multiply. In S/M it seems to be the ritual as much as the zone of the body that matters, the eroticisation of the situation as much as the orgasm. The whole body becomes a seat of pleasure, and the cultivation of roles and exotic practices the key to the attainment of pleasure. A degenitalisation of sex and of pleasure is taking place in these practices which disrupt our expectations about the erotic. In a curious, understated way, in this the extreme of lesbian sado-masochism thus meets up with the extreme of its greatest opponents. They too attempt to minimise the genital nature of sex. They too emphasise the importance of context, if in a differently understood way. The conclusions and prescriptions significantly differ, but both point to the qualitative shift that is taking place in the discussion of the erotic. Increasingly, it is not 'sexuality' as ordinarily understood that is the real object of debate, but 'the body' with its multitude of possibilities for pleasure—genital and non-genital. Whatever we think of the resulting practices—and surely they are more a question of aesthetics than of morals—it is important to register this profound move in preoccupations and concern. The meaning of sexuality is being transformed—and before our rather startled eyes.

Refusing to refuse the body

Any progressive approach to the question of sexuality must balance the autonomy of individuals against the necessity of collective endeavour and common cause. But where the exact parameters of the relationship should be is perhaps the most delicate and difficult problem for contemporary sexual politics. Inevitably, as Sue Cartledge has sensitively argued, there is a conflict between 'Duty and Desire' in which individual needs can all too readily become twisted and distorted to meet the constraints of obligation—to abstract cause or imagined ideal.[78] But, equally, the celebration of individual desires over all else can lead to the collapse of any collective activity, all social movements and any prospect of real change.

The recent history of sexual politics has seen the development of both tendencies as the utopian hopes of an ultimate resolution of the conflict between duty and desire have receded. The absolutisation of individual desires in a moral and political climate where marked social progress seems stymied can easily lead on the one hand to a partial or total retreat into privacy, into the narcissistic celebration of the body beautiful of the 'Perrier generation', regardless of the consequences. Sexual liberation becomes merely a synonym for individual self-expression, with scarcely a thought for the social relations in which all action must be embodied. This is the nadir of the libertarianism of the 1960s. On the other hand, a sense of embattlement, of hopes thwarted and 'dreams deferred', can as readily involve a search for new absolutes, for unifying norms which govern social movements and activities. Many feminists have found such a norm in the campaigns for sexual separatism, or against pornography where the female principle confronts, in a battle to an ever receding end, the male. Others committed to radical sexual change have sought a governing principle in a new morality or even a socialist eugenics, where the principle of collective need transparently hegemonises the desires of individuals.[79]

A radical pluralist approach starts with the recognition that certain conflicts of needs, desires and ambitions can never readily be resolved. Its governing principle is that no attempt should be made to reduce human sexual diversity to a uniform form of 'correct' behaviour. It does not argue, however, that all forms of sexual behaviour are equally valid, regardless of consequences, nor does it endorse the laissez-faire pluralism of the typical liberal approach, which is unable to think through values and distinctions. On the contrary, radical pluralism is sensitive to the workings of power, alive to the struggles needed to change the existing social relations which constrain sexual autonomy, and based upon the 'collective self-activity' of those oppressed by the dominant sexual order. The most significant development in sexual politics over the past generation has not been a new volubility of sexual need, nor the new sexual markets, nor the proliferation of sexual styles or practices. It has been the appearance of new sexual-political subjects, constituting new 'communities of interest' in political terms who have radically transformed the meaning of sexual politics. The sexually oppressed have spoken more explicitly than ever before on their own behalf: and if there is often confusion and ambiguity and contradictions between different groups, and even within single movements, this seems a small and possibly temporary price to pay for what is ultimately a major transformation of the political scene. There is a new sexual democracy struggling to be born and if its gestation seems over long, with a number of unforeseen complications, there is every indication that the neonate can still grow into a vigorous, healthy maturity.

'Democracy' seems an odd word to apply to the sexual sphere. 'Sexuality' as we have seen in this book is a phenomenon which is typically understood as being outside the rules of social organisation. We celebrate its unruliness, spontaneity and wilfulness, not its susceptibility to calculation and decision-making. But it is surely a new form of democracy that is called for when we speak of the right to control our bodies, when we claim 'our bodies are our own'.

The claim to bodily self-determination is an old one, that has roots in a number of different discourses: liberal, Marxist and biological. From liberal roots in the puritan revolution of the seventeenth century we can trace the ideal of 'property in one's own person'. From the Marxist tradition comes the ideal of a society in which human needs can be satisfied. And from the biological sciences comes an understanding of the body, its capacities and limitations, demarcating the boundaries of individual possibility.[80] None of these traditions, nor the contemporary form of the claim to determination, can resolve the ambivalences within the discourse of choice. If we just look at the claim for a woman's right to choose in relation to abortion we can see that the phrase itself cannot resolve problems: is a woman's right to abortion absolute? Even up to the final month of pregnancy? Whatever the consequences for the potential life or the life of the woman? Saying a woman should choose does not specify under what conditions she can choose and what she should choose. There are ultimately political decisions.

Nevertheless, the concept of the 'right to choose' is a powerful mobilising idea, is still, as Denise Riley argues, the 'chief inherited discourse' which fuels any demand for social reform.[81] It has a defensive ring to it against those who would subordinate women to moral control. But it can also have a powerful positive challenge if it is seen as a collective assertion of right in the demand for a new ordering of social possibility.

The willingness to discuss the principles and conditions of

sexual behaviour, of what we conventionally designate as 'personal life', is what marks the new political movements around sexuality from more orthodox political forms. It does not mean that there will be automatic agreement. On the contrary, conflicts of interpretation, conviction, orientation and behaviour are inevitable if we reject—as I believe we must—any idea of a mystical transcendence of difficulty and difference. The real task is to find mediations for the conflicts that will inexorably arise, to invent procedures for their settlement or discover resources for their acceptance by all parties in a spirit of mutual recognition.

The new sexual-social movements serve to disrupt the private/public dichotomy of liberal politics by their very nature, while specific campaigns (for, say, the rights of gay people at work, for the rights of lesbian parents, against sexual harassment at work) and the cultural politics of feminism and the gay movement can snap traditional distinctions between work and leisure, normal and abnormal sexualities. Feminism and radical sexual politics grow out of a recognition of people's needs and hence can begin to reunite the spheres of personal and political life. They provide a politics of people and not simply for people.

But what is this politics ultimately about? It is not about sexuality as generally understood. The starting points for the political movements around sex were the categorisations of the sexologists, that exotic profusion whose effects have been so defining and limiting. But the movements themselves offered, in Foucault's now famous phrase, a 'reverse affirmation', where first homosexuals and then others radically disqualified by the sexual tradition began to demand that their own legitimacy or 'naturality' be acknowledged.[82] But though beginning with the categories as they existed, the activities of the new movements gradually evacuated them of any meaning. For the elaborate taxonomies and distinctions existed in the end only to explain the variations in relationship to an assumed norm. Once the norm itself was challenged, then the category of the perverse became redundant, and with them the whole elaborate edifice of 'sexuality'—the belief that the erotic is a unified domain, governed by its own laws, organised around a norm and its variations—begins to crumble.

We are left with the body and its potentialities for pleasure. This is a peculiarly ambiguous phrase which states an ambition without specifying its means of attainment. I intend to take it as a metaphor for the subjectivisation of erotic pleasure, for the willingness to explore possibilities which may run counter to received definitions but which nevertheless, in context, with full awareness of the needs and limits of the situation, can be affirmed. Many of the new sexual subcultures, implicitly and explicitly, express this attitude. Richard Dyer sees in the subcultures of the gay world a new 'body culture' expressed in styles, physical expressiveness and body awareness, that 'refuses to refuse the body any more'.[83] This surely is the hallmark of the new politics of sexuality, and its organising principle is the celebration of pleasure. Pleasure, writes Frederic Jameson, 'is finally the consent of life in the body, the reconciliation—momentary as it may be—with the necessity of physical existence in a physical world.'[84] Pleasure, yes, but not pleasure selfishly attained: pleasure in the context of new codes and of new types of relationships. It is this that makes the new pluralism radical. The new relationships may not yet exist on a large scale. But in the inventiveness of the radical sexual movements in creating new ways of life lies the ultimate challenge to the power of definition hitherto enjoyed by the sexologists and the sexual tradition.

CHAPTER 10

Conclusion: beyond the boundaries of sexuality

> ... a socialism which could create, root and
> develop a transformation and renewal of that
> old friend of the people, democracy. Well,
> that would be worth the trouble.
>
> SHEILA ROWBOTHAM, *Dreams and Dilemmas*

'The subject of sex', Edward Carpenter, the great English socialist and (homo-)sexual radical, wrote in 1896 at the beginning of his key work, *Love's Coming of Age*, 'is difficult to deal with.'[1] As the years have passed and the mists and mystifications surrounding it have swirled and eddied and only partially lifted, the subject has not grown any less difficult: to a large degree it has become more complex and intractable as the rhetoric of sexuality has increased dramatically in volume, swelling to encompass contending forces largely unwished for and undreamt of by the pioneers. Two problems now seem particularly insistent, and their tortuous interconnections run like a tangled skein through the recent history of sexuality. The first is the question of 'sexual theory': the means by which we try to understand that bundle of sensual possibilities we know as our sex, and through which we claim to know ourselves. The second is the problem of what has universally become known as 'sexual politics': of how we can relevantly politicise what has conventionally been known as the most private of experiences, and of the articulation between this class of political endeavour and other struggles against power and domination. Each area today is in crisis and their complex interactions feed the general crisis of sexuality.

246

For Edward Carpenter, writing in the heady early years of 'sexology', there was no unsolvable difficulty with the first of these issues. The theory, or theories, were for someone like Carpenter the hopeful sign of a new age. The chief problem lay not in their pretensions but in their acceptability (or lack of it) to the established powers. In this country, a contemporary wrote of Britain in 1906, 'we have too long, from a sense of mock modesty, neglected the science relating to sex'.[2] For him, as for Carpenter and all the early sexologists, the new science, even with its contending explanations, was the cutting edge of enlightenment, the chief motor for rooting out prejudice, ignorance and false modesty. By the 12th edition of *Love's Coming of Age* in 1923 Carpenter was able to note some progress on this front. Times, he observed, had much changed. The subject of sex had been 'swept out into a larger orbit', and new conclusions had been reached and widely accepted. As revised, the book represented 'the most modern thought', and he freely and eclectically paid homage to those advanced thinkers: Ellis, Forel, Moll, Hirschfeld, Weininger, Geddes, Thomson, Ellen Key, even hints of Freud ... the luminaries of the first phase of the science of desire.[3] Since the 1920s few commentators of sexuality, even the most hardened supporters of social purity, have ventured forth without some backing from one or other of the schools of sexology.

Today, as this book has tried to argue, we can no longer be so certain of the verities of sexology. Our 'most modern' currents of thought tend to be a little more sceptical of some of those early claims. The crisis of sexual theory is a crisis in the certainty that once existed in the truth of sexology.

Let's take as an example the deployment of arguments from biology, a wide enough field stretching from natural history to molecular biology. In the wake of Darwin, as we have seen, arguments from this science came to hegemonise the study of sex. By the beginning of this century hereditarian theories, a particular appropriation of Darwinianism, seemed to have conquered all. The change in Krafft-Ebing's explanation of homosexuality from environmental factors ('seduction') to congenital is one significant mark of this shift. Even someone like Freud, who struggled valiantly to assert the autonomy of psychic processes, found himself time and time again drawn back to the seductive embrace of biology, while the adoption by later writers, partially in revulsion at the excesses of the determinism of eugenics, of a conditioning model of sexuality still failed to break the fundamental dichotomy inscribed in all accounts of sexuality: between 'sex' as the domain of the natural *and* 'society' as the source of sexual regulation. Part of the appeal of sociobiology is precisely that it ends the dichotomy, though in favour of a new genetic (that is, biological) determinism. Now the very pinnacles of human achievement can be revealed as little more than functional adaptations to the movement of molecules.

My aim has not been to demonstrate that 'biology' is irrelevant to an understanding of sexuality. No theory, however dependent it may be on 'social construction', can ignore the limits set by the possibilities of the body. The problem lies in the claim by sexology to find in biology *the* key to sexual, and hence social, life, and in the deployment by sexologists of biological arguments to explain and justify sexual divisions and differences which are transparently social in origins. Biology gives its exponents the power to naturalise their prejudices, and many sexologists have used this to the full. I have not attempted to criticise the sexological theories on the basis of their truth in correspondence with objective reality. I suspend that question—which is, in any case, largely outside my competence—in favour of a more urgent one: the question of the effects of believing the theories to be true regardless of other factors that might be taken into account in understanding human behaviour.

Those effects have been limiting and controlling in two crucial areas: the sexuality of women, and the diversity of human sexuality. Carpenter, again, embodies the problem. He was a genuine sexual radical, an advocate of homosexual rights at a time when a homosexual way of life was virtually unthinkable. He was a strong supporter of feminism, and was deeply admired by many of the most militant women of his day. Yet his views on women are clearly, by modern standards, normative and essentialist. He speaks of women as 'the more primitive, the more intuitive, the more emotional ... to her, sex is a deep and sacred instinct ... in a way she is nearer the child herself, and nearer to the savage ...'[4] Here all the then existing cultural assumptions about women are encoded into what was intended as, and to some extent was, an acceptable progressive discourse. In practice all the resources of scientific authority, the 'most modern' thought of the day, are adduced to sharpen ancient dichotomies and give them a new life as scientifically proved divisions. As contemporary sociobiologists now claim, the *is* of a biologically rooted sexual difference did not necessarily lead to the *ought* of sexual inequality, but it was relatively easy for Carpenter's contemporaries to slip from 'different but equal' to 'unequal because different'. Modern feminists have lost faith in the early sexologists precisely because of these arguments which relied on an apparently scientific insight.

It would be difficult to reject the salience of the different bodily potentials of men and women: the bodily differences are the irreducible sites for the inscription of sexual difference.[5] But the task of sexual theory ought to be the understanding of how these bodily differences become meaningful both at the level of the individual psyche and culturally, with the aim not of abolishing human divergences but of escaping from the trap of seeing all character and identity as emanating directly from the morphology of the body. It is not biology that is the real destiny in our culture but morphology.

Inevitably, the normative implications of this determinism are extended to the question of sexual diversity. Once it is demonstrated, by 'scientific proof', that body, reproductive capacity, desire and identity are part of an inevitable continuum, when heterosexuality is inscribed as the norm of behaviour because it is deeply rooted in the shape and reproductive potential of the body, then all other forms of sexual behaviour have to be explained as deviant. A similar closure of argument develops as with the issue of sexual difference. Because the variations are 'natural' they can on a certain level be accepted—this has always been the argument of sexual libertarians. But using the same evidence variations can also become seen as 'unnatural', beyond the pale, because they are not reproductive, or are with the wrong partner, or use the incorrect orifices. In the meantime the historical nature of the social privilege we grant to heterosexual genitality is never questioned, let alone challenged.

Various sexologists have struggled with the knot of these

complexities—Freud, particularly, with the question of sexual difference and his challenge to the idea of a pre-given identity, Kinsey with his catalogue of sexual diversity. But it is in the new social movements that have grown up around sexuality and gender that the radical import of their questions has been recognised. These new political subjects, working on the terrain demarcated by sexology, but challenging its more excessive claims to scientific insight and truth, have asserted new political priorities. This does not mean that the 'grass roots sexology' that has emerged in recent years can ignore the findings of sex research or adopt less stringent standards of scholarship or rational argument (indeed it needs to be better researched, more scholarly, more rational). We need to recognise and more or less humbly accept the limits of human potential as well as its possibilities, but this recognition, inevitably, takes place within the context of our political perspectives. This has always been the case, covertly. The difference today is that the perspectives are now overt, and can therefore be debated and assessed.

This brings us to the second major difficulty I referred to earlier: that of 'sexual politics'. In practice most of the early sexologists were progressive in their sympathies, whatever the normalising impact of their theories on individual lives. Sexologists such as Krafft-Ebing, Freud, Alfred Kinsey, Masters and Johnson were (or are) broadly liberal in their attitudes to law reform, sex education, state harassment of sexual minorities and the like, while others, such as Havelock Ellis in his early days, Carpenter, Hirschfeld, Federn, Adler, as well as the more familiar names of Reich, Marcuse and Fromm, had close socialist affiliations. Generally they all saw themselves as part of the historic sweep towards a more humane and generous and rational society, and felt themselves, to some degree, as oppositional to existing bastions of power. There was no great caesura between sexual theory and sexual politics. Many of the pioneers were involved in sex reform movements or provided the inspiration for radical sexual politics. The sex reformers relied on the sexual theorists to give scientific backing to their political campaigns and became in a real sense the political arm of the sexologists. This is clearly no longer the case.

But nor is it true that sexual politics is any longer necessarily radical and oppositional. The rise of the New Right, contending for dominance on territory historically mapped out by the left, has produced an acute crisis in the politics of sexuality. In the early years of sexology, the pioneers worked promiscuously alongside feminists, homosexual radicals, social hygienists, eugenicists and social purity leaders. There were tensions, differences of perspective, sharp debates, but no fundamental divide. Ellis, Carpenter, Hirschfeld, Ellen Key, Stella Browne, Margaret Sanger, Marie Stopes, all used eugenicist and social hygiene arguments at various times, while by the 1920s even the most ardent social purity groupings were distributing texts by many of the same people. Today feminists and sexual radicals confront the sexual politics of the right across a chasm which no common cause of health or hygiene or sexual enlightenment, or common pool of sexual knowledge, can bridge (which is why the flirtation of some radical feminists with New Right moralists over issues such as pornography is fundamentally more problematic than it ever was in the early twentieth century). Sexual theory in all its ever-growing abundance is now more a resource than a guide to activity. This is less true with regard to the New Right, whose programmes are at least 'validated' by reference to the writings (usually) of sociobiology. But on the left, especially in the wake of the theoretical deconstruction of 'sexuality' that has been undertaken by radical psychoanalysts, sociologists and historians, there can be no esoteric 'truth' of sex to be uncovered by diligent research; only perspectives on contending 'truths' whose evaluation is essentially political rather than scientific.

But what sort of politics? Edward Carpenter, with whom I started this chapter, had no doubt: the real 'coming of age' of love could only occur in a new, and fundamentally different, sort of society. He looked forward to 'a really free Society'[6] where the toils not only of sexual oppression and gender slavery but of (commercial) 'civilisation' itself would fall away in a socialist transformation. This ideal of 'sexual liberation' occurring as part of general human liberation in a socialist revolution is a powerful one whose resonance echoes through the radical sexual writings of the nineteenth and twentieth centuries. For Carpenter, as for his socialist predecessors, the association of sexual freedom and socialism was not an arbitrary coupling: they were essentially linked as part of the forward march of humanity. Many in the radical sexual politics that emerged out of the 1960s—including myself—have made the same connections and commitments and willed an identical end. The problem, as always, lies in specifying the processes by which this can be achieved.

Three distinct traditions are intertwined in this form of political commitment: that of socialism itself, the feminist tradition in all its diversity, and sexual radicalism. At certain moments these traditions have apparently come together in a common struggle. Engels noted that 'in all times of great agitation, the traditional bonds of sexual relations, like all other fetters, are shaken off.'[7] It is this perception which inspires the belief in a moment of revolutionary transcendence when the chains would indeed fall away like water from our backs. The reality has always been more mundane. Even in the radical groupings which have embraced in varying degrees all three traditions, as in the Owenite movement in England in the 1830s and 1840s, tensions inevitably arose, as Barbara Taylor has vividly described, between the socialist and the feminist commitments, or between the feminist and the radical sexual aims. Many men in the movement were unwilling to challenge their own patriarchal assumptions, while sexual freedom for men could, in nineteenth-century conditions, involve increased sexual exploitation for women.[8] Notoriously, the same has been true in recent years. Many women became feminists because of their bitter experiences in male-dominated progressive movements in the 1960s,[9] while many feminists today can find no common cause with the sexual radicalism of the gay movement. This is not said to negate the ambition but to underline the difficulty of its attainment. Socialism, feminism and sexual radicalism have different dynamics, embody contrary logics and have alternative definitions of their goals. Class struggle, gender conflicts and campaigns for sexual freedom have separate rhythms of development and contradictions between them inevitably arise. Will the adoption of radical sexual demands slow down the advance of socialism? Will full participation of women in the socialist struggle alienate patriarchally inclined working-class men? Will sexual freedom for men necessarily advance the cause of women? Such questions have resounded through the debates of even the most radical groupings during the most favourable conjunctures. In practice, during long, less amiable periods, the questions have not even been posed as the 'struggle for socialism' has been narrowly defined in terms of legislative and economic advance, and the fundamental issues raised by feminism and sexual radicals have been marginalised when they have not been ignored.[10]

I have spoken of three traditions: socialism, feminism and sexual radicalism. Each appeals to goals which transcend the immediate, the dogged but necessary task of piecemeal reform. Sexual radicalism involves an appeal for the end to sexual domination and exploitation; feminism demands the end of an age-old subordination of one gender to another; and socialism looks forward to resolution of class exploitation and the termination of the oppression of the unprivileged majority by a privileged minority. It is the socialist tradition which historically has claimed priority over the others as the most universalistic in its appeal, one which can and should embrace the others, both in its goals (the ending of all exploitation and oppression) and means (the alliance of all exploited and oppressed peoples). A further question that now arises, in the wake of the emergence of a mass feminism with its own universal claims, is whether that socialist appropriation of the concept of human liberation can have any current validity.

There are many socialisms, some of them ('democratic socialism', 'socialist-feminism') more appealing than others ('actually existing socialism'). But within these socialisms one strand of theory and political analysis stands out, both in its intellectual coherence and power and in its historical impact, that of Marxism. Of all the socialist approaches Marxism alone lays claim to being a general science of existing social relations and a political analysis which provides guidelines to their transcendence. If there is a crisis of socialist conviction today at the heart of that is a crisis in Marxism.

In a recent defence of orthodox Marxism, *In the Tracks of Historical Materialism*,[11] Perry Anderson has admitted the lacunae in, and underdevelopment of, Marxist theory in many areas, especially the question of women's oppression, war and peace, the meaning of 'Nature' and the possibilities of a socialist morality, but powerfully reaffirmed the validity and flexibility of the general approach as an indispensable guide to social transformation. But the real test of Marxism is whether it can meet the challenge of analysing and embracing the new social movements that have emerged out of the new and complex social antagonisms of the post-war world, movements which Anderson (representatively) barely mentions. As Paul Patton has put it, 'The assertion of the superiority of Marxism is also the (unargued) assertion of the priority of the problems which Marxism addresses.'[12] The ultimate focus of the crisis of historical materialism is its inability to transcend the reductionism which has been basic to it for most of its history. Mouffe has detected two forms of this: what she terms 'epiphenomenalism' and 'class reductionism'.[13] The first refuses any effectivity to the political and ideological levels of the social formation, for it sees these as simple expressions of an economic base, with its own laws and logic of movement. In effect this form of crude economic reductionism, with its tendency to a technological determinism, has been in crisis since Lenin's demonstration of the effectiveness of the political level in the Bolshevik seizure of power, though its effects linger on in many tracts. But the second form of reductionism is more subtle and potent, and still very influential: it sees the superstructures of ideology and politics as necessarily determined at the level of productive relations. Class relations are therefore the key to all social forms, which dictate an analysis (the irreducible class nature of all existing social relations) and a politics (the primacy of proletarian struggles) which necessarily place all other struggles as secondary.

Class conflict is endemic in western capitalist countries and I have no intention of minimising the crucial significance of working-class struggle in any strategy for socialist advance. But the outstanding issue that has to be addressed is whether the protocols of Marxism and in particular its emphasis on class antagonism are sufficient to help us understand the complex struggles of advanced capitalist societies. Rosalind Coward has shown how, historically, the Marxist tradition, though generous in its embrace of the cause of women's emancipation, has been unable to think through the question of women's subordination except in class terms, and hence has been resistant to the autonomy of women's struggles.[14] Similarly, the rise of black, gay and ecological politics in recent years has challenged some fundamental rigidities in Marxism. As Mouffe has argued:

> The emergence of new political subjects—women, national, racial and sexual minorities, anti-nuclear and anti-institutional movements, etc., are the expression of antagonisms that cannot be reduced to the relations of production.[15]

It may be that Marxism as a broad and still-developing tradition can meet the challenge. But it is its failure to do so hitherto that has opened the door to alternative modes of analysis, either in the form of alternative universalisms, as in feminist theories of patriarchy, or in microscopic investigations of specific modalities of domination, as in the work inspired by Michel Foucault. The latter approach has produced some of the most productive analysis of sexual subordination: it represents at its best a historically grounded analysis of local strategies of power which in their interlocking have produced the contemporary structures of sexuality.[16] The difficulty has lain not so much in the approach as in the inability of many self-declared Foucauldians to weld the multiplicity of local analyses into a coherent political project. I would argue, however, that such analyses are not incompatible with a broader concept of socialist politics.[17]

The significance of the demands of the women's movement and the radical sexual movements as they emerged in the late 1960s and early 1970s is that they put into question relations of power at levels largely unrecognised by the majority of socialists, and provided radically new insights into the complex and overlapping forms of domination of advanced capitalist societies. They thereby also signalled an enlargement of existing concepts of politics by proposing that what seemed microscopically personal (relations in the domestic sphere, individual sexual harassment at work, sexual practices and preferences, resistance to medicalisation or psychiatrisation) were all potentially political and politicisable, both because they were not ultimately personal in any essentialist sense, for they were all products of social processes and enmeshed in social relations, and because they engaged people's involvement in a way that conventional politics struggles could not. The sex-radical movements developed out of people's personal sense of subordination in a supposedly liberal-pluralist society; inevitably therefore they looked forward to a different sort of society. A libertarian socialism was reborn in the practices of the women's and radical sexual movements.

But of course not all activists in these new movements, let alone the constituencies for which they spoke, were radical or socialist, nor was the experience of domination and subordination similarly experienced across the spectrum. As we have seen, within the women's movement divisions over the importance of sexual pleasure erupted; different political priorities between lesbians and gay men have emerged, as have radically different attitudes towards sexual experimentation, sexual consumerism and the subcultures; the emergence of new 'sexual minorities' has produced an ambivalent response from the feminist and gay communities. Crisis-crossing these potential divisions, between men and women, heterosexuals and gays, the 'radical fringe' and more conventional 'variations', is the potent fact of institutionalised racism. 'Identity politics' is inevitably enmeshed in all the·contradictory and interlocking forms of oppression in modern society, and the new social movements are hardly immune from their effects. A group of black feminists has described how disillusionment with existing movements 'led to the need to develop, a politics that was anti-racist, unlike those of white women, and anti-sexist, unlike those of black and white men.' There are dense interconnections between racial and sexual oppression which lead to different priorities for black people as against white, black women as against men: 'We struggle together with Black men against racism, while we also struggle with Black men about sexism.'[18] The very definition of 'sexual freedom' in modern society has come largely from white men. In the new movements new definitions are emerging from women, and black people, which are asserting often contradictory definitions and new hierarchies of values.

In these circumstances the naturally fissiparous tendencies of the new movements are accentuated, and contradictory pulls of loyalty and commitment undermine the potential strength of the new communities of interest. There seems no common purpose, only the negative fact of a common marginalisation, and in a climate dominated by New Right rhetoric and governments, with the closure of oppositional space that inevitably follows this wave of conservatism, a tendency to avoid difficult alliances, to retreat into cultivating one's own garden—or body, or tastes—or even to surrender to political reaction at worst, or apoliticism at best, inevitably develops.

And yet, if there is no single common enemy, if there is no identifiable source of all our discontents in either capitalism or patriarchy or racism, there are common enemies, in the multiple forms of domination and subordination that flaw our society, and which the New Right seeks to reinforce. Many of these forms are more severe and ruthless than others, so it is notionally possible to draw up a 'hierarchy of oppression'. But the power of each is reinforced by the existence of the others, so they feed on one another incessantly, and in multifarious and polyvocal ways they work to limit self-determination and assert authority. If we accept this analysis, a common cause does, therefore, potentially exist, in the project of a thorough democratisation of contemporary society—extending and widening political democracy, democratising the processes of economic decision-making, opening up the different communities to popular involvement, and realising a sexual democracy. It is in such a project that the possibility exists of a new popular majority for social change extending from the working class and the poor through the traditional 'minorities' to the new social movements and the constituencies they speak for.

That there is a widespread dissatisfaction with the existing state of things in most advanced capitalist countries is signalled by the rise of the New Right, combining stringent economic liberalism with social authoritarian tendencies but apparently appealing via a populist rhetoric to wide constituencies. In countries like the United States and Britain New Right politicians captured, however temporarily, the seats of state power; in others they provide fuel for a vocal and ruthless opposition or are important partners in governing coalitions. Each national New Right has a different local configuration, and a varying combination of forces and priorities, but in all of them there is an appeal, subliminal or direct, to sexual dissatisfaction and for sexual orthodoxy. But an even more striking factor is that in none of these countries is there a popular majority for the more extreme of their prescriptions. Neither in the United States in 1980 and 1984, nor Britain in 1979 and 1983, which saw the return of right-wing governments, was there a majority of the total electorate behind even their most general policies. New Right policies on the family and sexual orthodoxy, though they have well-organised and militant constituencies behind them, have no popular legitimacy.

One reason for this is the very success of that commercialisation of sex in the post-war world which feeds the anxiety and militancy of the discrete constituencies of the right. We are most familiar with its excesses, in the form of degrading and objectifying imagery, the seediness of the sex areas of major cities, the romanticisation of sexual violence, the commodification of sexual pleasure. But for many millions of people escaping from social privation and sexual puritanism this new 'sexual freedom' has offered opportunity and even potentially a free space for the exploration of sexual desire. The priorities of this new sex field are not those of individual growth or collective self-activity, but those of the market place. Nonetheless the effect has been a reshaping of sexual needs and pleasure which make it extremely unlikely that the sexual restrictions of old can ever be fully restored. It is a recognition of this that has led many European radicals to worship at the altar of American sexual opportunity.[19]

The left, drawing on the huge reserves of its own puritanism, has signally failed to listen to this and has resorted to a deadening negativity and purism instead of engaging with the genuine if limited opportunities for personal growth that now exist. This is not an argument for accepting the commercialisation of sex, but it is an argument for coming to terms with the cultural changes of recent decades and recognising why they often do have popular support and legitimacy. People will only give up what they have—a tenuous freedom at best, but nonetheless something better than before—if they believe they are being offered a better future: a genuine freedom based on opportunity, equality and choice, in which individual pleasure can be integrated into social goals.

The key achievement of the new movements, of women and

of gay people and others, is that they have produced a politics that is closely geared to individual needs, growing out of a felt sense of oppression and offering the possibility of a 'collective self-help' through which some control over our life chances can be realised. There is no necessary push in these movements towards a commitment to general social change. The movements can as easily become the voice of new particularisms, of interests that can be partially at least accommodated within a liberal pluralist society. But the pluralistic nature of these movements also offers the opportunity for realising a new social vision, one in which freedom and individuality were guaranteed by the very autonomy of these movements.

This suggests a left project which is not organised in an authoritarian fashion, in serried ranks behind the leading role of a particular class or party, but one articulated around a politics which relates to individual and collective needs as felt and experienced, while simultaneously offering the hope of transforming their content into something new and better. The process of 'democratisation' is one such programme—perhaps the only realistic one—which can appeal to genuine revulsions against bureaucratisation, social and sexual authoritarianism and economic exploitation and bring together into an effective political alliance the working class, women, and the subordinate minorities, old and new.

On one level this is a matter of a political programme, of disparate policies that can bridge the gap between need and hope, and through whose development and operation a new popular majority for change can be organised. But this is the instrumental side of the socialist project. To succeed, it needs something more, a vision of an alternative society in which exploitation and oppression can be tamed, in which a real equality and genuine self-determination for all can be achieved. Today this seems a distant prospect, a bare hope to keep the flame of resistance flickering. But without such hope, no resistance or opposition is possible at all. In his discussion of the various forms of imaginative utopias that have existed throughout history Raymond Williams has pinpointed two that are still relevant today.[20] The first is the *systematic utopia*, which can envisage a different and practical way of life, thereby offering a belief that human beings can live in radically different ways, by radically different means. The significance of this, as we contemplate the pessimism and 'extending irrationalities' of the 1980s, is that it is based on the knowledge that societies have changed in the past, are changing now and can change in the future. That is a recognition of hope which gives meaning to the preparation of alternative policies and projects.

The second form of utopian hope is what Williams calls a *heuristic utopia*, an education of 'desire' in its widest sense, an imaginative encouragement to feel and relate differently in a better future. Williams, like other contemporary socialists, is referring to a wider idea of desire than is simply embraced in our definitions of sexuality. Such utopias have been the inspiration behind the visions of many socialists and sexual radicals from the Fourierists and Owenites of the early nineteenth century to the work of Carpenter and his fellow socialists in the early twentieth century, from the Bolshevik feminism of Alexandra Kollantai to the sexual politics of Reich, from the vivid writings of Marcuse to the hopes and aspirations of our contemporary sexual radicals. Much may be questioned and questionable in the details of their dreams. We must stay alert to their contradictions and tensions. But the vision of a freer, unalienated sexual world powerfully survives as an antidote and alternative to the meretriciousness, restrictions and oppressions of the present.

The majestic edifice of 'sexuality' was constructed in a long history, by many hands, and refracted through many minds. Its 'laws', norms and proscriptions still organise and control the lives of millions of people. But its unquestioned reign is approaching an end. Its intellectual incoherence has long been rumbled; its secular authority has been weakened by the practice and politics of those social-sexual movements produced by its own contradictions and excesses; now we have the opportunity to construct an alternative vision based on a realistic hope for the end of sexual domination and subordination, for new sexual and social relations, for new, and genuine, opportunities for pleasure and choice. We have the chance to regain control of our bodies, to recognise their potentialities to the full, to take ourselves beyond the boundaries of sexuality as we know it. All we need is the political commitment, imagination and vision. The future now, as ever, is in our hands.

NOTES

Chapter 1   Introductory: the subject of sex

1 Sue Cartledge, 'Bringing it All Back Home: Lesbian Feminist Morality' in Gay Left Collective (ed.), *Homosexuality: Power and Politics*, London, Allison & Busby, 1980, p. 102.

2 *Coming Out: Homosexual Politics in Britain from the Nineteenth Century to the Present*, London, Quartet Books, 1977.

3 I argue this in detail in 'Discourse, desire and sexual deviance: some problems in a history of homosexuality' in Kenneth Plummer (ed.), *The Making of the Modern Homosexual*, London, Hutchinson, 1981. For an alternative view see John Boswell, 'Revolutions, Universals and Sexual Categories', *Salmagundi*, nos. 58–59, Fall 1982–Winter 1983.

4 *Sex, Politics and Society: The Regulation of Sexuality Since 1800*, London, Longman, 1981.

5 'Havelock Ellis and the Politics of Sex Reform' in Sheila Rowbotham and Jeffrey Weeks, *Socialism and the New Life. The Personal and Sexual Politics of Edward Carpenter and Havelock Ellis*, London, Pluto Press, 1977.

6 See especially Michel Foucault, *The History of Sexuality*, Volume 1, *An Introduction*, London, Allen Lane, 1979, Volume 2, *L'Usage des plaisirs*, Volume 3, *Le Souci de soi*, Paris, Editions Gallimard, 1984, for the most important recent stimulant to the rethinking of the social history of sex.

7 I am here following the discussion in Bill Schwarz, '"The People" in history: the Communist Party Historians' Group, 1946–56' in Centre for Contemporary Cultural Studies, *Making Histories. Studies in History, Writing and Politics*, London, Hutchinson, 1983.

8 E.P. Thompson, *The Making of the English Working Class*, Harmondsworth, Pelican Books, 1968, p. 13.

9 For a bibliographical discussion of women's history see Elizabeth Fox-Genovese, 'Placing Women's History in History', *New Left Review*, no. 133, May–June 1982; for references for gay history see notes to Chapter 4 below.

10 Edmund Leach, *A Runaway World? The Reith Lectures 1967*, London, BBC Publications, 1968, pp. 47, 54.

261

Chapter 2 The 'sexual revolution' revisited

1 For a general discussion of this theme see Chapters 1–4 of my *Sex, Politics and Society*. For a defence of the myth of the 'golden age' see Christopher Lasch, *The Culture of Narcissism. American Life in An Age of Diminishing Expectations*, London, Abacus, 1980, p. xvii.

2 In Britain, for instance, Roy Jenkins, the reforming Home Secretary of the 1960s, and chief proponent of liberal reforms, disavowed the term.

3 27 March 1982, as reported in *New Socialist*, no. 13, p. 22.

4 For a representative view see Mary Whitehouse, *Whatever happened to sex?*, London, Hodder & Stoughton, 1978, Chapter 1.

5 Celia Haddon, *The Limits of Sex*, London, Corgi Books, 1983, p. 12. See also Germaine Greer, *Sex and Destiny*, London, Secker & Warburg, 1983.

6 See Oliver Gillie, 'Revenge on the Swinging Sixties', *The Sunday Times* (London), 5 December 1982, p. 13.

7 The representative advocate of this position is Andrea Dworkin: see her *Right-Wing Women. The Politics of Domesticated Females*, London, The Women's Press, 1983, pp. 88ff.

8 Though not for the first time: see Judith R. Walkowitz's discussion of the parallels between the late nineteenth century and today in the coalescence of social purity and feminist views: 'Male Vice and Feminist Virtue: Feminism and the Politics of Prostitution in Nineteenth Century Britain', *History Workshop Journal*, no. 13, Spring, 1982, p. 77ff.

9 Jon P. Alston and Francis Tucker, 'The Myth of Sexual Permissiveness', *Journal of Sex Research*, Vol. 9, no. 1, February 1973, pp. 34–40 shows the persistence of fairly conservative attitudes into the 1970s in the USA. But see also James Moneymaker and Fred Montanino, 'The New Sexual Morality: A Society comes of Age' in James M. Henslin and Edward Sagarin (eds), *The Sociology of Sex: An Introductory Reader*, New York, Schocken Books, 1978, pp. 27ff. For similar discussions of Britain, showing a gradually more liberal frame of mind, see Geoffrey Gorer, *Sex and Marriage in England Today*, London, Nelson, 1971; and discussion in my *Sex, Politics and Society*, Chapter 13. For an overview of changes in attitude from Kinsey to the 1980s see Paul H. Gebhard, 'The Galton Lecture, 1978: Sexuality in the Post-Kinsey Era' in W.H.G. Armytage, R. Chester and John Peel (eds), *Changing Patterns of Sexual Behaviour*, London, New York, Academic Press, 1980, pp. 45ff.

10 See references in note 2, Chapter 3 below.

11 Dennis Altman, *Homosexual: Oppression and Liberation*, New York, Outerbridge & Dienstfrey, 1971.

12 See the discussion in Ellen Ross, '"The Love Crisis": Couples Advice Books of the Late 1970s', *Signs*, vol. 6, no. 1, 1980, p. 110; for a discussion of British trends see Leslie Rimmer, *Families in Focus*, London, Study Commission on the Family, 1981.

13 I discuss this more fully in Chapter 13 of *Sex, Politics and Society*. For a theoretically convincing analysis of permissiveness see Stuart Hall, 'Reformism and the Legislation of Consent' in National Deviancy Conference (ed.), *Permissiveness and Control: The Fate of Sixties Legislation*, London, Macmillan, 1980.

14 See Chapter 7 below for a discussion of Marcuse.

15 *Sex, Politics and Society*, chs 2–4.

16 The general theme of this section is anticipated in Herbert Marcuse, *Eros and Civilization*, London, Sphere Books, 1969, and is developed in Reimut Reiche, *Sexuality and the Class Struggle*, London, New Left Books, 1970. An account, with particular reference to the effects of consumerism on homosexuality, can be found in Dennis Altman, *The Homosexualization of America, the Americanization of the Homosexual*, New York, St Martin's Press, 1982, chapter 3, 'Sex and the Triumph of Consumer Capitalism'.

17 Stan Cohen and Laurie Taylor, *Escape Attempts. The Theory and Practice of Resistance to Everyday Life*, Harmondsworth, Pelican Books, 1978, p. 106.

18 William Masters and Virginia Johnson, *Human Sexual Inadequacy*, Boston, Little, Brown, 1970; a point emphasised in Paul A. Robinson, *The Modernization of Sex*, London, Elek, 1976, p. 142.

19 Gay Talese, *Thy Neighbour's Wife. Sex in the World Today*, London, Collins, 1980, p. 28. Hefner is one of the heroes of this book which also successfully and unappealingly illustrates the effects of consumerised sex.

20 Barbara Ehrenreich, *The Hearts of Men. American Dreams and the Flight from Commitment*, London, Pluto Press, 1983, p. 46. On the growth of pornography see (for the USA) *The Report of the Commission on Obscenity and Pornography*, New York, Bantam Books, 1970 and (for the UK) Home Office, *Report of the Committee on Obscenity and Film Censorship*, Cmnd 7772, London, HMSO, 1979. The term 'pornocracy' is used in Mathilde and Mathias Vaerting, *The Dominant Sex: A Study in the Sociology of Sex Differentiation*, translated from the German by Eden and Cedar Paul, London, George Allen & Unwin, 1923, p. 89.

21 For a suggestive discussion of this see Jonathan Ned Katz, *Gay/ Lesbian Almanac. A New Documentary*, New York, Harper & Row, pp. 137–74; and John D'Emilio, *Sexual Politics, Sexual Communities: The Making of a Homosexual Minority in the United States 1940–1970*, Chicago and London, The University of Chicago Press, 1983, chapter 1.

22 On the evidence of sex manuals see Michael Gordon, 'From an Unfortunate necessity to a Cult of Mutual Orgasm: Sex in American Marital Education literature, 1830–1940' in Henslin and Sagarin (eds), *The Sociology of Sex*; Ellen Ross, '"The Love Crisis"', op. cit.; and Rosalind Brunt, '"An immense verbosity": Permissive Sexual Advice in the 1970s' in Rosalind Brunt and Caroline Rowan (eds), *Feminism, Culture and Politics*, London, Lawrence & Wishart, 1982. For a discussion of therapies see Helen Singer Kaplan, *The New Sex Therapy. Active Treatments of Sexual Dysfunctions*, New York, Brunner/Mazel, 1974, and P.T. Brown, 'The Development of Sexual Function Therapies after Masters and Johnson', in Armytage et al. (eds), *Changing Patterns of Sexual Behaviour*. For the growth of places like Plato's Retreat and Sandstone see Talese, *Thy Neighbour's Wife*, and Gebhard, op. cit.

23 See Altman, *The Homosexualization of America* and D'Emilio, *Sexual Politics, Sexual Communities*; and an article on 'Tapping the Homosexual Market', *New York Times*, 2 May 1982.

24 Alfred C. Kinsey, William B. Pomeroy and Clyde E. Martin, *Sexual Behavior in The Human Male*, Philadelphia, W.B. Saunders, 1948.

25 Elizabeth Wilson, 'The Context of "Between Pleasure and Danger": The Barnard Conference on Sexuality', *Feminist Review* no. 13, Spring 1983, p. 39.

26 For a suggestive discussion see Rosalind Coward, '"Sexual liberation" and the family', *M/F*, no. 1, 1978; and *Female Desire*, London, Paladin, 1984.

27 Gebhard, op. cit., pp. 47ff.

28 Deirdre English, Amber Hollibaugh and Gayle Rubin, 'Talking Sex. A Conversation on Sexuality and Feminism', *Socialist Review*, no. 58, July–August 1981, p.45.

29 Edmund S. Morgan, *The Puritan Family: Religion and Domestic Relations in Seventeenth Century New England*, New York, Harper & Row, 1966; William and Mallerville Haller, 'The Puritan Art of Love', *Huntington Library Quarterly*, vol. 5, no. 2, January 1942. Katz, *Gay/Lesbian Almanac*, pp. 43ff. challenges the validity of this view.

30 Randolph Trumbach, *The Rise of the Egalitarian Family*, Aristo-

cratic Kinship and Domestic Relations in Eighteenth Century England, New York, San Francisco, London, 1978. Ellen Ross, '"The Love Crisis"', op. cit., p. 113, and 'Survival Networks: Women's Neighbourhood Sharing in London before World War I', *History Workshop Journal* no. 15, Spring 1983; Carroll Smith-Rosenberg, 'The Female World of Love and Ritual: Relations between women in Nineteenth Century America', *Signs*, vol. 1, no. 1, Autumn 1975.

31 Ross, '"The Love Crisis"', p. 109.

32 *New York Times*, 29 October 1972.

33 Edwin Schur, *The Politics of Deviance: Stigma Contests and the Uses of Power*, Englewood Cliffs, N.J., Prentice-Hall, 1980, p. 138; see also Joseph R. Gusfield, *Symbolic Crusade: Status Politics and the American Temperance Movement*, Urbana, Chicago, London, University of Illinois Press, 1972, p. 4.

34 See Hall, 'Reformism and the legislation of consent'; and Christie Davies, 'Moralists, Causalists, Sex, Law and Morality' in Armytage et al., *Changing Patterns of Sexual Behaviour*.

35 On Britain see Victoria Greenwood and Jock Young, *Abortion in Demand*, London, Pluto Press, 1976; on the USA Zillah R. Eisenstein, 'The Sexual Politics of the New Right: Understanding the "Crisis of liberalism" for the 1980s', *Signs*, vol. 7, no. 3, 1982; and Rosalind Pollack Petchesky, 'Anti-Abortion, Anti-Feminism, and the Rise of the "New Right"', *Feminist Studies*; and for an example of a culture out of synch with the others, Gaullist France, see Anne Batiot, 'The Political Construction of Sexuality: The Contraception and Abortion Issues in France, 1965–1975', in Phil. G. Cerney, *Social Movements and Protest in France*, London, Francis Pinter, 1982.

36 George F. Gilder, *Sexual Suicide*, New York, Quadrangle, 1973; Mary Whitehouse, *Whatever happened to sex?*; and see discussion of the rise of the New Right, Chapter 3, pp. 33–44.

37 'Recasting Marxism: Hegemony and New Political Movements. Interview with Ernesto Laclau and Chantal Mouffe', *Socialist Review*, no. 66, Nov.–Dec. 1982, p. 109.

Chapter 3   The new moralism

1 The Briggs initiative had proposed to severely limit the rights of homosexuals to public position in education in California. It was defeated by a popular mobilisation which extended beyond normal political boundaries. Even the then ex-Governor Ronald Reagan opposed the proposed amendment. See Joseph R. Gusfield, 'Political Ceremony in California', *The Nation*, 9 Dec. 1978;

Schur, *The Politics of Deviance*, pp. 137-8; and Amber Holli-bough, 'Sexuality and the State: The Defeat of the Briggs Initia-tive and Beyond', *Socialist Review*, no. 45, May-June 1979. On liberalising popular attitudes in the USA see Altman, *The Homo-sexualization of America*, pp. 101-2.

2 Donald and Beth Wellman Granberg, in *Sociology and Social Research*, vol. 65, no. 4, p. 424, cited in *New Society*, 1 April 1982; Zillah R. Eisenstein, 'The Sexual Politics of the New Right'; Weeks, *Sex, Politics and Society*, pp. 275-6; and on the general liberalism of public opinion in Britain, see David Lipsey, 'Re-forms People Want', *New Society*, 4 October 1979. For a more cautious assessment see J.G. Pankhurst and S.K. Homeknecht, 'The Family, Politics and Religion in the 1980s: In fear of the New Individualism', *Journal of Family Issues*, vol. 4, no. 1, March 1983, pp. 5-34.

3 This account is indebted to the following: Alan Wolfe, 'Sociology, Liberalism and the Radical Right' and Mike Davis, 'The New Right's Road to Power', *New Left Review*, no. 128, July-August 1981; Kevin Phillips, 'Post-Conservative America', *The New York Review of Books*, vol. XXIX, no. 8, 13 May 1982; Linda Gordon and Allen Hunter, 'Sex, Family and the New Left: Anti-Feminism as a Political Force', *Radical America*, vol. 11, no. 6, vol. 12, no. 1, November 1977-February 1978; and the special edition on the New Right of *Radical America*, vol. 15, nos 1-2, Spring 1981; Zillah R. Eisenstein, 'The Sexual Politics of the New Right', and 'Anti-Feminism in the Politics and Election of 1980', *Feminist Studies*, vol. 7, no. 2, 1981; and David Edgar, 'Reagan's hidden agenda: racism and the new American right', *Race and Class*, vol. XXII, no. 3, Winter 1981.

4 'The New Right: A Special Report', *Conservative Digest*, June 1979.

5 Whitehouse, *Whatever happened to sex?*, p. 241.

6 Gusfield, op. cit., p. 635; and Pankhurst and Homeknecht, op. cit., pp. 7-12.

7 Whitehouse, op. cit, chapter 1.

8 Allen Hunter, 'In the Wings: New Right Organization and Ideol-ogy', *Radical America*, vol. 15, nos 1-2, p. 124.

9 Lynne Segal (ed.), *What is to be Done about the Family?*, Har-mondsworth, Penguin, 1983, p. 9.

10 Dworkin, *Right-Wing Women*, p. 34. See also Pamela Johnston Conover and Virginia Gray, *Feminism and the New Right. Con-flict over the American Family*, New York, Praeger, 1983.

11 David Morrison and Michael Tracey, 'Beyond Ecstasy: Sex and Moral Protest' in Armytage et al., *Changing Patterns of Sexual*

Notes 267

Behaviour, and Barbara Ehrenreich, 'The Women's Movements: Feminist and Anti-Feminist', *Radical America*, vol. 15, nos 1–2, Spring 1981.

12 Linda Gordon and Ellen DuBois, 'Seeking Ecstasy on the Battlefield: Danger and Pleasure in Nineteenth Century Feminist Sexual Thought', *Feminist Review*, no. 13, Spring 1983, p. 42 and in Carole S. Vance (ed.), *Pleasure and Danger: Exploring Female Sexuality*, London and Boston, Routledge & Kegan Paul, 1984. See also Ellen Willis, 'Abortion: which side are you on?' *Radical America*, vol. 15, nos 1–2, p. 90.

13 Deirdre English, 'The War against Choice', *Mother Jones*, February/March 1981.

14 Ehrenreich, *The Hearts of Men*, chapter 10; Petchesky, op. cit.; Andrew Merton, *Enemies of Choice. The Right-to-Life Movement and its Threat to Abortion*, Boston, Beacon Press, 1981; and Linda Gordon, 'The Long Struggle for Reproductive Rights', *Radical America*, vol. 15, nos 1–2, Spring 1981.

15 See Judith R. Walkowitz, op. cit.; Gordon and Dubois, op. cit., and David J. Pivar, *Purity Crusades, Sexual Morality and Social Control 1868–1900*, Westport, Conn., Greenwood Press, 1973, p. 254.

16 Linda Gordon, 'The Long Struggle', p. 88. See also Gay Left Collective, 'Democracy, Socialism and Sexual Politics', *Gay Left*, no. 10, Summer 1980, also printed in *Radical America*, vol. 15, nos 1–2, Spring 1981; comments in the Laclau and Mouffe Interview, *Socialist Review*, no. 66, p. 109; and Sheila Rowbotham, Lynne Segal and Hilary Wainwright, *Beyond the Fragments. Feminism and the Making of Socialism*, London, Merlin Press, 1979.

17 Allen Hunter, op. cit., pp. 116ff, offers a very clear outline of these tendencies. On anti-gay mobilisation, see Anita Bryant, *The Anita Bryant Story: The Survival of Our Nation's Families and the Threat of Militant Homosexuality*, Old Tappan, N.J. Fleming Revell, 1977. For a representative example of neo-conservatism see Irving Kristol, *On the Democratic Idea in America*, New York, Harper & Row, 1973.

18 Jim O'Brien, 'The New Terrain of American Politics', *Radical America*, vol. 15, nos 1–2, Spring 1981, p. 14. For a wider discussion, with British examples, see especially articles by Stuart Hall and Andrew Gamble in Stuart Hall and Martin Jacques (eds), *The Politics of Thatcherism*, London, Lawrence & Wishart, 1983.

19 Quoted in Altman, *The Homosexualization of America*, p. 86.

20 Alan Macfarlane, *The Rise of English Individualism*, Oxford, Blackwell, 1978; Christopher Lasch, *Haven in a Heartless World*, New York, Basic Books, 1977, and *The Culture of Narcissism*; Ferdinand Mount, *The Subversive Family*, London, Cape, 1982;

George F. Gilder, *Wealth and Poverty*, New York, Basic Books, 1981.

21 Jacques Donzelot, *The Policing of Families. Welfare versus the State*, London, Hutchinson, 1979; Rayna Rapp, Ellen Ross and Renate Bridenthal, 'Examining Family History', *Feminist Studies*, vol. 5, no. 1, Spring 1979.

22 Daniel Patrick Moynihan, 'The Negro Family, the Case for National Action' in Lee Rainwater and William Yancey (eds), *The Moynihan Report and the Politics of Controversy*, Cambridge, Mass., MIT Press, 1967; Hunter, op. cit., p. 131.

23 For discussions of the relationship between sexism and racism see: Errol Lawrence, 'Just plain common sense: the roots of racism' and other essays in Centre for Contemporary Cultural Studies, *The Empire Strikes Back. Race and Racism in 70s Britain*, London, Hutchinson, 1983; Charles Herbert Stember, *Sexual Racism: The Emotional Barrier to an Integrated Society*, New York, Harper & Row, 1965.

24 Phillips, op. cit., p. 32; on 'authoritarian populism' see Hall and Jacques, op. cit.

25 Whitehouse, *Whatever happened to sex?*, p. 257—which makes references to George F. Gilder's *Sexual Suicide:* chapter 10 of her book is in fact given his title.

26 Roger Scruton, 'The Case against Feminism', *The Observer*, 22 May 1983.

27 Phyllis Schlafly, *The Power of the Positive Woman*, New Rochelle, Arlington House, 1977; George F. Gilder, *Wealth and Poverty*, p. 69.

28 Leach, *A Runaway World?*, p. 49.

29 Michèle Barrett and Mary McIntosh, *The Anti Social Family*, London, NLB and Verso, 1982.

30 Ellen Ross, ' "The Love Crisis" ', p. 121.

31 Paul Hirst, 'The Genesis of the Social', Fran Bennett, Beatrix Campbell, Rosalind Coward, 'Feminists—the Degenerates of the Social?' and Paul Hirst, 'Reply', *Politics and Power*, no. 3: *Sexual Politics, Feminism and Socialism*, London, Routledge & Kegan Paul, 1981; Betty Friedan, *The Second Stage*, London, Michael Joseph, 1981; and on the pro-family left see Michael Lerner, 'A new Pro-Family group really belongs on the Left', in *These Times*, 30 Sept.–6 Oct. 1981; Michael Lerner, Laurie Zoloth and Wilson Riles Jnr, *Bringing it All Back Home: A Strategy to Deal with the Right*, Oakland, Friends of the Family n.d.; and see comments in Barrett and McIntosh, op. cit. and Barbara Epstein and Kate Ellis, 'The Pro-Family Left in the United States: Two Comments', *Feminist Review*, no. 14, Summer 1983.

32 Gusfield, *Symbolic Crusade*, pp. 171, 172.

33 Gayle Rubin, 'The Leather Menace: Comments on Politics and S/M' in Samois (ed.), *Coming to Power. Writings and Graphics on Lesbian S/M*, Berkeley, Ca, Samois, 1981.

34 For a discussion of various eighteenth-century and nineteenth-century moral panics over sex see Edward J. Bristow, *Vice and Vigilance: Purity Movements in Britain since 1700*, Dublin, Gill & Macmillan, 1977; Gusfield, op. cit., Pivar, op. cit., and Schur, op. cit.

35 I follow here the account in Stan Cohen, *Folk Devils and Moral Panics*, London, MacGibbon & Kee, 1972, p. 9. For a powerful account of the political effects of moral panic see Georges Lefebvre, *The Great Fear of 1789, Rural Panics in Revolutionary France*, London, New Left Books, 1973; and for their contemporary significance, Stuart Hall et al., *Policing the Crisis*, London, Macmillan, 1978.

36 Altman, op. cit., p. 214.

37 Susan Sontag, *Illness as Metaphor*, New York, Farrer, Strauss & Giroux, 1978, London, Allen Lane, 1979; *New Republic*, 4 August 1983.

38 *New York Times*, 3 July 1981. The most comprehensive coverage has been in the gay press, especially *New York Native*. See the summary of the information as of mid-1983 in Jonathan Lieberson, 'Anatomy of an Epidemic', *New York Review of Books*, vol. XXX, no. 13, 18 August 1983; and Kevin M. Cahill (ed.), *The AIDS Epidemic*, New York, St Martin's Press, 1983.

39 *New York*, 31 May 1982.

40 Harry Coen, 'AIDS scare now becomes a phobia', *Sunday Times* (London), 14 August 1983, p. 4. See also Duncan Fallowell, 'AIDS is here', *The Times*, 27 July 1983. *The Times*, 21 November 1984, delivered its opinion that gay promiscuity was to blame. This reflected a moral panic in the British press; see especially newspapers for February 1985, *passim*.

41 Joe Dolce, 'The Politics of Fear: Haitians and AIDS', *New York Native*, 1–14 August 1983, p. 16.

42 Norman Podhoretz, *Breaking Ranks*, New York, Harper, 1979, p. 363.

43 Nathan Fain, 'Is our "lifestyle" hazardous to our health? Part II', *The Advocate*, 1 April 1982, p. 19.

44 'Sexual Choice, Sexual Act: An Interview with Michel Foucault', *Salmagundi*, no. 58–59, Fall 1982–Winter 1983, p. 20.

45 See Gayle Rubin, 'The Leather Menace', op. cit., p. 201, for a discussion of the documentary.

46 Midge Decter, 'The Boys on the Beach', published in *Commen-*

tary, and quoted in Gore Vidal, *Pink Triangle and Yellow Star, and other Essays*, London, Heinemann, 1982, p. 180.

47 *New York Post*, 24 May 1983.

48 Reported in *New York Native*, 1–14 August 1983, p. 9, as having been said at a 12 July news conference.

49 Judith R. Walkowitz, *Prostitution and Victorian Society: Women, Class and the State*, Cambridge, London, New York, Cambridge University Press, 1980, part II.

50 Konstantin Berlandt, quoted in *The Observer* (London), 26 June 1983. 'Social-psychological and moral containment' is the first of 8 'modes of containment' described by Schur (*The Politics of Deviance*, pp. 90ff). The others are interpersonal containment (shunning), economic containment (job discrimination), poverty, ghettoisation of work opportunities), visual containment; geographical containment and physical containment. Only the Falwell lunatic fringe hopefully goes to this extreme.

51 Nathan Fain, 'More on AIDS', *The Advocate*, 26 May 1983, p. 20.

52 Sontag, *Illness as Metaphor*, p. 18. On 'Machoisation' see Gregg Blachford, 'Male dominance and the gay world' in Kenneth Plummer (ed.), *The Making of the Modern Homosexual*.

53 Larry Kramer, '1,112 AND COUNTING', *New York Native*, no. 59, 14–27 March 1983, pp. 1, *et seq*. See also Bill Lewis, 'The real gay epidemic: Panic and paranoia', *Body Politic*, November 1982, pp. 38–40.

54 Michael L. Callen, letter, *Body Politic*, April 1983, p. 6.

55 Ken Popert, 'Public sexuality and social space', *Body Politic*, July/August 1982, p. 30.

56 Michael Lynch, 'Living with Kaposi's', *Body Politic*, November 1982, p. 31. See also Charles Shively, 'Are you ready to Die for Sexual Liberation', *Fag Rag*, no. 40, 1983, p. 1.

57 Arnie Kantrowitz, 'Till death us do part? Reflections on community', *The Advocate*, 17 March 1983, p. 26.

58 Ibid., p. 56.

59 Quoted in *Body Politic*, July/August 1983, p. 19. *The Advocate* reflected the new preoccupation by starting a regular health column, 26 May 1983: see Ken Charles, 'Shape up', p. 59. He suggests that exercise is as good as promiscuous sex in achieving a sense of well-being.

60 This threefold division is suggested by John Ellis, 'Pornography', *Screen*, Summer 1980.

61 Jane Caplan, review of *Sex, Politics and Society*, *Feminist Review*, no. 11, Summer 1982, p. 103.

62 Home Office, Scottish Home Department, *Report of the Committee on Homosexual Offences and Prostitution*, Cmnd 247,

London, HMSO, 1957. There is a discussion of its implications
in Weeks, *Sex, Politics and Society*, pp. 239–44. See also the debate following the publication of the *Report of the Committee on
Obscenity and Film Censorship* in 1979, which was in the Wolfenden mould: Beverley Brown, 'Private Faces in Public Places',
I & C, no. 7, Autumn 1980 discusses this. On the separation of
private and public see Richard Sennett, *The Fall of Public Man*,
Cambridge University Press, 1976; Marshall Coleman, *Continuing Excursions: Politics and Personal Life*, London, Pluto Press,
1982; Elie Zaretsky, *Capitalism, The Family and Personal Life*,
London, Pluto Press, 1976.

63 Ernesto Laclau and Chantal Mouffe, 'Socialist Strategy: where
next?', *Marxism Today*, January 1981.

Chapter 4 'Nature had nothing to do with it'

1 Havelock Ellis, *Psychology of Sex*, London, William Heinemann,
1946 (first published 1933), p. 3; Michel Foucault, *The History of
Sexuality*, vol. 1, *An Introduction*.

2 Richard von Krafft-Ebing, *Psychopathia Sexualis. A Medico-Forensic Study, with especial reference to the Antipathic Sexual Instinct*, Brooklyn, New York, Physicians and Surgeons Book Com-
pany, 1931 (English adaptation of the 12th German edition of
1906), 'Preface to the First Edition', p. v.; Alfred C. Kinsey, Wardell B. Pomeroy, Clyde E. Martin, *Sexual Behavior in the Human
Male*, Philadelphia and London, W.B. Saunders, 1948, p. 21. Magnus Hirschfeld, perhaps the presiding genius of the political and
organisational aspects of early sexology, attributes the main im-
petus to the development of sexology c. 1900 as stemming from
the impact of three works, Havelock Ellis's *Studies in the
Psychology of Sex*, August Forel's *The Sexual Question* and Iwan
Bloch's *Sexual Life of Our Time*: see Hirschfeld's 'Presidential
Address: The Development of Sexology' in World League for
Sexual Reform, *Proceedings of the Third Sexual Reform Con-
gress*, ed. Norman Haire, London, Kegan Paul, 1930. For an
'over-view' of sex research see: Edward Brecher, *The Sex Re-
searchers*, Boston, Little, Brown, 1969; and Edward Sagarin, 'Sex
Research and Sociology: Retrospective and Prospective' in James
M. Henslin and Edward Sagarin (eds), *The Sociology of Sex: An
Introductory Reader*, New York, Schocken Books, 1978.

3 Krafft-Ebing, *Psychopathia Sexualis*; August Forel, *The Sexual
Question, A Scientific Psychological, Hygienic and Sociological
Study for the Cultured Classes*, New York, Robman, 1908, Pre-
face to first edition.

4 *Psychopathia Sexualis*, p. vi. For examples of the responses of early sociologists to sexology see Mike Brake (ed.), *Human Sexual Relations. A Reader in Human Sexuality*, Harmondsworth, Penguin Books, 1982, pp. 35ff.

5 See Foucault, *The History of Sexuality*, vol. 1.

6 *The Kama Sutra of Vortsyayana*, translated by Sir Richard Burton and F.F. Arbuthnot, edited with a Preface by W.G. Archer, introduction by K.M. Panikkar, London, George Allen & Unwin, 1963, Dedication.

7 The three published volumes of Foucault's *The History of Sexuality* are the most powerful evocation of the Christian influence in constructing the 'Man of desire'.

8 S. Tissot, *On Onania or a Treatise Upon the Disorders Produced by Masturbation* first published in Lausanne in 1758, and in London in 1760; see Richard Sennett's discussion in Michel Foucault and Richard Sennett, 'Sexuality and Solitude', R. Dworkin et al., *Humanities in Review*, vol. 1, New York and Cambridge, New York Institute for the Humanities, and Cambridge University Press, 1982, pp. 16-21. See also G.B. Boucé, *Sexuality in Eighteenth-century Britain*, Manchester University Press, 1982. On the general situation see Henri F. Ellenberger, *The Discovery of the Unconscious. The History and Evolution of Dynamic Psychiatry*, New York, Basic Books, 1970, pp. 291-303, who also discusses the Christian literature.

9 See E.H. Hare, 'Masturbatory Insanity: The History of an Idea', *The Journal of Mental Science*, vol. 108, no. 452, Jan. 1962; Robert H. MacDonald, 'The Frightful Consequences of Onanism. Notes on the History of a Delusion', *Journal of the History of Ideas*, vol. XXVIII, no. July-September 1967; R.P. Neuman, 'Masturbation, Madness and the Modern Concepts of Childhood and Adolescence', *Journal of Social History*, Spring 1975.

10 Kinsey et al., *Sexual Behavior in the Human Male*, p. 202.

11 Henricus Kaan, *Psychopathia Sexualis* (ipsiae voss 1844). See Ellenberger, op. cit., p. 296ff. On childhood sexuality see Stephen Kern, 'Freud and the Discovery of Child Sexuality', *History of Childhood Quarterly*, vol. 1, 1973, pp. 117-41. Youth sex was debated in some dozen publications between 1870 and 1905. For a summary to, and overview of, the debate see Albert Moll, *The Sexual Life of the Child*, London, George Allen & Unwin, 1912. Chapter I explored contemporary researches.

12 Karl Heinrich Ulrichs, *Forschungen über das Ratsel der Mann Mannlichen Liebe*, 12 volumes in one, New York, Arno Press, 1975, originally Leipzig, 1898; see Hubert C. Kennedy, 'The

"Third Sex" Theory of Karl Heinrich Ulrichs' in Salvatore J. Licata and Robert P. Petersen (eds), *Historical Perspectives on Homosexuality*, New York, The Haworth Press and Stein & Day, 1981 (hardback version of *Journal of Homosexuality*, vol. 6, no. 5, 1/2, Fall/Winter 1980–81), pp. 103–11. Carl Westphal, 'Die Conträre Sexualempfindung', *Archiv für Psychiatrie*, vol. 11, 1870, pp. 73–108. Krafft-Ebing, *Psychopathia Sexualis*.

13 Charles Darwin, *On the Origin of Species by Means of Natural Selection, or, The Preservation of Favoured Races in the Struggles for Life*, London, John Murray, 1859; *The Descent of Man, and Selection in Relation to Sex*, 2 vols, London, John Murray, 1871, revised and enlarged edition 1874. For commentaries on the importance of Darwin's work see: Rosalind Coward, *Patriarchal Precedents: Sexuality and Social Relations*, London, Routledge & Kegan Paul, 1983, pp. 76–8, Janet Sayers, *Biological Politics, Feminist and Anti-Feminist Perspectives*, London and New York, Tavistock, pp. 31–3, Frank J. Sulloway, *Freud, Biologist of the Mind*, London, Burnett Books, 1979, pp. 238–76.

14 Sulloway, *Freud, Biologist of the Mind*, p. 283; Magnus Hirschfeld, *Sexual Anomalies and Perversions, Physical and Psychological Development and Treatment. A Summary of the Works of the Professor Dr. Magnus Hirschfeld, Compiled as a Humble Memorial by his Pupils*, London, Torch, 1948, p. 226.

15 Sigmund Freud, 'Three Essays on the Theory of Sexuality' in James Strachey (ed.), *The Standard Edition of the Complete Psychological Works of Sigmund Freud*, 24 vols, 1953–74, London, Hogarth Press and The Institute of Psychoanalysis (hereafter *S.E*), vol. 7.

16 See Iwan Bloch, *Beiträge zur Aetiologie der Psychopathia Sexualis*, 2 vols, Dresden, H.R. Dohm, 1902–3; Charles Féré, *L'Instinct sexuel: Evolution et dissolution*, Paris, Felix Alcan, 1899; Albert Moll, *Perversions of the Sex Instinct*, Newark, N.J., Julian Press, 1933 (original German 1891) and *Libido Sexualis—Studies in the Psychosexual Laws of Love*, New York, American Ethnological Press, 1933 (original 1897); Hirschfeld, *Sexual Anomalies and Perversions* for a summary of his views and Magnus Hirschfeld, *Sex in Human Relationships*, London, John Lane the Bodley Head, 1935, for an autobiographical survey of his life and work; and Havelock Ellis, *Studies in the Psychology of Sex*, Philadelphia, F.A. Davis, 1905–10, 1928, with a summary of his views in *Psychology of Sex*, 1933.

17 Havelock Ellis, *Man and Woman*, London, Walter Scott, 1894. Robert Latou Dickinson, *Human Sexual Anatomy*, Baltimore,

Williams and Wilkins, 1949 (1st edition 1933) was an early compilation of data on 'normal' sexuality.

18 *Psychopathia Sexualis*, p. 1.

19 On this see Jonathan Ned Katz, *Gay/Lesbian Almanac*, New York, Harper & Row, 1983, General Introduction.

20 Wardell B. Pomeroy, *Dr. Kinsey and the Institute for Sex Research*, New York, Harper & Row, 1972, pp. 68–70. See also Kinsey, *Sexual Behavior in the Human Male*, p. 34.

21 For a discussion on Ellis see my essay in Sheila Rowbotham and Jeffrey Weeks, *Socialism and the New Life*, pp. 139–85, and my discussion in *Sex, Politics and Society*, pp. 148–52. See also Vincent Brome, *Havelock Ellis: Philosopher of Sex*, London, Routledge & Kegan Paul, 1979, who discusses the Ellis-Freud relationship in chapter 17, and Phyllis Grosskurth, *Havelock Ellis: A Biography*, London, Allen Lane, 1980.

22 Kinsey, *Sexual Behavior in the Human Male*, p. 41. See also his comments about the need to accumulate 'scientific fact completely divorced from questions of moral value and social custom' (p. 3).

23 Kenneth Plummer, *Sexual Stigma. An Interactionist Account*, London, Routledge & Kegan Paul, 1975, p. 4. For a clear statement of the deep-seated belief in the continuous evolution to objectivity and pure science in sex research see Ira L. Reiss, 'Personal Values and the Scientific Study of Sex' in Hugo G. Beigel (ed.), *Advances in Sex Research. A Publication of the Society for the Scientific Study of Sex*, New York, Holber Medical Division, Harper & Row, 1963, p. 3: 'One of the most recent and most crucial advances in the study of human sexual relations is the emerging development of an impartial and objective approach'.

24 Katz, *Gay/Lesbian Almanac*, p. 156.

25 Hirschfeld, *Sex in Human Relationships*, p. xx. On Hirschfeld's works see James Steakley, *The Homosexual Emancipation Movement in Germany*, New York, Arno Press, 1975. For a brief discussion of the World League see my *Sex, Politics and Society*, pp. 184–6.

26 See Rowbotham and Weeks, *Socialism and the New Life*.

27 Kinsey, *Sexual Behavior in the Human Male*, p. 224

28 G. Bachelard, *L'Activité Rationaliste de la physique contemporaine*, Paris, PUF, 2nd edn 1965.

29 The following is drawn from chapter 2 of my *Sex, Politics and Society*.

30 Michel Foucault, *The History of Sexuality*, vol. 1.

31 *The History of Sexuality*, vol. 1, p. 146. Charles Webster notes the English concern with population throughout the nineteenth century in Webster (ed.), *Biology, Medicine and Society, 1840-*

1940, Cambridge University Press, 1981, p. 4, and points to a piquant coincidence, the introduction of civil registration of births, marriages and deaths occurred within a year of Charles Darwin's first notebook on the transmutation of species. Concern with population and species being marched together.

32 See notes 9 and 11 above. Also G. Stanley Hall, *Adolescence: Its Psychology, and its Relation to Physiology, Anthropology, Sociology, Sex Crimes, Religion and Education*, 2 vols, New York, D. Appleton, 1904.

33 See particularly the discussions in Ellis's *Man and Woman*, and in *Studies in the Psychology of Sex*, vol. 1. *The Evolution of Modesty, the Phenomena of Sexual Periodicity and Auto-Erotism*, 1st published Philadelphia, F.A. Davis, 1900, 3rd revised edn 1927.

34 See the discussion of Wilhelm Fliess, Freud's early mentor and early theorist of bisexuality, in Sulloway, *Freud, Biologist of the Mind*, pp. 135ff. See also discussion of Freud on bisexuality below. On transvestism, see Magnus Hirschfeld, *Die Transvestiten: Eine Untersuchung über den Erotischen Verkleidungstrieb*, Berlin, 1910; and Havelock Ellis, *Studies in the Psychology of Sex*, vol. VII, *Eonism and other supplementary studies*, Philadelphia, F.A. Davis, 1928.

35 *Psychopathia Sexualis*, p. vii. All the early sexologists dealt with homosexuality, though Hirschfeld's work was the most substantial contribution. See *Die Homosexualität des Mannes und des Weibes*, Berlin, Louis Marcus, 1914; also Ellis, *Sexual Inversion*, Watford University Press, 1897, later vol. II of *Studies in the Psychology of Sex*. For a committed discussion by a homosexual see Edward Carpenter, *The Intermediate Sex*, London, George Allen & Unwin, 1908; Sulloway, *Freud*, pp. 309–12 discusses the conceptual shifts involved in breaking from the degeneration model. By the early part of this century the congenital model was dominant, signified by a shift in Krafft-Ebing's accounts—though differences persisted over the nature of this congenitality.

36 Havelock Ellis, *Psychology of Sex*, p. 1. On his connection with eugenics see his *The Task of Social Hygiene*, London, Constable, 1912.

37 Ellenberger, *The Discovery of the Unconscious*, p. 298.

38 For a brief but suggestive discussion of this see Jane Caplan, 'Review' of *Sex, Politics and Society*, *Feminist Review*, no. 11, pp. 101–104.

39 *Psychopathia Sexualis*, p. vii.

40 See Rowbotham and Weeks, *Socialism and the New Life*, pp. 154–5; Grosskurth, *Havelock Ellis*, chapters 12 and 13. The English

translation of Iwan Bloch, *The Sexual Life of Our Time in its relations to modern civilisation* (London, Robman, 1908) explicitly addressed itself to a lay public (Prefatory note by its translator M. Eden Paul). It consequently was forced to confront public controversy. On Edward Carpenter's difficulties see my *Coming Out: Homosexual Politics in Britain from the Nineteenth Century to the Present*, London, Quartet, 1977, chapter 6.

41 Katz, *Gay/Lesbian Almanac*, p. 510.

42 Ibid., p. 156.

43 Pomeroy, *Alfred Kinsey*, p. 262; the subsequent reference is on p. 275.

44 Ruth and Edward Brecher (eds), *An Analysis of Human Sexual Response*, London, Andre Deutsch, 1967, p. 42. See William H. Masters and Virginia E. Johnson, *Homosexuality in Perspective*, Boston, Little, Brown, p. 6, where they note the 'extreme social and professional pressures to discontinue the research programs that existed during the original heterosexual study'—though these had been 'markedly reduced' by the start of the homosexual study in the 1960s.

45 Ernest Jones, *The Life and Work of Sigmund Freud*, vol. 1, New York, Basic Books, 1981, p. 27.

46 See Michel Foucault, *The Birth of the Clinic: An Archeology of Medical Perception*, New York, Vintage Books, 1975. See also Georges Canguilhem on the significance of medical normalisation: *Le Normal et le pathologique*, Paris, PUF, 1972. Foucault, 'Georges Canguilhem: Philosopher of Error' and Colin Gordon, 'The normal and the biological: a note on Georges Canguilhem', *Ideology and Consciousness*, no. 7, Autumn 1980; and Mike Shortland, 'Disease as a way of Life', *Ideology and Consciousness*, no. 9, Autumn 1981.

47 See F.P. Cobbe, 'The Little Health of Ladies', *Contemporary Review*, January 1878, when she argues that the medical profession occupies 'the position of the priesthood of former times'. For a discussion of the role of the medical profession in England see Jean L'Esperance, 'Doctors and Women in Nineteenth Century Society: Sexuality and Role'; in John Woodward and David Richards, *Health Care and Popular Medicine in Nineteenth Century England*, London, Croom Helm, 1977; Lorna Duffin, 'The Conspicuous Consumptive: Woman as an Invalid' in Sara Delamont and Lorna Duffin (eds), *The Nineteenth Century Woman. Her Cultural and Physical World*, London, Croom Helm, 1978; Brian Harrison, 'Women's Health and the Women's Movement in Britain: 1840–1940' in Charles Webster (ed.), *Biology, Medicine and Society*; on the United States experience see Carroll Smith-

Rosenberg, 'The Hysterical Woman: Sex Roles and Role Conflict in Nineteenth Century America', *Social Research*, no. 39, 1972, Charles Rosenberg and Carroll Smith-Rosenberg, 'The Female Animal: Medical and Biological Views of Women', *Journal of American History*, no. 60, 1973, and Ann Douglas Wood, ' "The Fashionable Diseases": Women's Complaints and Their Treatment in Nineteenth Century America' in Mary S. Hartman and Lois Banner (eds), *Clio's Consciousness Raised*, New York, Harper Colophon Books, 1974.

48 Ivan Illich, *Gender*, London, Martin Robertson, 1983, pp. 123–5; Otto Weininger, *Sex and Character*, London, Heinemann, part II, chapter 2; Ellis *Studies*, vol. 3, part 1, p. vi.

49 Kenneth Plummer, *Sexual Stigma*, p. 4.

50 Weeks, *Sex, Politics and Society*, p. 212.

51 William H. Masters and Virginia E. Johnson, *Human Sexual Response*, Boston, Little, Brown, 1966.

52 See for example Sagarin, 'Sex Research and Sociology'; and Laud Humphreys, *Tearoom Trade*, 'Postscript: A Question of Ethics', London, Duckworth, 1970. See also the discussion about methods in Kinsey et al., *Sexual Behavior in the Human Male*; and Alfred Kinsey, Wardell B. Pomeroy, Clyde E. Martin, Paul H. Gebhard, *Sexual Behavior in the Human Female*, Philadelphia and London, W.B. Saunders, 1953. For contemporary sociological approaches see J.H. Gagnon and William Simon, *Sexual Conduct. The Social Sources of Human Sexuality*, London, Hutchinson, 1974; John H. Gagnon, *Human Sexualities*, Glenview, Illinois, Scott, Foresman, 1977.

53 *Psychology of Sex*, p. 3.

54 Ibid., p. 7. See Sulloway, *Freud*, p. 261, for early discussion on origins of sexuality.

55 Krafft-Ebing, *Psychopathia Sexualis*, p. 25, Ellis, *Psychology of Sex*, pp. 302–3.

56 *Psychopathia Sexualis*, p. 2.

57 Michel Foucault and Richard Sennett, 'Sexuality and Solitude', in Dworkin et al., *Humanities in Review*, vol. 1, p. 13; Katz, *Gay/Lesbian Almanac*, p. 71.

58 Kinsey, *Sexual Behavior in the Human Male*, p. 269.

59 See Ronald Fletcher, *Instincts in Man. In the light of Recent Work in Comparative Psychology*, London, George Allen & Unwin, 1957.

60 'Ontogeny' repeats 'phylogeny': this was crucial to Freud's work—see below. But it was not unique. See Ernst Haeckel, *The Evolution of Man*, vol. 1, *Human Embryology, or Ontogeny*, vol. 2. *Human Stem—History, or Phylogeny*, London, Watts,

1906 (translation of 5th revised edn; 1st published 1874), for the original formulation. It was common ground among early sexologists. See Charles Samson Féré, *Sexual Degeneration in Mankind and in Animals*, New York, Anthropological Press, 1932, p. 14 (first English edition 1904): 'Every animal in its embryonic period sums up the history of the evolution of the race', and Forel, *The Sexual Question*, p. 192. See Sulloway, *Freud*, p. 274 for the implications of this neo-Lamarckianism.

61 See the description of the significance of this, especially with regard to the development of eugenics, in my *Sex, Politics and Society*, chapter 7. For the implications of Mendelism see Ruth Hubbard's 'The Theory and Practice of Genetic Reductionism— From Mendel's Laws to Genetic Engineering' in The Dialectics of Biology Group (General Editor Steven Rose), *Towards a Liberatory Biology*, London, Allison & Busby, 1982.

62 See Fletcher, *Instincts*, pp. 71, 91. See references in note 9, p. 156, *Sex, Politics and Society*. The subtle changes in definition become apparent if we examine two editions of the English translation of Féré's *L'Instinct Sexuel*. The first English version of 1904 (*The Evolution and Dissolution of the Sexual Instinct*, Paris, Charles Carrington) defined instinct as 'characterised by a definite hereditary activity, which is not acquired by personal experience; it thus differs from habit, which is the result of individual acquisition'.

The 1932 edition, translated as *Sexual Degeneration in Mankind and in Animals*, has the following (my emphasis): 'Instinct is *popularly believed to be* some definite hereditary activity, which is not acquired by any personal experience, and so differs from habit, which is the result of individual acquisition. But further research proved it to be a tendency to act in some fixed way, guided by trial and error.'

63 Ellis summarises the debate in *Studies in the Psychology of Sex*, vol. 3, *Analysis of the Sexual Impulse*, Philadelphia, F.A. Davis, pp. 1ff.

64 Masters and Johnson's four-fold pattern of sexual response for men and women rediscovered Moll's four phases in his *Sexual Life of the Child*. His 'ascending climb, the equable voluptuous sensation, the acme, and the rapid decline' appeared more prosaicly in *Human Sexual Response* as the excitement phase, the plateau, the orgasm and the resolution.

65 Krafft-Ebing, *Psychopathia Sexualis*, p. 25.

66 Jill Conway, 'Stereotypes of Femininity in a Theory of Sexual Evolution' in Martha Vicinus (ed.), *Suffer and Be Still*, Bloomington, University of Indiana Press, 1977, p. 14. See also Janet Sayers, *Biological Politics*.

67 Patrick Geddes and J.A. Thomson, *The Evolution of Sex*, London, Contemporary Science Series, 1st edn, 1889, and Geddes and Thomson, *Sex*, London, 1914. For Ellis's analogous views see *Sex, Politics and Society*, pp. 148–52. Jane Lewis has pointed out to me that Geddes and Thomson's views were still in circulation in the 1940s, when Simone de Beauvoir found it necessary to criticise them.

68 Geddes and Thomson, *Sex*, pp. 148, 162, 185. See a similar discussion in my *Sex, Politics and Society*, pp. 144–5. Compare Bloch, *Sexual Life of our Times*, p. 14: 'it is only for normal heterosexual love between a normal man and a normal woman that it is possible to find any unimpeachable sanction'.

69 Kinsey et al., *Sexual Behavior in the Human Male*, p. 567.

70 Geddes and Thomson, *Sex*, p. 203.

71 Lynda Birke, 'Cleaving the Mind: Speculations on Conceptual Dichotomies' in Dialectics of Biology Group (General Editor Steven Rose), *Against Biological Determinism*, London, Allison & Busby 1982, p. 72.

72 Ludmilla Jordanova, 'Natural facts: a historical perspective on science and reality', in Carol MacCormack and Marilyn Strathern (eds), *Nature, Culture and Gender*, Cambridge University Press, 1980, p. 44.

73 Frank Mort, 'The Domain of the Sexual', *Screen Education*, no. 36, Autumn 1980, pp. 69–84, and Lucy Bland, 'The Domain of the Sexual: A Response', *Screen Education*, no. 39, Summer 1981, pp. 56–67. For a discussion of the nature/culture, male/female divide see: MacCormack and Strathern, *Nature, Culture and Gender*; a review of this work by Beverley Brown, 'Displacing the Difference', *M/F*, no. 8, 1983; Carolyn Merchant, *The Death of Nature*, New York, Wildwood, 1982; and a review of this by Lynda Birke, *New Scientist*, 25 Nov. 1982, pp. 516–17.

74 An overview of the literature on this issue can be found in Daniel G. Brown, 'Female Orgasm and Sexual Inadequacy' in Ruth and Edward Brecher, *An Analysis of Human Sexual Response*. As the article suggests denials of female orgasmic potential or of clitoral sexuality were by no means universal; but then interest was not high. He states (p. 127): 'In a span of thirty-six years from 1928–1963 the number of specific references to female orgasm in *Psychological Abstracts* was under thirty, an average of less than one per year, and the number of references to female frigidity was under forty, an average of about one per year.'

75 E. Bergler and W.S. Kroger, *Kinsey's Myth of Female Sexuality*, New York, Grune & Stratton, 1954, quoted in Brown, op. cit., p. 137. See also E. Bergler, 'Frigidity in the Female: Misconcep-

tions and Facts', *Marriage Hygiene*, vol. 1, 1947, pp. 16–21; 'The Problem of Frigidity', *Psychiatric Quarterly*, vol. 18, 1944, pp. 374–90. A more balanced view can be found in Helena Wright, 'A Contribution to the Orgasm Problem in Women' in A.P. Pillay and Albert Ellis (eds), *Sex, Society and the Individual*, Bombay, International Journal of Sexology Publication, 1953. Ironically, in view of Bergler's criticisms, Kinsey was himself busy pathologising the sexually frustrated single woman: Kinsey et al., *Sexual Behavior in the Human Female*, pp. 526–7.

76 *Sexual Behavior in the Human Male*, p. 7.

77 The following discussion is based on: Weeks, *Coming Out*, and chapter 6, 'The Construction of Homosexuality' in *Sex, Politics and Society*; the essays in Kenneth Plummer (ed.), *The Making of the Modern Homosexual*, London, Hutchinson, 1981, especially Mary McIntosh, 'The Homosexual Role' and my own 'Discourse, Desire and Sexual Deviance'; Michel Foucault, *The History of Sexuality*, vol. 1; Katz, *Gay/Lesbian Almanac* and his earlier *Gay American History*, New York, Thomas Crowell, 1976.

78 Plummer, *Sexual Stigma*, p. 97; Kinsey et al., *Sexual Behavior in the Human Male*, pp. 638–41; Alan P. Bell and Martin S. Weinberg, *Homosexualities: A Study of Diversity among Men and Women*, London, Mitchell Beazley, 1979, pp. 132–8.

79 *Psychology of Sex*, p. 126. Kinsey et al., *Sexual Behavior in the Human Male*, p. 638.

80 See footnote 77 above, to which general accounts should be added a host of specialised studies, especially on homosexual subcultures: John Boswell, *Christianity, Social Tolerance and Homosexuality*, Chicago and London, University of Chicago Press, 1980; Alan Bray, *Homosexuality in Renaissance England*, London, Gay Men's Press, 1983; Randolph Trumbach, 'London's Sodomites: Homosexual Behaviour and Western Culture in the 18th Century', *Journal of Social History*, vol. 11, no. 1, Fall 1977–78; Lillian Faderman, *Surpassing the Love of Men*, London, Junction Books, 1982; and the Lesbian History number of *Frontiers: A Journal of Women's Studies*, vol. V, no. 3, Fall 1979.

81 Faderman, and Carroll Smith-Rosenberg, 'The Female World of Love and Ritual', *Signs*, vol. 1, no. 1, 1975, argue for the absence of a distinct lesbian identity in the nineteenth century. But see the critique of Faderman by Sonja Ruehl, *History Workshop Journal*, no. 14, Autumn 1982, pp. 157–9. On the male identity my argument in *Coming Out* that the late nineteenth century was a crucial period in the emergence of a male homosexual identity has been challenged by Bray, pp. 134–7. The issue is exhaustively discussed in the proceedings of the conference on 'Homosocial

and Homosexual Arrangements', University of Amsterdam, June 1983.

82 Foucault, *The History of Sexuality*, vol. 1; Faderman, *Surpassing the Love of Men*.

83 Boswell and Trumbach appear to see a continuous homosexual subculture during the Christian era, as if homosexuals were a distinct species with particular needs. Bray challenges this, and follows McIntosh, 'The Homosexual Role', in dating the change from sexual acts to sexual identities in distinct subcultures to the early eighteenth century in England. Katz distinguishes the 'Age of Sodomitical Sin' of the pre-eighteenth century in America from the period of 'The Invention of the Homosexual' post-1880. All agree on the different histories of male and female homosexual networks and identities.

84 Katz, *Gay/Lesbian Almanac*.

85 Kinsey et al., *Sexual Behavior in the Human Male*, p. 37.

86 See Katz, *Gay/Lesbian Almanac*, p. 354.

87 John D'Emilio makes a related point, by suggesting that though the impact of sexology on 'homosexuals' was very negative, its ostensibly scientific mode did encourage empirical research which served to undermine the model. At the same time, by treating homosexuality as an inherent quality, it actually helped people to define themselves positively around an assumed natural identity: D'Emilio, *Sexual Politics, Sexual Communities. The Making of a Homosexual Minority in the United States 1940–1970*, Chicago and London, University of Chicago Press, 1983, pp. 18–19. See also Ann Ferguson, 'On "Compulsory Heterosexuality and Lesbian Existence": Defining the Issues: Patriarchy, Sexual Identity, and the Sexual Revolution', *Signs*, vol. 7, no. 1, 1981, pp. 158–72.

88 Gayle Rubin, 'Sexual Politics, the New Right, and the Sexual Fringe', in Daniel Tsang (ed.), *The Age Taboo*, Boston, Alyson Publications, 1981, p. 109.

Chapter 5 'A never-ceasing duel'? 'Sex' in relation to 'society'

1 Havelock Ellis, *Studies in the Psychology of Sex*, vol. VI, *Sex in Relation to Society*, 1910, Philadelphia, F.A. Davis, originally the final volume of the series. (There was in fact an additional volume, *Eonism and Other Related Studies*, published in 1927.)

2 Rosalind Coward, *Patriarchal Precedents*, p. 294.

3 Krafft-Ebing, *Psychopathia Sexualis*, p. 5. Compare Charles Féré: 'there is no physiological reason why sexual instinct should not be controlled like other instincts, and that utilitarian morality and hygiene teach the necessity of restraining it': Féré, 1932, p. 305.

4 Susan Griffin, *Pornography and Silence: Culture's Revenge Against Nature*, New York, Harper & Row, 1981, p. 255. The debate on the corrupting force on sex of 'civilisation' is discussed in the Preface to V.F. Calverton and S.D. Schmalhausen, *Sex In Civilisation* (with an introduction by Havelock Ellis), London, George Allen & Unwin, 1929. For representative examples see J.J. Rousseau, *The Social Contract*, 1st published 1762, in various editions; Jonathan Beecher and Richard Bienvenu, *The Utopian Vision of Charles Fourier. Selected Texts on Work, Love and Passionate Attraction*, London, Jonathan Cape, 1975; Edward Carpenter, *Civilisation: Its Cause and Cure, and Other Essays*, London, 1889; and *Love's Coming of Age;* Freud, *Civilisation and its Discontents*, S.E. 21; see chapter 6 for a discussion of Reich and Herbert Marcuse; René Guyon, *Sex Life and Sex Ethics*, London, John Lane, 1933; and *Sexual Freedom*, London, John Lane, 1939. For a discussion of the theme see Paul Hirst and Penny Woolley, *Social Relations and Human Attributes*, London and New York, Tavistock Publications, 1982, p. 132. They make the point that this metaphysics of the 'person' is as much a vogue on the right or the left; the liberatory dialectics of, for example, a Ronald Laing in the 1960s were balanced by the conservative libertarianism of a Thomas Szasz. The libertarian theme is also of course present in a large range of other writers on sex, from Havelock Ellis to Kinsey.

5 Havelock Ellis, 'Preface' in Bronislaw Malinowski, *The Sexual Life of Savages in North-Western Melanesia*, London, Routledge & Kegan Paul, 1932, 3rd edn, p. vii. Ruth Benedict, *Patterns of Culture*, London, Routledge & Kegan Paul, 1980, first published, 1935, p. 12.

6 See the discussion in Coward, *Patriarchal Precedents*, chs 1–3.

7 See his 'special Foreword' to the third edition of *Sexual Life of Savages*, pp. xxii–xxiii, where he recants lingering evolutionism; or rather, suggests that while he does not disavow evolution, he no longer believes it useful to speculate on how things started or how they followed one another.

8 *Sexual Life of Savages*, p. xix.

9 See his discussion of the work of Edward Westermarck in 'Pioneers in the Study of Sex and Marriage' in *Sex, Culture and Myth*, London, Rupert Hart-Davis, 1963, p. 119; and his reviews of Robert Briffault's *The Mothers* and Ernest Crawley's *The Mystic Role* (first published 1902), pp. 122–9. Here he endorses (p. 125) Crawley's rejection of the doctrine of survivals, and agrees with him in postulating a basic human nature, quoting him to the effect that 'Human nature remains fundamentally

primitive', which Malinowski approves of as 'physiological thought'.

10 Malinowski endorsed Edward Westermarck's break with evolutionary theories of the family. For Westermarck the family was a natural monogamous union of men and women, paralleling that of the animal world: Edward Westermarck, *The History of Modern Marriage*, London, 5th edn 1922 (first published 1891). For Malinowski's views see *Sex, Culture and Myth*, pp. 117–18, p. 120. Havelock Ellis similarly endorsed the idea of a natural family: See Ellis, *Psychology of Sex*, p. 79: 'The substance of the family is biological but its forms are socially moulded.' For a discussion of the importance of the call on natural history to explain family history, made possible by the break-up of Henry Maine's view of the patriarchal family as a political unit, via an appropriation of Darwin, see Coward, *Patriarchal Precedents*, p. 56.

11 *Sex, Culture and Myth*, p. 116. The fullest discussion of Freud's theories is in *Sex and Repression in Savage Society*, London, Routledge & Kegan Paul, 1960, first published 1927. See ibid., p. 182: 'It will be my aim to show that the beginning of culture implies the repression of instincts, and that all the essentials of the Oedipus complex or any other "complex" are necessary by-products in the process of the gradual formation of culture.'

12 See his essay on Ellis, in *Sex, Culture and Myth*, p. 129, p. 130 and ibid., p. 167 and p. 206.

13 Ibid., p. 127.

14 *Sex and Repression*. The following discussion draws on this book.

15 Adam Kuper, *Anthropology and Anthropologists. The British School 1922–72*, Harmondsworth, Penguin Books, 1978, p. 36.

16 Benedict, *Patterns of Culture*, p. 35. Malinowski's riposte was just as sharp. He criticises Benedict and her mentor Franz Boas for being anti-determinists, averting their eyes from generalisations, and for not being scientific enough. He wrote majestically: 'Many of the younger generation are drifting into mystical pronouncements, avoiding the difficult and painstaking search for principles; they are cultivating rapid cursory field work, and developing their impressionistic results into brilliantly dramatised film effects, such as the New Guinea pictures of Dr Margaret Mead in her *Sex and Temperament* (1935)': 'Culture as a Determinant of Behaviour', *Sex, Culture and Myth*, p. 172.

17 Benedict, *Patterns of Culture*, p. 9.

18 See Derek Freeman, *Margaret Mead and Samoa. The Making and Unmaking of an Anthropological Myth*, Cambridge, Mass.,

and London, Harvard University Press, 1983, pp. 54–5, on Watson's influence; and Coward, *Patriarchal Precedents*, pp. 247–50, on the appropriation of Freud via the anthropological work of Geza Roheim. Freeman, p. 40, quotes Boas in 1911 as defining culture as a result not of innate mental qualities but 'a result of varied external conditions acting upon general human characteristics'.

19 For a discussion of eugenics in a British context see my *Sex, Politics and Society*, chapter 7; in the German context, Paul Weindling, 'Theories of the Cell State in Imperial Germany' in Charles Webster (ed.), *Biology, Medicine and Society*, pp. 99–155; and Loren R. Graham, 'Science and Values: the Eugenics Movement in Germany and Russia in the 1920s', *American Historical Review*, vol. 82, no. 5, Dec. 1977; and in the United States, Freeman, op. cit., chapter 1.

20 Margaret Mead, *Coming of Age in Samoa. A Study of Adolescence and Sex in Primitive Societies*, Harmondsworth, Penguin Books, 1977, first published 1928. See Freeman, *Margaret Mead*, pp. 96–7, for 1920s hopes of a new sexual enlightenment. For an early taking up of Mead's work by sexologists see Havelock Ellis, *Psychology of Sex*, pp. 88–9.

21 Freeman, *Margaret Mead*, an incisive academic hatchet-job. For a defence of Mead see Marilyn Strathern, 'The Punishment of Margaret Mead', *London Review of Books*, 5–18 May 1983, pp. 5–6.

22 Margaret Mead, *Sex and Temperament in Three Primitive Societies*, London, Routledge & Kegan Paul, 1948, first published 1935, pp. 279–80.

23 Margaret Mead, *Male and Female. A Study of the Sexes in a Changing World*, London, Victor Gollancz, 1949, pp. 7, 163.

24 Mead, *Sex and Temperament*, pp. 313–16.

25 *Male and Female*, chapter XVIII, the quotations are from pp. 372 and 370. On 1940s attitudes to the family see my *Sex, Politics and Society*, chapter 11.

26 *Male and Female*, p. 194.

27 Coward, *Patriarchal Precedents*, pp. 116, 130.

28 On this theme see Coward, *Patriarchal Precedents*, p. 124; Hirst and Woolley, *Social Relations and Human Attributes*, pp. 138; and pp. 178–9 above.

29 There are obvious affinities between the anthropologists enwrapping themselves in primitive cultures and modern investigators 'down there on a visit' in contemporary sexual subcultures. See John H. Gagnon and William Simon, *The Sexual Scene*, New Brunswick, N.J., Transaction Books, 1973.

30 A point made by Dominique Lecourt, 'Biology and the Crisis of the Human Sciences', *New Left Review*, no. 125, Jan.–Feb. 1981, pp. 90–6.

31 Janna L. Thompson, 'Human Nature and Social Explanation' in The Dialectics of Biology Group (General Editor Steven Rose), *Against Biological Determinism*, London and New York, Allison & Busby, 1982, p. 31.

32 E.O. Wilson, *Sociobiology: The New Synthesis*, Cambridge, Mass., and London, The Belknap Press of Harvard University Press, 1975.

33 David Barash, *Sociobiology: The Whisperings Within*, London, Fontana, 1981, p. 240; E.O. Wilson, *On Human Nature*, Cambridge, Harvard University Press, 1978.

34 See Richard Dawkins, *The Selfish Gene*, St Albans, Granada, 1978, p. 12.

35 The award of the Nobel Prize for Medicine to Lorenz, Tinbergen and Karl von Frisch in 1973 has been seen as the 'coming of age' of ethology; Lecourt, op. cit., p. 92. On the emergence of the 'Modern synthesis' in biology see E.O. Wilson, *Sociobiology*, pp. 63–4; Ronald Fletcher, *Instinct in Man*, pp. 111ff., 279; John R. Durant, 'Innate Character in Animals and Man: A perspective on the Origins of Ethology' and Daniel J. Kerles, 'Genetics in the United States and Great Britain 1890–1930: A Review with Speculations' in Charles Webster (ed.), *Biology, Medicine and Society*.

36 Konrad Lorenz, *Studies in Animal and Human Behaviour*, London, Methuen, vol. I, 1970, vol. II, 1971; N. Tinbergen, *The Study of Instinct*, Oxford, Clarendon Press, 1969, first published 1951, and *Social Behaviour in Animals*, London, Methuen, 1953.

37 Desmond Morris, *The Naked Ape*, London, 1967; Konrad Lorenz, *On Aggression*, London, Methuen, 1966; Robert Ardrey, *The Social Contract*, London, Collins, 1970; and *The Territorial Imperative*, London, Collins, 1967; Lionel Tiger and Robin Fox, *The Imperial Animal*, New York, Holt, Rinehart & Winston, 1971; and Lionel Tiger, *Men in Groups*, New York, Random House, 1969.

38 Wilson, *Sociobiology*, p. 551.

39 Barash, *Sociobiology*, p. 159.

40 E.O. Wilson, *On Human Nature*, p. 3. For a more cautious statement see Glenn Wilson, *Love and Instinct*, London, Temple Smith, 1981, p. 9.

41 Charles Darwin, *On the Origin of Species*, London, Watts, 1950, p. 290.

42 Wilson, *Sociobiology*, p. 3.

43 Dawkins, *The Selfish Gene*, p. 7, p. x. Sociobiologists are less definite on what exactly is a 'gene'. Dawkins (p. 30) notes that there is no universally agreed definition of a gene. Wilson, *On Human Nature*, p. 216, makes a brave attempt at definition: 'A basic unit of heredity, a portion of the giant DNA molecules that affects the development of any trait at the most elementary biochemical level. The term gene is often applied more precisely to the cistron, the section of DNA that carries the codes for the formulation of a particular portion of a protein molecule.'

44 R.L. Trivers, Foreword to Dawkins, p. vii.

45 H.J. Eysenck and G.D. Wilson, *The Psychology of Sex*, London, Dent, 1979, p. 43.

46 E.O. Wilson, *Sociobiology*, p. 314.

47 E.O. Wilson, *On Human Nature*, p. 122; *Sociobiology*, p. 316.

48 Eysenck and Wilson, *The Psychology of Sex*, p. 9.

49 Steven Goldberg, response to E. Leacock's review of *The Inevitability of Patriarchy*, in Eleanor Leacock, *Myths of Male Dominance. Collected Articles on Women Cross Culturally*, New York and London, Monthly Review Press, 1981, p. 9. (Goldberg's *The Inevitability of Patriarchy*, London, Temple Smith, 1977, takes sociobiological arguments to their logical anti-feminist conclusion); Wilson, *On Human Nature*, pp. 129, 132, 133, *Sociobiology*, p. 553.

50 Donald Symons, *The Evolution of Human Sexuality*, Oxford University Press, 1979, p. v. For a critical appraisal of this work see Clifford Geertz, 'Sociosexuality', *New York Review of Books*, 24 January 1980, pp. 3–4.

51 Symons, op. cit. pp. 286ff.

52 Lynda Birke, 'Cleaving the Mind' in *Against Biological Determinism*, p. 64. See also John Money, *Love and Love Sickness. The Science of Sex, Gender Difference and Pair-Bonding*, Baltimore and London, Johns Hopkins University Press, 1980, p. 133. For a recent synthesis of evidence see John Archer and Barbara Lloyd, *Sex and Gender*, Harmondsworth, Penguin, 1982.

53 R.C. Lewontin, 'Sociobiology: Another Biological Determinism', *International Journal of Health Services*, vol. 10, no. 3, 1980.

54 Marshall Sahlins, *The Use and Abuse of Biology: An Anthropological Critique of Sociobiology*, London, Tavistock, 1976, p. 75.

55 E.O. Wilson, *On Human Nature*, p. 38.

56 Tiger and Fox, *The Imperial Animal*. On this theme see Joan Smith, 'Sociobiology and Feminism. The very strange courtship of competing paradigms', *The Philosophical Forum*, vol. XIII, nos 2–3, Winter–Spring 1981-2, pp. 226–43.

57 Barash, *Sociobiology*, pp. 231ff; Glenn Wilson, *Love and Instinct*,

p. 18. See Joan Smith, op. cit., p. 235, for the desire of E.O. Wilson and his followers to have it both ways: 'he can deplore sexism or racism but at the same time warn of possible dire consequences that may attend their eradication.'

58 For a particularly extreme, neo-fascist use of sociobiology see Richard Verrall, 'Technique of the "Race Equality" Charlatans', *Spearhead*, no. 113, January 1978; 'Karl Marx's Piltdown Men', no. 114, February 1978; and 'Sociobiology: the instincts in our genes', March 1979. *Spearhead* was the magazine of the British National Front, a neo-Nazi party.

59 Barash, *Sociobiology*, p. 239. See Donna Haraway, 'The Biological Enterprise: Sex, Mind and Profit from Human Engineering to Sociobiology', *Radical History Review*, no. 20, Spring/Summer 1979.

60 Joe Crocker, 'Sociobiology: The Capitalist Synthesis', *Radical Science Journal*, no. 13; for a different emphasis see Richard Lewontin, Steven Rose and Leo Kamin, 'Bourgeois ideology and the origins of biological determinism', *Race and Class*, vol. XXIV, no. 1, 1982.

61 For an overview of the popular reception of sociobiology see Marion Lane and Ruth Hubbard, 'Sociobiology and Biosociality: Can Science Prove the biological basis of sex differences in behaviour?' in Ruth Hubbard and Marion Lane (eds), *Genes and Gender: II: Pitfalls in Research on Sex and Gender*, New York, Gordian Press, 1979. The popular dissemination of sociobiology extended from articles in the popular press to films: for example, 'A genetic defence of the free market', *Business Week*, 10 April 1978, pp. 103-4; and S. Morris, 'Darwin and the Double Standard', *Playboy*, August 1978, advertised on the cover as 'Do men *need* to cheat on their women? A new science says yes'; and a film for high schools, 'Sociobiology: Doing what comes Naturally', Documents Associates 1976.

62 Sebastiano Timpanaro, *On Materialism*, London, New Left Books, 1975, pp. 13ff. For a discussion of the relation of Marxism to biology see Kate Soper, 'Marxism, Materialism and Biology' and Ted Benton, 'Natural Science and Cultural Struggle' in J. Mepham and D.H. Ruben (eds), *Issues in Marxist Philosophy*, vol. 2. *Materialism*, Brighton, Harvester Press, 1979, pp. 61-137.

63 A good example of this is the work of the *soi-disant* Marxist art critic, Peter Fuller. See his defence of the 'biological Marxism' of Timpanaro in 'Putting the individual back into Socialism', *New Society*, 18 September 1980. Here biology becomes more than a limit; it assumes once again absolute (and absolutist) status.

64 *New York Times*, 30 November 1977.

65 See, for example, A.S. Rossi, 'A Biosocial Perspective on Parenting', *Daedalus*, vol. 106, 1977, pp. 1–31, and 'The Biosocial Side of Parenthood', *Human Nature*, vol. 1, no. 6, June 1973, pp. 72–9. Compare Lowe and Hubbard, op. cit., p. 93. For other feminist readings of sociobiology see Donna Haraway, 'Viewpoint: In the Beginning was the Word: The Genesis of Biological Theory', *Signs*, vol. 6, no. 3, 1981; and Adrienne L. Zihlman, 'Women in Evolution, Part II: Subsistence and Social organisation among early Primates', *Signs*, vol. 4, no. 1, Autumn 1978. Zihlman in effect revises the anti-feminist appropriation of sociobiology, in favour of her own. Women choose mates who can help bring up children, ensuring reproductive success (p. 4). But she rejects (p. 11) the 'sex-contract' theory, as set out in Helen Fisher, *The Sex Contract*, St Albans, Granada, 1982, which argues that pair-bonding evolved from male jealousy over female attentions.

66 See Weeks, *Coming Out*. On the theme of 'natural rights' see Lecourt, op. cit., p. 95.

67 Wilson, *On Human Nature*, p. 142.

68 Wilson, *Sociobiology*, p. 555.

69 See, for example, Michael Ruse, Review of *On Human Nature*, *The Advocate*, no. 266, 3 May 1979. An influential work which uses sociobiology to back up its pro-gay sentiments is John Boswell, *Christianity, Social Tolerance and Homosexuality*. For a less scholarly appropriation of the same theme see the publications of the small group of gay activists around the work of 'Charlotte Bach': Bob Mellors (ed.), *Extracts from an unpublished Work. An Outline of Human Ethology by Charlotte M. Bach*, 4 Pamphlets, London, Another Orbit Press, n.d.; and Don Smith, *Why are there 'gays' at all? Why hasn't evolution eliminated 'gayness' millions of years ago?*, London, Quantum Jump Publication, no. 6, n.d. See also discussion in Michael Ruse, 'Are there Gay Genes? Sociobiology and Homosexuality', *Journal of Homosexuality*, vol. 6, no. 4, Summer 1981, Glenn D. Wilson, *The Child-Lovers: A Study of Paedophiles in Society*, London and Boston, Peter Owen, 1983; and Chris Gosselin and Glenn Wilson, *Sexual Variations. Fetishism, Transvestism and Sado-Masochism*, London and Boston, Faber & Faber, 1980.

70 Alan P. Bell, Martin S. Weinberg and Sue Kiefer Hammersmith, *Sexual Preference. Its Development in Men and Women*, Bloomington, Indiana University Press, 1981, pp. 191–2.

71 The sixth of Marx's 'Theses on Feuerbach': 'Feuerbach resolves the essence of religion into the essence of *man*. But the essence of man is no abstraction inherent in each single individual. In its reality it is the ensemble of the social relations.' For a textual

analysis of this, and ultimate rejection of the idea that Marx had no concept of human nature, see Norman Geras, *Marx and Human Nature—Refutation of a Legend*, London, Verso, 1983.

72 Marcel Mauss, 'A Category of the Human Mind: The Notion of Person, the Notion of Self' in *Sociology and Psychology*, London, Routledge & Kegan Paul, 1979; compare Hirst and Woolley, *Social Relations*, p. viii: 'Many important mental and physical capacities of human beings and also their very forms of existence as persons are constructed through social categories'; Michel Foucault, *The Order of Things: An Archaeology of the Human Sciences*, London, Tavistock, 1980, p. xxiii; and Julian Henriques *et al.*, *Changing the Subject: Psychology, social regulation and subjectivity*, London, Methuen, 1984.

73 See Herbert L. Dreyfus and Paul Rabinow, *Michel Foucault: Beyond Structuralism and Hermeneutics*, Brighton, Harvester Press, 1982.

74 Steven Rose, *The Guardian* (London), 6 May 1982, p. 20. The Dialectics of Biology Group, *Towards a Liberatory Biology* is notably vague on what a new synthesis of biological and historical understanding would be.

75 Plummer, *Sexual Stigma*, p. 5.

Chapter 6 Sexuality and the unconscious

1 See Rosalind Coward, *Patriarchal Precedents*, p. 188.

2 Sigmund Freud, *On Aphasia: A Critical Study*, translated, with a critical Introduction by E. Stengel, London, Imago Publishing, 1953; 'Project for a Scientific Psychology' first published in English in *The Origins of Psychoanalysis, Letters to Wilhelm Fliess, Drafts and Notes: 1887–1902*, edited by Marie Bonaparte, Anna Freud and Ernst Kris, London, Imago, 1954. See John Forrester, *Language and the Origins of Psychoanalysis*, London, Macmillan, 1980; and Colin MacCabe (ed.), *The Talking Cure. Essays in Psychoanalysis and Language*, London, Macmillan, 1981.

3 Sigmund Freud, *An Outline of Psycho-Analysis* (1940, written 1938), S.E. 23, pp. 141–207. Compare Forrester, op. cit., p. 223.

4 Sigmund Freud, *The Interpretation of Dreams* (1900), S.E. 5.

5 'The Unconscious', S.E. 14, p. 195; *New Introductory Lectures on Psycho-Analysis* (1933), S.E. 22., Lecture 31, p. 73.

6 Freud, *Introductory Lectures on Psychoanalysis* (1916–17), S.E. 16, Lecture 13, p. 210.

7 See, for example, Jacques Lacan, 'The agency of the letter in the unconscious or reason since Freud', *Ecrits. A Selection*, London, Tavistock Publications, 1977, p. 147.

8 Ferdinand de Saussure, *Course in General Linguistics*, edited by Charles Bally and Albert Sechehaye in collaboration with Albert Reidlinger, translated from the French by Wade Barkin, London, Fontana/Collins, 1974; Anthony Wilden, *System and Structure, Essays in Communication and Exchange*, London, Tavistock, 2nd edn, 1980.

9 *Introductory Lectures*, Lecture 18, *S.E.* 16.

10 *Dreams*, *S.E.* 5, p. 621.

11 See Juliet Mitchell, op. cit., p. 14: cf. Jacques Lacan, 'The Mirror Stage as Formative of the Function of the I as revealed in the psychoanalytic experience' in *Ecrits*.

12 Freud, *Dreams*, *S.E.* 5, pp. 965-6. See discussion in J. Laplanche and J.B. Pontalis, *The Language of Psycho-Analysis*, London, The Hogarth Press and the Institute of Psycho-Analysis, 1980, pp. 481-3.

13 See, for example, *Introductory Lectures*, Lecture 22, *S.E.* 16, p. 351.

14 *An Outline*, *S.E.* 23, p. 186.

15 See *Three Essays on the Theory of Sexuality* (1905), *S.E.* 7, p. 190 and *Introductory Lectures*, Lecture 23, *S.E.* 16, p. 370 for his later views on the seduction theory.

16 For Freud's own evaluation of the significance of the rejection of the seduction theory see section 1 of his 'On the History of the Psycho-Analytic Movement' (1914), *S.E.* 14; chapter 3 of *An Autobiographical Study* (1925), *S.E.* 20; and *New Introductory Lectures*, Lecture 33, *S.E.* 22, p. 120.

17 Letter of 7 April 1907, quoted in Ernest Jones, *The Life and Work of Sigmund Freud*, vol. 2, New York, Basic Books, 1981, p. 436. For the break with Jung, see 'On the History . . .', *S.E.* 14, pp. 60-6; cf. Sulloway, *Freud*, p. 259.

18 *Three Essays*, *S.E.* 7, pp. 147-8.

19 Ibid.

20 The emergence of the concept is discussed by the *Standard Edition* Editors in a note added to 'Instincts and their Vicissitudes' (1915), *S.E.* 14, p. 114. I have followed convention and used the term 'instinct' while quoting from Freud. Otherwise I shall use the term 'drive' in the rest of this section.

21 'Instincts . . .', *S.E.* 14, pp. 121-2.

22 'On the Sexual Theories of Children' (1908), *S.E.* 9, pp. 207-26; 'Analysis of a Phobia in a Five-Year-Old Boy' (hereafter 'Little Hans'), *S.E.* 10, pp. 3-147.

23 *An Outline of Psychoanalysis*, *S.E.* 23, p. 152.

24 *Introductory Lectures*, Lecture 21, *S.E.* 16, p. 323. For the difficulties of defining 'the sexual nature of a process' see ibid., p. 320.

25 Ibid., p. 311.

26 Ibid., pp. 324–6.

27 *Three Essays*, *S.E.* 7, p. 223. He cites Havelock Ellis as a source and collaboration of these 'sacrilegious' views (note 1, pp. 233–4). See the discussions on the origins of sexuality in J. Laplanche and J.B. Pontalis, 'Fantasy and the Origins of Sexuality', *The International Journal of Psychoanalysis*, vol. 49, no. 19, p. 196; Jean Laplanche, *Life and Death in Psychoanalysis*, Baltimore, Johns Hopkins, 1976; and Laplanche and Pontalis, op. cit., p. 421.

28 *Introductory Lectures*, *S.E.* 16, p. 328; *Three Essays*, *S.E.* 7, p. 192; and 'The Claims of Psycho-Analysis to Scientific Interest' (1913), *S.E.* 13, p. 180.

29 See *Introductory Lectures*, op. cit., pp. 207–8, 329ff; for ideas of parallelism, and for accounts of the emergence of Oedipus between 1907–10 see John Forrester, *The Language of Psychoanalysis*, pp. 90–1, and Gilles Deleuze and Felix Guattari, *Anti-Oedipus, Capitalism and Schizophrenia*, New York, Viking Press, 1977, pp. 60–6.

30 'The Dissolution of the Oedipus Complex' (1924), *S.E.* 19, pp. 172–9.

31 *Three Essays*, *S.E.* 7, p. 195, point added 1915. See also 'On the Sexual Theories of Children' (1908) and 'Family Romances' (1908), *S.E.* 9, pp. 205–26, 235–44.

32 'The Infantile Genital Organisation: An Interpolation into the Theory of Sexuality' (1923), p. 144, note 2.

33 *An Outline*, *S.E.* 23, p. 193.

34 Ibid., p. 194.

35 'Some Psychical Consequences of the Anatomical Distinction Between the Sexes' (1925), *S.E.* 19, p. 257.

36 Ernest Jones, *The Life and Work of Sigmund Freud*, vol. 3, p. 258.

37 Ernest Jones, 'Early Female Sexuality', chapter XVII in *Papers on Psychoanalysis*, 5th edn, London, Baillière, Tindall & Cox, 1950, p. 492.

38 'The Psychogenesis of a Case of Homosexuality in a Woman' (1920), *S.E.* 18, pp. 146–72; 'Some Psychical Consequences ...', *S.E.* 19; 'Female Sexuality' (1931), *S.E.* 21, pp. 223–43; 'Femininity', Lecture 33, *New Introductory Lectures*, *S.E.* 22.

39 For a summary of the debate see Juliet Mitchell, *Psychoanalysis and Feminism*, pp. 121–31, and Janice Chasseguet-Smirgel, *Female Sexuality. New Psychoanalytic Views*, London, Virago, 1981, pp. 1–46. For the views of a major participant see Karen Horney, *Feminine Psychology*, New York and London, W.W. Norton, 1973.

40 Luce Irigaray, *Speculum de l'Autre Femme*, Paris, Les Editions de

Minuit, 1974; see also Jacques Lacan and *The École Freudienne*, *Feminine Sexuality*, edited by Juliet Mitchell and Jacqueline Rose, London, Macmillan, 1982.

41 See the comments of Nancy Chodorow, *The Reproduction of Mothering—Psychoanalysis and the Sociology of Gender*, Berkeley and Los Angeles, Ca., and London, 1978, p. 117.

42 Rosalind Coward and John Ellis, *Language and Materialism*, London, Routledge & Kegan Paul, 1977, p. 3.

43 For the criticisms of feminist analysts and their supporters, see Irigaray, op. cit.; *Le Sexe qui n'en est pas un*, Paris, Les Editions de Minuit, 1977, and 'Women's exile. Interview with Luce Irigaray', *Ideology and Consciousness*, no. 1, May 1977, pp. 62–76; Monique Plaza, ' "Phallomorphic power" and the psychology of "woman" ', *Ideology and Consciousness*, no. 4, Autumn 1978, pp. 51–112.

For feminist appropriations of Freud see Mitchell, *Psychoanalysis and Feminism*; the introductions by Mitchell and Rose to Lacan, *Feminine Sexuality*, op. cit.; Rosalind Coward, 'Rereading Freud. The Making of the Feminine', *Spare Rib*, no. 70, May 1978, pp. 43–6, and 'Sexual Politics and Psychoanalysis: Some notes on their relation' in Rosalind Brunt and Caroline Rowan (eds), *Feminism, Culture and Politics*; and Gayle Rubin, 'The Traffic in Women: notes on the "Political Economy" of Sex', in Rayna Reiter (ed.), *Towards an Anthropology of Women*, New York, Monthly Review Press, 1975. There are critical comments on such approaches in Elizabeth Wilson, 'Psychoanalysis: Psychic Law and Order', *Feminist Review*, no. 8, Summer 1981, pp. 63–78; the debate is continued in subsequent issues.

44 Jacqueline Rose, 'Femininity and its Discontents', *Feminist Review*, no. 14, p. 9.

45 Chodorow, op. cit.; Rose, op. cit. p. 9.

46 *S.E.* 19, p. 178.

47 Michel Foucault, *The History of Sexuality*, vol. 1, *An Introduction;* Deleuze and Guattari, *Anti-Oedipus*; Robert Castel, *Le Psychoanalysme: L'ordre psychoanalytique et le pouvoir*, Paris, François Maspero, 1973; Colin Gordon, 'The Unconsciousness of psychoanalysis', *Ideology and Consciousness*, no. 2, Autumn 1977, pp. 109–27. For the context of this critique see Sherry Turkle, *Psychoanalytic Politics. Freud's French Revolution*, London, Burnett Books in association with Andre Deutsch, 1979.

48 'Fragment of an Analysis of a Case of Hysteria' (1905; hereafter 'Dora'), *S.E.* 7.

49 Lacan, *Ecrits*, p. 91.

50 *S.E.* 7, p. 28.

51 For feminist readings of the Dora case, see Toril Moi, 'Representations of Patriarchy, Sexuality and Epistemology in Freud's Dora', *Feminist Review*, no. 9, Autumn 1981; Maria Ramas, 'Freud's Dora, Dora's Hysteria: The negation of a Woman's Rebellion', *Feminist Studies*, Fall 1980, also printed in Judith L. Newton, Mary P. Ryan and Judith R. Walkowitz, *Sex and Class in Women's History*, London, Routledge & Kegan Paul, 1983; Jacqueline Rose, 'Dora-fragment of an analysis', *M/F* no. 2, 1978; and Suzanne Gaerhart, 'The Scene of Psychoanalysis: The Unanswered Questions of Dora', *Diacritics*, Spring 1979.

52 See 'Little Hans', *S.E.* 10, p. 15.

53 Ibid., p. 62.

54 Ibid., p. 87.

55 Mia Campioni and Elizabeth Gross, 'Little Hans: The Production of Oedipus', in Paul Foss and Meaghan Morris (eds), *Language, Sexuality and Subversion*, Darlington, Australia, A Feral Publication, 1978, p. 105. For a similar critical account of the social significance of Little Hans' accession to masculinity see 'The Oedipus Complex: Comments on the Case of Little Hans', in Erich Fromm, *The Crisis of Psychoanalysis. Essays on Freud, Marx and Social Psychology*, Harmondsworth, Penguin Books, 1973.

56 Mitchell, *Psychoanalysis and Feminism*, p. 82.

57 Campioni and Gross, op. cit., p. 104.

58 For the impact of this on the development of American ego psychology, see Turkle, *Psychoanalytic Politics*, and Russell Jacoby, *Social Amnesia. A Critique of Contemporary Psychology from Adler to Laing*, Boston, Beacon Press, 1975. For the disastrous impact on contemporary feminist attitudes the modern *locus classicus* is Kate Millett, *Sexual Politics*, London, Abacus, 1972, pp. 176–220; see discussion of this and other related works in Mitchell, *Psychoanalysis and Feminism*, pp. 295–355.

59 A recent publication on homosexuality which sharply attacks psycho-analysis is Katz, *Gay/Lesbian Almanac*. Dennis Altman has made use of Freudian concepts in his pioneering *Homosexual: Oppression and Liberation*, New York, Outerbridge & Dienstfrey, 1971, in *Coming Out in the Seventies*, Boston, Alyson Publications, 1981; and in *The Homosexualization of America, the Americanization of the Homosexual*. David Fernbach has also deployed a form of Freudian theory in his 'Towards a Marxist Theory of Gay Liberation', republished in Pam Mitchell (ed.), *Pink Triangles*, Boston, Alyson Publications, 1981. See also Fernbach, *The Spiral Path. A Gay Contribution to Human Survival*, London, Gay Men's Press, 1981; and Martin Dannecker, *Theories of Homosexuality*, London, Gay Men's Press, 1981, which un-

usually among pro-gay publications goes overboard for psychoanalysis. Mario Mielli, *Homosexuality and Liberation. Elements of a Gay Critique*, London, Gay Men's Press, 1980, attempts to use both Freud and Jung. See my critique in *Gay Left*, no. 10, Winter 1980. For other psychoanalytic texts which ignore or put down lesbianism (by Jean Baker Miller, Dorothy Dinnerstein and Nancy Chodorow) see Adrienne Rich, 'Compulsory Heterosexuality and Lesbian Existence', *Signs*, vol. 5, no. 4, 1980, pp. 634–9. Feminist psychoanalytic works which do deal with lesbianism include Charlotte Wolff, *Love Between Women*, London, Duckworth, 1971; J. McDougall, 'Homosexuality in Women' in J. Chasseguet-Smirgel (ed.), *Female Sexuality. New Psychoanalytic Views*, pp. 171–212.

60 C.W. Socarides, 'The psychoanalytic theory of homosexuality, with special reference to therapy' in I. Rosen (ed.), *Sexual Deviation*, Oxford University Press, 1979, p. 246; *Homosexuality*, New York, Jason Aranson, 1978; I. Bieber, 'Clinical Aspects of Male Homosexuality' in J. Marmor (ed.), *Sexual Inversion: The Multiple Roots of Homosexuality*, New York, Basic Books, 1965. For a penetrating discussion of the fate of Freud in the USA see Henry Abelove, 'Freud, Male Homosexuality, and the Americans' (unpublished 1982). It is noticeable that liberal psychoanalytically inclined writers have not returned to Freud's 'polymorphous perversity', but have simply reversed the terms of the Socarides position: homosexuality is a natural variation, good rather than bad (e.g. Judd Marmor).

61 Socarides, 'The Psychoanalytic Theory of Homosexuality', p. 264.

62 'Psychogenesis of a case of homosexuality in a woman', *S.E.* 18, p. 151.

63 Hocquenghem, *Homosexual Desire*, pp. 44–7. See 'Psychoanalytic notes on an Autobiographical Account of a Case of Paranoia (Dementia Paranoides)' (1911), *S.E.* 12, pp. 3–79.

64 Ellenberger, *The Discovery of the Unconscious*, pp. 598, 617; Ernest Jones, *The Life and Work of Sigmund Freud*, vol. 2, p. 279.

65 'An Autobiographical Study', *S.E.* 20, p. 38.

66 *Three Essays*, *S.E.* 7, p. 149, note 1, added 1910.

67 'Homosexuality in a Woman', *S.E.* 18, p. 151.

68 *Three Essays*, *S.E.* 7, p. 146, note 1, added 1915.

69 *Leonardo da Vinci and a Memory of His Childhood* (1910), *S.E.* 11, p. 99, footnote added in 1919.

70 *Group Psychology and the Analysis of the Ego* (1921), *S.E.* 18, pp. 67–143.

71 See *Three Essays*, *S.E.* 7, pp. 138–9.

72 'Homosexuality in a Woman', *S.E.* 18, p. 154.

73 See the discussion in the 'Wolfenden Report' of 1978: Weeks, *Coming Out*, chapter 14.
74 *Leonardo*, S.E. 11, p. 98.
75 'Homosexuality in a Woman', *S.E.* 18, p. 170.
76 *Three Essays*, S.E. 7, p. 145.
77 Ibid., p. 146.
78 'Homosexuality in a Woman', *S.E.* 18, p. 153.
79 Ernst Freud (ed.), *Letters of Sigmund Freud 1873–1939*, London, Hogarth Press, 1961, p. 277.
80 Laplanche and Pontalis, *The Language of Psychoanalysis*, p. 308.

Chapter 7 Dangerous desires

1 On Freud's attitude to Jung see, for example, Larry David Nachman, 'Psychoanalysis and Social Theory: The Origin of Society and of Guilt', *Salmagundi*, nos 92–93, Spring–Summer 1981, pp. 65–106. For an overview of neo-Freudianism see Jacoby, *Social Amnesia* and Mark Poster, *Critical Theory of the Family*, New York, the Seabury Press, London, Pluto Press, 1978, ch. 3. On Erich Fromm see his *The Sane Society*, London, Routledge & Kegan Paul, 1963. For other sociological Freudians see Patrick Mullahy, *Psychoanalysis and Interpersonal Psychiatry—The Contribution of Harry Stack Sullivan*, New York, Science House, 1970; on Heinz Hartman, *Ego Psychology and the Problem of Adaptation*, New York, 1958, *Essays on Ego Psychology: Selected Problems in Psychoanalytic Theory*, New York, 1964.
2 *Totem and Taboo* (1913), S.E. 13, p. 141. See also *Moses and Monotheism: Three Essays* (1939), *S.E.* 23, and *Group Psychology*, S.E. 18.
3 Juliet Mitchell, *Psychoanalysis and Feminism*, p. 376. See C. Lévi-Strauss, *Elementary Structures of Kinship*, Boston, Beacon Press, 1969.
4 See the discussion in Coward, *Patriarchal Precedents*, ch. 7.
5 For an extreme statement of the confinement of the role of Marxism to the economic see Mark Cousins, 'Material arguments and Feminism', *M/F*, no. 2, pp. 62–70. For Freud's hostility to radical appropriations of his work see *New Introductory Lectures*, Lecture 35, pp. 176 ff.
6 Jacoby, *Social Amnesia*, pp. 21, 84–5, 172, note 46.
7 For the essential background see Martin Jay, *The Dialectical Imagination: A History of the Frankfurt School and the Institute of Social Research, 1923–1950*, London, Heinemann, 1973; Paul A. Robinson, *The Sexual Radicals, Reich, Roheim, Marcuse*,

London, Paladin, 1972; also Perry Anderson, *Considerations on Western Marxism*, London, New Left Books, 1976. For a recent discussion of Habermas see Russell Keat, *The Politics of Social Theory. Habermas, Freud and the Critique of Positivism*, Oxford, Basil Blackwell, 1981.

8 For the social framework of Reich's work see Atina Grossman, ' "Satisfaction is Domestic Happiness": Mass Working Class Sex Reform Organizations in the Weimar Republic' in M.N. Dobkowski and I. Wallinan, *Towards the Holocaust*, Westport, Greenwood, 1984, and Mitchell, *Psychoanalysis and Feminism*, pp. 137–52. On Marcuse, see Vincent Geoghegan, *Reason and Eros: The Social Theory of Herbert Marcuse*, London, Pluto Press, 1981.

9 Wilhelm Reich, *The Function of the Orgasm. Sex-Economic Problems of Biological Energy*, London, Panther Books, 1972, p. 114. (*Note*: this is not the same work as the book of the same title just mentioned in the text. This is more of an intellectual autobiography, covering the development of Reich's work.)

10 Ibid., p. 179.

11 Freud, *Introductory Lectures*, Lecture 37, *S.E.* 16, pp. 432–3.

12 Reich, *The Function*, p. 231.

13 Wilhelm Reich, *Dialectical Materialism and Psychoanalysis*, London, Socialist Reproduction, n.d., p. 49.

14 Wilhelm Reich, *The Mass Psychology of Fascism*, Harmondsworth, Pelican Books, 1975.

15 Wilhelm Reich, *The Sexual Revolution. Towards a Self-Governing Character Structure*, New York, Ferrar, Straus & Giroux, 1970.

16 See Gilles Deleuze and Felix Guattari, *Anti-Oedipus*; Kate Millett, *Sexual Politics*; Mitchell, *Psychoanalysis and Feminism*, pp. 227–92.

17 Gad Horowitz, *Repression, Basic and Surplus Repression in Psychoanalytic Theory: Freud, Reich and Marcuse*, Toronto and Buffalo, University of Toronto Press, 1977, p. 141.

18 Robert Kronemeyer, *Overcoming Homosexuality*, New York, Macmillan, London, Collier-Macmillan, 1980; Bertell Ollman, *Social and Sexual Revolution. Essays on Marx and Reich*, London, Pluto Press, 1979, pp. 159–203; William Masters and Virginia Johnson, *Human Sexual Response*.

19 Herbert Marcuse, *Eros and Civilization*, London, Sphere Books, 1969, p. 190.

20 Ibid., pp. 203–14.

21 Compare Horowitz, *Repression*, p. 27.

22 Marcuse, *Five Lectures*, London, Allen Lane, 1970, p. 19.

23 See the critique of Norman O. Brown, *Life Against Death. The Psychoanalytic Meaning of History*, London, Sphere Books, 1968.

24 *Eros and Civilization*, pp. 132-9.

25 Herbert Marcuse, *One-Dimensional Man*, London, Abacus, 1972.

26 Reimut Reiche, *Sexuality and Class Struggle*, London, New Left Books, 1979, p. 46.

27 Herbert Marcuse, *An Essay on Liberation*, Harmondsworth, Pelican, 1969. For critical assessment of Marcuse see Alasdair MacIntyre, *Marcuse*, London, Fontana, 1970.

28 Jacoby, *Social Amnesia*, p. 30; Christopher Lasch, 'The Freudian Left and Cultural Revolution', *New Left Review*, no. 129, September-October 1981, pp. 23-4.

29 Reiche, op. cit.; Jacoby, op. cit.; Lasch, op. cit.; and in *The Culture of Narcissus*. Reiche modifies his attitudes to homosexuality in subsequent works: R. Reiche and M. Dannecker, 'Male homosexuality in West Germany—a sociological investigation', *Journal of Sex Research*, vol. 13, no. 1, pp. 35-53.

30 See Turkle, *Psychoanalytic Politics*, and Rose, 'Femininity and its Discontents' for discussions of Lacan's crusades against egopsychology from the late 1930s.

31 See Louis Althusser, 'Ideology and Ideological State Apparatuses' in *Lenin and Philosophy*, for his use of the concept of the imaginary.

32 For articles by Kristeva, Cixous and Irigaray see Elaine Marks and Isabelle de Courtivron (eds), *New French Feminisms*, Brighton, Harvester Press, 1981. See also Juliet Mitchell, op. cit.; Coward, *Patriarchal Precedents* and Jane Gallop, *Feminism and Psychoanalysis. The Daughter's Seduction*, London, Macmillan, 1982.

33 Rosalind Coward, *Female Desire. Women's Sexuality Today*, London, Granada, 1984, p. 14.

34 Ann Rosalind Jones, 'Julia Kristeva on femininity—the limits of a semiotic politics', *Feminist Review*, no. 18, Winter 1984.

35 Michel Foucault, 'Preface' to Deleuze and Guattari, *Anti-Oedipus*, p. xi.

36 Deleuze and Guattari's *Anti-Oedipus*, Jean-François Lyotard, *Dérive à Partir de Marx et Freud*, Paris, 1973 and *Economie Libidinale*, Paris, Les Editions des Minuits, 1974.

37 See comments in Jacques Donzelot, 'An Aetiology', *Semiotext(e) Anti-Oedipus*, vol. 11, no. 3. 1977, p. 30.

38 Deleuze and Guattari, *Anti-Oedipus*, p. 33. See also Guy Hocquenghem, *Homosexual Desire*.

39 *Anti-Oedipus*, p. 29.

40 Perry Anderson, *Arguments within English Marxism*, London, Verso, 1980, p. 161.

41 Frederic Jameson, 'Pleasure: A Political Issue' in *Formations of Pleasure*, London, Routledge & Kegan Paul, 1983, p. 4. For samples of this politics of desire see Felix Guattari, *Molecular Revolution. Psychiatry and Politics*, Harmondsworth, Penguin, 1984.

42 For example, Gagnon and Simon, *Sexual Conduct*, and Plummer, *Sexual Stigma*.

43 Michel Foucault, *The History of Sexuality*. For a recent critique which simultaneously relates him to, but distinguishes him from, the philosophies of desire, see Peter Dews, 'Power and Subjectivity in Foucault', *New Left Review*, 144, March/April, 1984.

44 *L'Usage des Plaisirs* and *Le Souci de Soi*.

45 Foucault, *The History of Sexuality*, vol. 1, p. 153.

46 Maria Black and Rosalind Coward, 'Linguistics, Social and Sexual Relations: A Review of Dale Spencer's *Man-Made Language*' in *Screen Education*, Summer 1981, no. 39, p. 80. On the background to structural linguistics see Rosalind Coward and John Ellis, *Language and Materialism*.

47 Hirst and Woolley, *Social Relations*, p. 134; Ernesto Laclau, 'Populist Rupture and Discourse', *Screen Education*, no. 34, Spring 1980, pp. 87–93; Ernesto Laclau and Chantal Mouffe, *Hegemony and Socialist Strategy*, London, Verso, 1985, ch 3.

48 Gayle Rubin, 'The Traffic in Women' in Rayna Reiter (ed.), *Towards an Anthropology of Women*, New York, Monthly Review Press, 1979, pp. 197–210.

49 *Sex, Politics and Society*, pp. 11ff.

Chapter 8 'Movements of affirmation': identity politics

1 Dennis Altman, *The Homosexualization of America*, pp. 73, 74.

2 Pat Califia, *Sapphistry. The Book of Lesbian Sexuality*, New York, The Naiad Press, 1980, p. 165.

3 Lisa Steele, 'Freedom, Sex and Power': interview with Charlotte Bunch, *Fuse*, January/February 1983, p. 233.

4 Pat Califia, 'Gay Men, Lesbians and Sex. Doing it Together', *The Advocate*, 7 July 1983, pp. 26–7.

5 Gayle Rubin, 'The Leather Menace' in Samois (ed.), *Coming to Power. Writings and Graphics on Lesbian S/M*, Berkeley, Ca., Samois, 1981, p. 195.

6 For the emergence of transvestism and transexuality as political categories see Dave King, 'Gender Confusions: psychological and psychiatric conceptions of transvestism and transexualism' in

Plummer (ed.), *The Making of the Modern Homosexual*, and Janice C. Raymond, *The Transsexual Empire*, Boston, Beacon Press, 1979; for paedophiles, see Daniel Tsang (ed.), *The Age Taboo: Gay Male Sexuality, Power and Consent*, Boston, Alyson Publications, 1981, and Ken Plummer, '"The paedophile's" progress: a view from below' in Brian Taylor (ed.), *Perspectives on Paedophilia*, London, Batsford, 1981; on sado-masochists see Samois (ed.), *Coming to Power*, and on bisexuals see the work of Philip W. Blumstein and Pepper Schwartz, especially 'Lesbianism and Bisexuality' in Erich Goode and Richard R. Troiden, *Sexual Deviance and Sexual Deviants*, New York, William Morrow, 1974; 'Bisexuality in Women', *Archives of Sexual Behaviour*, no. 5, March 1976, pp. 171–81; and 'Bisexuality in Men' in C. Warren (ed.), *Sexuality: Encounters, Identities and Relationships*, New York, Sage Contemporary Science Issues, No. 35, 1977.

7   For an outstanding impressionistic account of the US gay male scene at the end of the 1970s see Edmund White, *States of Desire. Travels in Gay America*, New York, E.P. Dutton, 1980.

8   D'Emilio, *Sexual Politics, Sexual Communities*, p. 248.

9   Michel Foucault (ed.), *Herculine Barbin: Being the Recently Discovered Memoirs of a Nineteenth Century French Hermaphrodite*, New York, Pantheon, 1980, pp. xiii, viii.

10   Barry D. Adam, *The Survival of Domination. Inferiorization and Everyday Life*, New York, Elsevier, 1978, p. 12.

11   Erik H. Erikson, *Identity, Youth and Crisis*, London, Fuser, 1968. See comments in Richard Sennett, *The Uses of Disorder. Personal Identity and City Life*, New York, Alfred A. Knopf, 1970.

12   Dennis H. Wrong, 'Identity—Problem and Catchword', in *Sceptical Sociology*, New York, Columbia University Press, 1976, p. 81.

13   Stan Cohen and Laurie Taylor, *Escape Attempts*, p. 27. For a discussion of the relation of this background debate to modern sexual identities see Altman, *The Homosexualization of America*, pp. 93 ff, Plummer (ed.), *The Making*, Adam, *The Survival of Domination* and Laud Humphreys, 'Exodus and Identity: The Emerging Gay Culture' in Martin P. Levine (ed.), *Gay Men. The Sociology of Male Homosexuality*, New York, Harper & Row, 1979.

14   Jonathan Ned Katz, *Gay/Lesbian Almanac*, p. 406.

15   Plummer, op. cit., p. 29. See also Humphreys, op. cit., p. 145, Adam, pp. 60-1, and Martin S. Weinberg and Colin J. Williams, *Male Homosexuals, their Problems and Adaptations*, New York, Oxford University Press, 1974, for documentation of the relationship between a secure sense of self and the alleviation of guilt, anxiety and shame.

16 Ethel Spector Person, 'Sexuality as the Mainstay of Identity: Psychoanalytic Perspectives', *Signs*, vol. 5, no. 4, 1980, p. 629. Despite its methodological inadequacies there is a useful documentation of male insecurities in Shere Hite, *The Hite Report on Male Sexuality*, New York, Alfred A. Knopf, 1981. For interesting speculations on the history of masculinity see Andrew Tolson, *The Limits of Masculinity*, London, Tavistock, 1977; Paul Hoch, *White Hero, Black Beast. Racism, Sexism and the Mask of Masculinity*, London, Pluto Press, 1979; Peter N. Stearns, *Be a Man! Males in Modern Society*, New York, Holmes & Meier, 1979; David Fernbach, *The Spiral Path. A Gay Contribution to Human Survival*, London, Gay Men's Press, 1981; Emmanuel Reynaud, *Holy Virility. The Social Construction of Masculinity*, London, Pluto Press, 1983. For thoughts on the history of heterosexuality see Jonathan Katz, 'The invention of heterosexuality, 1892–1982' in Supplement II, papers of the conference 'Among Men, Among Women', University of Amsterdam, 1983.

17 Spector Person, op. cit., p. 629. See also Eric Carlton, *Sexual Anxiety: A Study of Male Impotence*, Oxford, Martin Robertson, 1980.

18 Richard Dyer, 'Getting over the Rainbow: Identity and Pleasure in Gay Cultural Politics' in George Bridges and Rosalind Brunt (eds), *Silver Linings: Some Strategies for the Eighties*, London, Lawrence & Wishart, 1981, p. 61. The classic statement on camp is Susan Sontag, 'Notes on Camp' in *Against Interpretation*, New York, Dell, 1970. For a critique (and also implicitly of Dyer's position) see Andrew Britton, 'For Interpretation: Notes Against Camp' in *Gay Left*, no. 7, Winter 1978/9, pp. 11–14. On use of an effeminate style amongst gay men in the 1960s see Gagnon and Simon, *Sexual Conduct*, p. 147. With regards to lesbianism, Kinsey et al., *Sexual Behavior in the Human Female*, p. 486, note 38, cites numerous references for the 'statistically unsupported opinion that females with homosexual histories frequently and usually exhibit masculine physical characters, behavior, or tastes'.

19 Dyer, op. cit., p. 61. On the general phenomenon of gay macho styles see articles by John Marshall, and Gregg Blatchford, in Plummer (ed.), *The Making* and Altman, *The Homosexualization of America*, pp. 13–15, 34. The 'guerrilla warfare' phrase is used by Dick Hebdige, *Subcultures: The Meaning of Style*, London, Tavistock, 1979. See also M.D. Storms, 'Attitudes toward Homosexuality and Femininity in Men', *Journal of Homosexuality*, vol. 3, no. 3, Spring 1979.

20 Adam, *The Survival of Domination*, p. 123.

21 References are from Katz, *Gay/Lesbian Almanac*, pp. 147, 324.

For analogous developments, and a discussion of wider issues about subcultures, see George Chauncey's paper in the conference collection *Among Men, Among Women*, 1983: 'Fairies, Pogues and Christian Brothers: The Newport (Rhode Island) Homosexuality Scandal, 1919-1920'. On British developments see Weeks, *Coming Out*, ch. 3. For a more general discussion of the significance of urbanisation in producing gay communities see Joseph Harvy and William B. De Vall, *The Social Organisation of Gay Males*, New York, Praeger, 1978, ch 8; and on subcultural organisation see Plummer, *Sexual Stigma*, ch 8.

22 Altman, *The Homosexualization*, p. 21; D'Emilio, op. cit., p. 33.

23 Edwin Schur, *The Politics of Deviance*, p. 191.

24 On this see the discussion in John Marshall, ch. 6, 'The Politics of Tea and Sympathy' in Gay Left Collective (ed.), *Homosexuality: Power and Politics*.

25 D'Emilio, op. cit., p. 25. See D'Emilio throughout for the wider post-war shift.

26 Judd Marmor (ed.), *Sexual Inversion: The Multiple Roots of Homosexuality*, New York, Basic Books, 1965; Evelyn Hooker, 'The Adjustment of the Male Overt Homosexual', *Journal of Protective Techniques*, no. 21, 1957, pp. 18-31; 'The Homosexual Community' in J.H. Gagnon and W. Simon, *Sexual Deviance*, New York, Harper & Row, 1967, and 'Final Report of the Task Force on Homosexuality', *Homophile Studies*, no. 8, 1969, pp. 5-12; Howard S. Becker, *Outsiders: Studies in the Sociology of Deviance*, New York, Free Press, 1963; Edwin M. Schur, *Crimes without Victims: Deviant Behavior and Public Policy*, Englewood Cliffs, N.J., Prentice-Hall, 1965; Erving Goffman, *Stigma: Notes on the Management of Spoiled Identity*, Englewood Cliffs, N.J., Prentice-Hall, 1963. For British developments during the same period see Michael Schofield, *Sociological Aspects of Homosexuality*, London, Longman, 1965. See also Martin Hoffman, *The Gay World: Male Homosexuality and the Social Creation of Evil*, New York, Basic Books, 1968. For an overview of the aetiological view see Bell and Weinberg, *Homosexualities*, pp. 195-6. W. Simon and J.H. Simon criticised the aetiological approach in 1967 as 'simplistic and homogeneous': 'Homosexuality: The Formulation of a Sociological Perspective', *Journal of Health and Social Behavior*, no. 8, 1967, pp. 177-85; see also Gagnon and Simon, *Sexual Conduct*, ch. 5; a call for a new sociological approach was made by David Sonnenschein, 'The Ethnography of Male Homosexual Relationships', *Journal of Sex Research*, vol. 4, no. 2, May 1968, pp. 69-83.

27 In her researches into the gay male S/M subculture Gayle Rubin

has found that Kinsey had a direct organising impact; he introduced his interviewees who were sado-masochists to one another thus encouraging network formation (private communication).

28 See Weeks, *Coming Out*, and D'Emilio, op. cit.

29 Kinsey et al., *Sexual Behavior in the Human Female*, pp. 474–5, sums up his statistical conclusion: the 37 per cent of men who enjoyed homosexual contact to orgasm compares with 13 per cent of women; see also *Sexual Behavior in the Human Male*, pp. 656–7, and p. 617 for his dislike of the concept of bisexual or homosexual persons.

30 For a summary of figures see Adam, *The Survival of Domination*, p. 92. More recent surveys suggest a substantial drop in this flight: Spada found that 85 per cent of his sample said they would rather *not* be straight: and 80 per cent felt good about their lives: James Spada, *The Spada Report. The Newest Survey of Gay Male Sexuality*, New York, New American Library/Signet, 1979, pp. 297, 310. On what they call 'preference denial' see also William Masters and Virginia Johnson, *Homosexuality in Perspective*. On 'homosocial' relationships see Universiteit van Amsterdam, *Among Men, Among Women: Sociological and historical recognition of homosocial arrangements*, conference papers 1983.

31 Barry M. Dank, 'Coming Out in the Gay World', in Levine (ed.), *Gay Men*, p. 130. On drifting into identity see Plummer, *Sexual Stigma*, ch. 7, Plummer (ed.), *The Making of the Modern Homosexual*, chs 1 and 3, and John Hart and Diane Richardson, *The Theory and Practice of Homosexuality*, London, Routledge & Kegan Paul, 1981, chs 3–5. For a concise study of the drift into another 'deviant' sexual identity, that of prostitute, see Nanette J. Davis, 'Prostitution; Identity, Career and Legal—Economic Enterprise' in Henslin and Sagarin (eds), *The Sociology of Sex*.

32 Bell and Weinberg, *Homosexualities*, p. 217; see also *The Spada Report* and White, *States of Desire*, for this diversity.

33 D'Emilio, op. cit., p. 9.

34 Donald Webster Cory, *The Homosexual in America*, New York, Peter Nevill, 1951, p. 14. The chapter in which this appears is called 'The Unrecognised Minority'. 'Cory' was the pseudonym of the sociologist/sexologist Edward Sagarin. He was later to explicitly reject his earlier political positions, and the idea of a homosexual minority: see his *Deviants and Deviance*, New York, Praeger, 1975, pp. 144–54. Also E. Sagarin (ed.), *The Other Minorities: Non ethnic Collectivities Conceptualized as Minority Groups*, Mass., Waltham, 1971.

35 Altman, *Homosexual: Oppression and liberation*. See also Simon

Watney, 'The Ideology of GLF' in Gay Left Collective (ed.), *Homosexuality, Power and Politics.*

36 Kenneth Plummer, ch. 3 in Plummer (ed.), *The Making of the Modern Homosexual*, p. 55.

37 F. Whitham, 'The prehomosexual male child in three societies: the United States, Guatemala, Brazil', *Archives of Sexual Behavior*, vol. 9, no. 2, pp. 87–99; see also Whitham, 'The homosexual role: a reconsideration', *Journal of Sex Research*, vol. 13, pp. 1–11, and subsequent issues for the debate.

38 Kinsey et al., *Sexual Behavior in the Human Male*, p. 168, found a mean age of first homosexual outlet at 9 years 2½ months. Twenty-one per cent of Spada's sample (*The Spada Report*, p. 30) had their first experience before 9. Bell, Weinberg, Kiefer, Hammersmith, *Sexual Preference*, p. 211, found exclusive homosexuality fixed by the end of adolescence. None of this, however, invalidates the fact that feelings, needs and desires, and experiences are different from identity. See the critique of the orientation model in Plummer, op. cit., pp. 69–72.

39 See Guy Hocquenghem, *Homosexual Desire;* Kinsey et al., *Sexual Behavior in the Human Male;* for a reification of the scale see Masters and Johnson, *Perspectives on Homosexuality.* For a debate on Mary McIntosh's concept of a historically constructed 'homosexual role', building on Kinsey's continuum, see Plummer (ed.), *The Making of the Modern Homosexual*, passim.

40 See *Polysexuality: Semiotext (e)*, vol. IV, no. 1, 1981.

41 For a scepticism about 'coming out', based on a rather scholastic reading of Foucault, see Jeff Minson, 'The Assertion of Homosexuality', in *M/F*, nos 5–6, 1981, pp. 19–40.

42 Lillian Faderman, *Surpassing the Love of Men*, pp. 142, 17. See also the various discussions of the homosocial arrangements of women in *Among Men, Among Women*, op. cit.

43 Joan Nestle, 'Butch-Fem Relationships', *Heresies*, no. 12, 1981, 'Sex Issue', p. 23.

44 See Elizabeth Wilson, 'I'll Climb the Stairway to Heaven: Lesbianism in the Seventies' in Sue Cartledge and Joanna Ryan, *Sex and Love.* The NOW declaration is reproduced in *Heresies*, no. 12, p. 92, with feminist responses p. 93.

45 For a critical appraisal of the literature see Annabel Faraday, 'Liberating lesbian research' in Plummer (ed.), *The Making of the Modern Homosexual.* An overview of recent work is provided in Susan Krieger, 'Lesbian Identity and Community: Recent Social Science Literature', *Signs*, vol. 8, no. 1, Autumn 1982, pp. 91–108. See also E.M. Ettorre, *Lesbians, Women and Society*, London, Routledge & Kegan Paul, 1980. See also D. Tanner, *The Lesbian*

Couple, New York, Lexington, 1978; D.G. Wolfe, *The Lesbian Community*, San Francisco, University of California Press, 1979; and Masters and Johnson, *Perspectives on Homosexuality*. Compare Gagnon and Simon, ch. 6, and Faraday, op. cit.

46 Adrienne Rich, 'Compulsory Heterosexuality and Lesbian Existence', *Signs*, vol. 5, no. 4, 1980, p. 648.

47 Ibid., p. 650.

48 Cora Kaplan, 'Wild Nights: Pleasure/Sexuality/Feminism' in *Formations of Pleasure*, London, Boston, Henley, Routledge & Kegan Paul, 1983, p. 31.

49 Paula Webster, 'Pornography and Pleasure', *Heresies*, no. 12, 'Sex Issue', p. 50.

50 Margaret Jackson, 'Sex and the Experts ... or Male Sexuality Rules OK', *Scarlet Woman*, no. 13, part 2, 'Sexuality', July 1981, p. 5.

51 Leeds Revolutionary Feminists, *Love Your Enemy? The Debate between Heterosexual Feminism and Political Lesbianism*, London, Only Women Press, 1981, p. 6.

52 Pat Califia, 'Feminism and Sadomasochism', *Heresies*, no. 12, p. 34.

53 Ann Ferguson, 'On "Compulsory Heterosexuality and Lesbian Existence"', *Signs*, vol. 7, no. 1, 1981, p. 160.

54 Beatrix Campbell, 'A Feminist Sexual Politics: Now you see it, now you don't', *Feminist Review*, no. 5, 1980, p. 2. Kinsey et al., *Sexual Behavior in the Human Male* and *Sexual Behavior in the Human Female*; Masters and Johnson, *Human Sexual Response*; Mary Jane Sherfey, *The Nature and Evolution of Female Sexuality*, New York, Random House, 1972. For an overview of the sexological debate see Seymour Fisher, *The Female Orgasm: Psychology, Physiology, Fantasy*, London, Allen Lane, 1973; and for its political appropriation see Anne Koedt, 'The Myth of the Vaginal Orgasm' (1968), reprinted in Leslie Tanner (ed.), *Voices from Women's Liberation*, New York, New American Library/ Mentor, 1970.

55 Masters and Johnson, *Perspectives on Homosexuality*, p. 208.

56 Shere Hite, *The Hite Report. A Nation-Wide Study of Female Sexuality*, New York, Macmillan, 1976, pp. 57–60.

57 See the essays in A. Snitow, C. Stansell and Sharon Thompson, *Desire: The Politics of Sexuality*, London, Virago, 1984; and Carole S. Vance (ed.), *Pleasure and Danger: Explaining Female Sexuality*, Boston and London, Routledge & Kegan Paul, 1984. Also Linda Gordon, *Woman's Body, Woman's Right: A Social History of Birth Control in America*, New York, Grossman, 1976; Judith R. Walkowitz, *Prostitution and Victorian Society*; Sheila Jeffreys,

' "Free from all Uninvited Touch of Man": Women's campaigns around sexuality, 1880-1914' in Elizabeth Sarah (ed.), *Reassessment of 'First Wave Feminism'*, Oxford and New York, Pergamon Press, 1983; and Weeks, *Sex, Politics and Society*, ch. 9.

58 Lisa Orlando, ' "Bad Girls" and "Good" Politics', *Village Voice Literary Supplement*, Dec. 1982, p. 18. See also *Diary of a Conference on Sexuality*, p. 6. The work of Andrea Dworkin hits the characteristic tone: *Pornography* and *Right Wing Women*. See also references below in the anti-pornography and anti S/M polemics.

59 Gayle Rubin and Pat Califia talk about 'Sadomasochism: Fears, Facts, Fantasies', *Gay Community News* (Boston), vol. 9, no. 5, 15 August 1981, p. 7

60 The *Diary of a Conference on Sexuality* gives the essential background to the theme of the conference. It was part of 'The Scholar and the Feminist' series, sponsored by the Helena Rubinstein Foundation, and held at Barnard College, New York on 24 April 1982, with 750 women attending. The controversy was so heated that the college withheld the *Diary* from distribution, and the Foundation subsequently withdrew support from the series. For conflicting feminist responses see: Orlando, op. cit., 'Conference Report: Towards a Politics of Sexuality', *Off Our Backs*, vol. XII, no. 6, June 1982, pp. 2ff; and Elizabeth Wilson, 'The Context of "Between Pleasure and Danger": The Barnard Conference on Sexuality', *Feminist Review*, no. 13, Spring 1983. The papers of the conference have been published in Vance (ed.), *Pleasure and Danger*.

61 Beatrix Campbell, op. cit., and Anna Coote and Beatrix Campbell, *Sweet Freedom. The Struggle for Women's Liberation*, London, Pan/Picador, 1982, ch. 8; and Angela Hamblin, 'Is a Feminist Heterosexuality Possible?' in Cartledge and Ryan (eds), *Sex and Love*.

62 Ann Ferguson, op. cit., p. 166. See also Sharon McDonald, 'My body or my politics', *The Advocate*, 9 Dec. 1982, and Wendy Clark, 'The Dyke, The Feminist and The Devil', *Feminist Review*, no. 11, Summer 1982, pp. 30-9.

63 Bell and Weinberg, *Homosexualities*, p. 115; Michel Foucault, 'Friendships as a Lifestyle', *Gay Information*, no. 7, Spring 1981.

64 Foucault, 'Sex, Power and the Politics of Identity'; An Interview by Bob Gallagher and Alexander Wilson, *The Advocate*, 7 August 1984. The most recent comprehensive discussion of the whole question of homosexual identities is *Bisexual and Homosexual Identities: Critical Theoretical Issues*, edited by John P. De Cecco and Michael G. Shively, New York, Haworth Press, 1984.

Chapter 9 The meaning of diversity

1 Kinsey et al., *Sexual Behavior in the Human Male*, p. 263.

2 Robert J. Stoller, *Perversion. The Erotic Form of Hatred*, London, Quartet Books, 1977, pp. xiii, xii. But see Gayle Rubin, 'Thinking Sex' in Vance (ed.), *Pleasure and Danger*, p. 317.

3 Ronald Bayer, *Homosexuality and American Psychiatry*, New York, Basic Books, 1981.

4 For references on the debates about pornography, intergenerational sex, sado-masochism and promiscuity see below. On transsexuality as a feminist issue see Janice G. Raymond, *The Transsexual Empire*, Boston, Beacon Press, 1979; and a response from a transsexual, Carol Riddell, *Divided Sisterhood: A Critical Review of Janice Raymond's 'The Trans-sexual Empire'*, Liverpool, News from Nowhere, 1980.

5 D'Emilio, *Sexual Politics, Sexual Communities*, p. 213. The original ACLU hostility was on the grounds that homosexuality was not enshrined constitutionally. In 1967 it reversed its position and challenged government regulation of private consensual sexual behaviour on the ground that it infringed the constitutional right of privacy.

6 John Stuart Mill, *On Liberty*; H.L.A. Hart, *Law, Liberty and Morality*, Oxford University Press, 1963.

7 Stuart Hall, 'Reformism and the Legislation of Consent' in National Deviancy Conference (ed.), *Permissiveness and Control*, pp. 13–14; Weeks, *Sex, Politics and Society*, ch. 13. Frank Mort, 'Sexuality: Regulation and Contestation' in Gay Left Collective (ed.), *Homosexuality: Power and Politics*. On pornography see Rosalind Coward, 'Sexual Violence and Sexuality', *Feminist Review*, no. 11, Summer 1982, p. 14.

8 Pat Califia, *Sapphistry*, p. xiii.

9 Charles Shively, 'Introduction', *Meat: How Men Look, Act, Walk, Talk, Dress, Undress, Taste and Smell*, San Francisco, Gay Sunshine Press, 1980.

10 Samois (ed.), *Coming to Power, Writings and Graphics on Lesbian S/M*, San Francisco, Up Press, 1981, p. 7.

11 Tim McCaskell, 'Untangling emotions and eros', *Body Politic*, July/Aug, 1981, p. 22.

12 Tim Carrigan and John Lee, 'Male homosexuals and the capitalist market', *Gay Changes* (Australia), vol. 2, no. 4, 1979, pp. 39–42; Vito Russo, 'When it comes to gay money—Gay Lib takes care of the pennies: Will Big Business take care of the pounds?' *Gay News* (England), no. 212, April 1981, pp. 16–17; Altman, *The*

Homosexualization of America, ch. 3; $\bar{Z}\bar{G}$, no. 2, 'Sado-maso-chism: Its Expression and Style' (London), n.d. (1982).

13 Alvin Gouldner, *For Sociology*, London, Allen Lane, 1973, p. 295.

14 *Heresies*, no. 12, p. 92.

15 Gouldner, op. cit., p. 296.

16 Diana E.H. Russell with Laura Lederer, 'Questions we get asked most often' in Laura Lederer (ed.), *Take Back the Night. Women on Pornography*, New York, William Morrow, 1980, p. 29. See also Irene Diamond, 'Pornography and Repression: A Reconsideration', *Signs*, vol. 5, no. 4, 1980.

17 *Diary of a Conference on Sexuality*, p. 72.

18 Michel Foucault, 'Sexual Choice, Sexual Acts', *Salmagundi*, nos 58–59, p. 12.

19 The earliest coherent advocacy of this was Alastair Heron (ed.), *Towards a Quaker View of Sex: An Essay by a Group of Friends*, London, Friends Home Services Committee, 1963.

20 Deirdre English, Amber Hollibaugh and Gayle Rubin, 'Talking Sex', p. 43; Michel Foucault, 'Friendship as a lifestyle: An Interview with Michel Foucault', *Gay Information*, Spring 1981; first published in French in *Le Gai Pied*, no. 25, April 1981.

21 Weeks, *Sex, Politics and Society*, ch. 6. See especially the discussion of the 1885 Criminal Law Amendment Act (which applied to most of the United Kingdom apart from Scotland) which outlawed all male homosexual activities in *private* as well as in public as part of a measure designed to control prostitution and *public* vice.

22 See, for example, Dennis Altman, 'Sex: The New Front Line for Gay Politics', in *Gay News* (London), no. 223, 3–16 September 1981, pp. 22–3 and *Gay Community News* (Melbourne), vol. 3, no. 6, August 1981, pp. 22–5.

23 Kinsey et al., *Sexual Behavior in the Human Male*, p. 259; Bell and Weinberg, *Homosexualities*, pp. 69–72; Altman, *The Homosexualization of America*, pp. 174–6; Spada, *The Spada Report*, p. 63.

24 Spada, op. cit., p. 63. See also Joseph Harvey and William B. De Vall, *The Social Organisation of Gay Males*, p. 83; Bell and Weinberg, *Homosexualization*, pp. 219ff.

25 Altman, *The Homosexualization*, pp. 79–80. See also Martin S. Weinberg and Colin J. Williams, 'Gay Baths and the Social Organisation of Impersonal Sex' in Martin P. Levine, *Gay Men*; and Edward William Delph, *The Silent Community: Public Homosexual Encounters*, Beverly Hills and London, Sage, 1978.

26 Spada, *The Spada Report*, p. 113, Sylvere Lotringer, 'Defunkt

Sex', *Semiotext(e): Polysexuality*, p. 279. Cf. Weinberg and Williams, op. cit., p. 179.

27 Laud Humphreys, *Tearoom Trade*, p. 162. The general discussions is pp. 154ff.

28 See *Action: A Publication of the Right to Privacy Committee*, Toronto, 1981–2; *Body Politic*, 1981–2; and submission of The Right to Privacy Committee to the City of Toronto and Ontario Provincial Legislature 1981 (in my possession; I would like to thank Bob Gallagher for information and documents).

29 See, for example, Daniel Tsang, 'Struggling Against Racism' in Tsang (ed.), *The Age Taboo*, pp. 161–2.

30 Ibid., p. 8. There are plentiful examples of the automatic association made between male homosexuality and child molesting. In the year I write this, 1983, there has been a rich crop of them in Britain, with the low point being reached in the Brighton rape case, August 1983, where a deplorable assault on a young boy led to a rapacious press attack on the local gay community and legal action against members of the Paedophile Information Exchange, who were in no way connected with the case. The moral panic had found its victims; calm was restored; but the three men who actually assaulted the child were never found.

31 Kinsey et al., *Sexual Behavior in the Human Female*, p. 117, note 16; Mary Whitehouse, *Cleaning-up TV. From Protest to Participation*, London, Blandford Press, 1967, and *A Most Dangerous Woman?*, Tring, Herts, Lion Publishing, 1982; Anita Bryant, *The Anita Bryant Story*. For general commentaries on events see the articles in Tsang, *The Age Taboo*; Altman, *The Homosexualization of America*, pp. 198ff; Mitzel, *The Boston Sex Scandal*, Boston, Glad Day Books, 1980; Tom O'Carroll, *Paedophilia: The Radical Case*, London, Peter Owen, 1980, ch. 12; Ken Plummer, 'Images of Paedophilia' in M. Cook and G.D. Wilson (eds), *Love and Attraction: An International Conference*, Oxford, Pergamon, 1979; Major events included the Revere 'Sex Scandal' in Boston, the raid on *Body Politic* following its publication of the article 'Men Loving Boys Loving Men' in Dec. 1977; the 'kiddie porn' panic of 1977; the trial of Tom O'Carroll and others in England for conspiracy to corrupt public morals in 1981.

32 Pat Califia, 'The age of Consent; An Issue and its Effects on the Gay Movement', *The Advocate*, 30 October 1980, p. 17. See also Florence Rush, 'Child Pornography' in Lederer (ed.), *Take Back the Night*, pp. 71–81; Illinois Legislative Investigating Commission, *Sexual Exploitation of Children*, Chicago, The Commission, 1980 (see further references in Tsang, op. cit., pp. 169–70); and

on similar events in Britain Whitehouse, *A Most Dangerous Woman?*, ch. 13, 'Kiddie Porn', pp. 146ff.

33 Roger Scruton, *The Times* (London), 13 September 1983.

34 Kinsey et al., *Sexual Behavior in the Human Female*, p. 121.

35 Interview by Guy Hocquenghem with David Thorstad in *Semiotext(e) Special: Large Type Series: Loving Boys*, Summer 1980, p. 34; Tom O'Carroll, *Paedophilia*, p. 153.

36 See, for example, ' "Lesbians Rising" Editors Speak Out' in Tsang, op. cit., pp. 125–32; Stevi Jackson, *Childhood and Sexuality*, Oxford, Basil Blackwell, 1982, ch. 9. See also, Elizabeth Wilson's comments on the debate about proposals to lower the age of consent in England in *What is to be Done about Violence against Women?* p. 205.

37 Theo Sandfort, *The Sexual Aspects of Paedophile Relations: The Experience of twenty-five Boys*, Amsterdam, Pan/Spartacus, 1982, p. 81.

38 Kenneth Plummer, 'The Paedophile's Progress' in Brian Taylor (ed.), *Perspectives on Paedophilia*. See J.Z. Eglinton, *Greek Love*, London, Neville Spearman, 1971 for a classic statement of the first legitimation, and O'Carroll, *Paedophilia*, especially chs 2 and 5 for the second.

39 For an overview of these stereotypes (and the facts which rebut them) to which I am very much indebted, see Plummer, 'Images of Paedophilia'.

40 Glenn D. Wilson and David N. Cox, *The Child-Lovers. A Study of Paedophiles in Society*, London and Boston, Peter Owen, 1983; Peter Righton, ch. 2: 'The Adult' in Taylor, *Perspectives in Paedophilia*; Parker Rossman, *Sexual Experiences between Men and Boys*, London, Maurice Temple Smith, 1976.

41 Tom Reeves, 'Loving Boys' in Tsang, op. cit., p. 27; the age range given on p. 29. On PIE members' interests see Cox and Wilson, op. cit., ch. II.

42 Krafft-Ebing, *Psychopathia Sexualis*, p. 552: 'By violation of sexually immature individuals, the jurist understands all the possible immoral acts with persons under fourteen years of age that are not comprehended in the term "rape".'

43 On paedophilia as abuse see Florence Rush, *The Best Kept Secret: Sexual Abuse of Children*, Englewood Cliffs, N.J., Prentice-Hall, 1980; Robert L. Geiser, *Hidden Victims: The Sexual Abuse of Children*, Boston, Beacon Press, 1979. For alternative opinions: Sandford, op. cit., pp. 49ff; cf. Morris Fraser, ch. 3, 'The Child' and Graham E. Powell and A.J. Chalkley, ch. 4, 'The Effects of paedophile attention on the child' in Taylor (ed.), *Perspectives on Paedophilia*.

44 See interview with the then 15-year-old Mark Moffat in *Semiotext(e)*, loc. cit, p. 10; cf. Tom Reeves's account of being cruised by two 14-year-olds in Tsang, op. cit., p. 30; and O'Carroll, ch. 4, 'Paedophilia in Action' in *Paedophilia*.

45 Taylor (ed.), *Perspectives on Paedophilia*, 'Introduction', p. xiii. In the rest of the discussion I shall, however use the term 'paedophile' to cover all categories as this is the phrase adopted most widely as a *political* description: 'Boy lover' is specific, but exclusive.

46 On offences see P.H. Gebhard, J.H. Gagnon, W.B. Pomeroy and C.V. Christenson, *Sex Offenders*, New York, Harper & Row, 1965; J. Gagnon, 'Female child victims of sex offences', *Social Problems*, no. 13, 1965, pp. 116–92. On identity questions see Plummer, 'The paedophile's progress'.

47 O'Carroll, *Paedophilia*, pp. 120, 118.

48 Ibid., ch. 6, 'Towards more Sensible Laws', which examines various proposals, from Israel to Holland, for minimising the harmful intervention of the law; compare Speijer Committee, *The Speijer Report*, advice to the Netherlands Council of Health concerning homosexual relations with minors, English Translation, London, Sexual Law Reform Society, n.d.

49 Interview with Kate Millett by Mark Blasius in *Semiotext(e) Special*, loc. cit, p. 38 (also printed in Tsang (ed.), op. cit.).

50 Carole Pateman, 'Women and Consent', *Political Theory*, vol. 8, no. 2, May 1980, pp. 149–68.

51 Deirdre English et al., 'Talking Sex', p. 51. Laura Lederer (ed.), *Take Back the Night* gives the most comprehensive coverage of the various American campaigns. The most passionate polemics are in Andrea Dworkin, *Pornography: Men Possessing Men* and Susan Griffin, *Pornography and Silence*. For an excellent general critical comment on the feminist politics of pornography see Lesley Stern, 'The Body as Evidence: A Critical Review of the Pornography Problematic' in *Screen*, vol. 23, no. 5, Nov./Dec. 1982, pp. 38–60.

52 Rosalind Coward, 'Sexual Violence and Sexuality', *Feminist Review*, no. 11, p. 11.

53 John Ellis, 'Pornography', *Screen*, 1980, p. 96. See also Elizabeth Wilson, *What is to be Done About Violence Against Women?* p. 160.

54 Califia, *Sapphistry*, p. 15; Lisa Orlando, ' "Bad" Girls and "good" politics', *Village Voice Literary Supplement*, Dec. 1982, p. 1.

55 The quotes are from Elizabeth Wilson, 'Interview with Andrea Dworkin', *Feminist Review*, no. 11, Summer 1982, p. 26; Helen E. Longino, 'Pornography, Oppression and Freedom: A Closer Look', in Lederer (ed.), *Take Back the Night*, p. 44; 'Interview

with Andrea Dworkin', p. 25; Susan Brownmiller, *Against Our Will*, New York, Simon & Schuster, 1975; Robin Morgan, *Going too Far*, New York, Random House, 1977; Gloria Steinam, 'Erotica and Pornography. A Clear and Present Difference' in Lederer (ed.), *Take Back the Night*, p. 38.

56 Deirdre English et al., 'Talking Sex', p. 57.

57 The absolutist position is expressed clearly in the Longford Committee, *Pornography: The Longford Report*, London, Coronet Books, 1972. 'Scientific' evidence supporting it can be found in H. J. Eysenck, *Sex and Personality*, London, Open Books, 1976, pp. 235–6, in H. J. Eysenck and D. K. B. Nias, *Sex, Violence and the Media*, London, Maurice Temple Smith, 1978, while the debate is assessed in Maurice Yaffe and Edward Nelson (eds), *The Influence of Pornography on Behaviour*, London, Academic Press, 1983. The liberal scepticism about such findings is best found in *The Report of the Commission on Obscenity and Pornography*, New York, Random House, 1970: the *Report of the Committee on Obscenity and Film Censorship* and in the liberal-feminist work by Beatrice Faust, *Women, Sex and Pornography*, Harmondsworth, Penguin Books, 1981; the radical feminist rejection of these positions is clearly expressed in Diamond, op. cit., pp. 691–7.

58 Susan Barrowclough, 'Not a Love Story', *Screen*, vol. 23, no. 5, Nov./Dec. 1982, p. 32.

59 Ellen Willis, 'Who is a Feminist? A Letter to Robin Morgan', *Village Voice Literary Supplement*, December 1982, p. 17; Lisa Orlando, ' "Bad" Girls and "Good" Politics', p. 16. Compare Angela Carter, *The Sadeian Woman: An Exercise in Cultural History*, London, Virago, 1979.

60 Gregg Blachford, 'Looking at Pornography: Erotica and the Socialist Morality', *Gay Left*, no. 6, Summer 1978, pp. 16–20 and (in a slightly different version) *Screen Education*, no. 29, Winter 1978–9, pp. 21–8; Chris Bearchall, 'Art, Trash and Titillation. A Consumer's Guide to Lezzy Smut', *Body Politic*, no. 93, May 1983, p. 33; *Diary of a Conference on Sexuality*, p. 19.

61 B. Ruby Rich, 'Anti Porn: Soft Issue, Hard World', *Feminist Review*, no. 13, Spring 1983.

62 Lesley Stern, 'The Body as Evidence', p. 42.

63 On the general point see Coward, op. cit; on romance see Ann Barr Snitow, 'Mass Market Romance: Pornography for Women is Different', *Radical History Review*, no. 20, Spring/Summer 1979, pp. 141–63, and Valerie Hey, *The Necessity of Romance*, Canterbury, England, University of Kent at Canterbury, Women's Studies Occasional Papers, no. 3, 1983.

64 See Altman, *The Homosexualization of America*, pp. 190ff. Ian Young, John Stoltenberg, Lyn Rosen and Rose Jordan, 'Forum on Sado-Masochism' in Karla Jay and Allen Young (eds), *Lavender Culture*, New York, A Jove HBJ Book, 1978; Samois, *What Color is Your Handkerchief? A Lesbian S/M Sexuality Reader*, Berkeley, CA., Samois, 1979; Samois, *Coming to Power*, Samois, a lesbian and feminist S/M group active between 1979 and 1983 became the most notorious of the political S/M groupings, provoking the reply *Against Sadomasochism* (see note 70 below).

65 Pat Califia, 'Unraveling the sexual fringe. A secret side of lesbian sexuality', *The Advocate*, 27 Dec. 1979, p. 19.

66 Ibid., pp. 19–21. See also Califia, *Sapphistry*, pp. 118–32.

67 Mark Thompson, 'To the Limits and Beyond', *The Advocate*, 8 July 1982, p. 31. On the theatrical metaphor see Paul Gebhard, 'Fetishism and Sado Masochism' in Martin S. Weinberg (ed.), *Sex Research: Studies from the Kinsey Institute*, New York, London, Toronto, Oxford University Press, 1976, p. 164. For the views of sexologists see Havelock Ellis, *Studies in the Psychology of Sex*, vol. III, Philadelphia, F.A. Davis, 1920, pp. 66–188; Gerald and Caroline Greene, *S-M: The Last Taboo*, New York, Ballantine Books, 1978; T. Weinberg and G.W. Levi Kamel (eds), *S and M Studies in Sadomasochism*, Buffalo, NY, Prometheus Books, 1983.

68 Califia, 'Unraveling the Sexual Fringe', p. 22; *Sapphistry*, p. 119; 'Feminism and Sadomasochism', *Heresies*, no. 12, p. 32.

69 Susan Ardill and Nora Neumark, 'Putting Sex Back into Lesbianism. Is the Way to a Woman's Heart Through her Sadomasochism?', *Gay Information*, no. 11, Spring 1982, p. 11.

70 Karen Sims, 'Racism and Sadomasochism. A conversation with two black lesbians', in Robin Ruth Linden, *Against Sadomasochism. A Radical Feminist Analysis*, East Palo Alto, Ca., Frog in the Well, 1982, pp. 99–105.

71 Pat Califia, 'Unraveling the sexual fringe', p. 22.

72 Quoted in Mariana Valverde, 'Feminism meets fist-fucking: getting lost in lesbian S&M', *Body Politic*, Feb. 1982, p. 43.

73 Ardill and Neumark, op. cit., p. 9.

74 Califia, *Sapphistry*, p. 10.

75 Califia, 'Feminism and Sado Masochism', p. 32.

76 'Our Statement' in Samois, *What Color is your Handkerchief?*, p. 2; Mark Thompson, 'To the Limits and Beyond', p. 28.

77 Ellen Willis, *Diary of a Conference on Sexuality*, p. 72. For a critique of this position from a socialist, not radical, feminist position see: Elizabeth Wilson, 'A New Romanticism?' in Eileen Philips (ed.), *The Left and the Erotic*, London, Lawrence & Wishart, 1983, pp. 37–52.

78 Sue Cartledge, 'Duty and Desire: Creating a Feminist Morality' in Sue Cartledge and Joanna Ryan (eds), *Sex and Love*, p. 167.

79 See, for example, David Fernbach, *The Spiral Path. A Gay Contribution to Human Survival*, London, Gay Men's Press, 1981; see my review in *Gay News* (London), September 1981.

80 I am here following Rosalind Pollack Petchesky, 'Reproductive Freedom: Beyond "A Woman's Right to Choose"', *Signs*, vol. 5, no. 4, 1980, pp. 661–87.

81 Denise Riley, 'Feminist Thought and Reproductive Control: the State and the "right to choose"' in The Cambridge Women's Studies Group (eds), *Women in Society: Interdisciplinary Essays*, London, Virago, 1981. See also Michèle Barrett and Mary McIntosh, *The Anti-social Family*, pp. 135–7, who also cite Riley.

82 Michel Foucault, *The History of Sexuality*, vol. 1, p. 101.

83 Richard Dyer, 'Getting Over the Rainbow'.

84 Frederic Jameson, 'Pleasure: A Political Issue', in *Formations of Pleasure*, p. 10.

Chapter 10   Conclusion: beyond the boundaries of sexuality

1 Edward Carpenter, *Love's Coming of Age. A Series of Papers on the Relation of the Sexes*, London, George Allen & Unwin, 1948 (first published 1896). For a discussion of Carpenter see Part 1 of Rowbotham and Weeks, *Socialism and the New Life* and Weeks, *Coming Out*, ch. 6. For a modern collection of relevant material see Edward Carpenter, *Selected Writings Volume I: Sex*, London, GMP, 1984.

2 James Burnet in *The Medical Times and Hospital Gazette*, vol. XXXIV, no. 1497, 10 Nov. 1906, quoted in Edward Carpenter, *The Intermediate Sex*, London, George Allen & Unwin, 1952 (first published 1908), p. 133.

3 Carpenter, *Love's Coming of Age*, Prefatory Note to Twelfth Edition (1923).

4 Ibid., p. 64.

5 See Moira Gatens, 'A Critique of the Sex/Gender Distinction' in Judith Allen and Paul Patton (eds), *Beyond Marxism. Interventions after Marx*, Leichhardt, New South Wales, Intervention Publications, 1983.

6 Carpenter, op. cit., p. 171.

7 Karl Marx and Friedrich Engels, *On Religion*, Moscow, People's Publishing House, 1957, p. 329.

8 Barbara Taylor, *Eve and the New Jerusalem*, London, Virago, 1983, especially pp. 40–8, and 213–16.

9 Compare Sara Evans, *Personal Politics. The Roots of Women's Liberation in the Civil Rights Movement and the New Left*, New York, Vintage Books, 1980.

10 Compare Rowbotham and Weeks, *Socialism and the New Life*, and Weeks, *Sex, Politics and Society*, ch. 9.

11 Perry Anderson, *In the Tracks of Historical Materialism. The Welleck Library Lectures*, London, Verso Editions, 1983.

12 Paul Patton, 'Marxism in Crisis: No Difference' in Allen and Patton (eds), *Beyond Marxism?* p. 58. See also Paul Hirst, *On Law and Ideology*, London, Macmillan, 1979, p. 2.

13 Chantal Mouffe, 'Hegemony and the Integral State in Gramsci: Towards a New Concept of Politics' in George Bridges and Rosalind Brunt (eds), *Silver Linings. Some Strategies for the Eighties*, London, Lawrence & Wishart, 1981, p. 183.

14 See Coward, *Patriarchal Precedents*.

15 Mouffe, op. cit., p. 167. Compare a similar interrogation of Marxism in Stanley Aronowitz, *The Crisis in Historical Materialism. Class, Politics and Culture in Marxist Theory*, New York, J.F. Bergin in Association with Praeger, 1981.

16 See, for example, Gay Left (ed.), *Homosexuality: Power and Politics* for essays which creatively use Foucault; and Dave Sargent, 'Reformulating (Homo)sexual politics: radical theory and practice in the gay movement' in Allen and Patton (eds), *Beyond Marxism?* For a critique of such positions see Craig Johnston, 'Foucault and Gay Liberation', *Arena* (Australia), no. 61, 1982, pp. 54–70. For feminist deployments of Foucault-influenced analysis see the journal *M/F* passim, and Coward, *Patriarchal Precedents*, 'Conclusion: Sex and Social Relations'.

17 See, for example, Stuart Hall, 'Reformism and the Legislation of Consent' in National Deviancy Conference (ed.), *Permissiveness and Control;* Mouffe, op. cit. and Chantal Mouffe (ed.), *Gramsci and Marxist Theory*, London, Routledge & Kegan Paul, 1979.

18 The Combahee River Collective, 'A Black Feminist Statement' in Gloria T. Hull, Patricia Bell Scott and Barbara Smith, *But Some of Us Are Brave: Black Women's Studies*, Old Westbury, NY, The Feminist Press, 1982, pp. 14, 16. Compare Carole Vance, *Diary of a Conference on Sexuality*, p. 1: 'it is likely that women of different communities (based on sexual preference, race, class, and ethnicity) have not only different things to say but different ways they want to say them'. The relationship between black and white feminism is powerfully discussed in *Feminist Review*, vol. 17, Autumn 1984, on 'Black Feminist Perspectives'.

19 See, for example, the comments by Frederic Jameson, 'Pleasure: A Political Issue' in *Formations of Pleasure*.

20 Raymond Williams, *Towards 2000*, London, Chatto & Windus, 1983, pp. 12–15.

Index*

317